Pharmacology Made Simple

Pharmacology Made Simple

An Introduction for the Health Professions

Anthony Guerra, MHCI, PharmD

Chemistry Instructor
Pre-Pharmacy Advisor
Former Chair, Pharmacy Technician Program
Des Moines Area Community College
Ankeny, Iowa

ELSEVIER

Elsevier
3251 Riverport Lane
St. Louis, Missouri 63043

PHARMACOLOGY MADE SIMPLE, FIRST EDITION
Copyright © 2022 by Elsevier, Inc. All rights reserved.

ISBN: 978-0-323-69544-2

ISBN: 978-0-323-69544-2

Content Strategist: Kristin Wilhelm
Content Development Specialist: Jeannine Carrado
Publishing Services Manager: Deepthi Unni
Project Manager: Haritha Dharmarajan
Design Direction: Patrick Ferguson

Printed in India

Last digit is the print number: 9 8 7 6 5 4 3 2

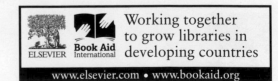

To Mindy, Brielle, Rianne, and Teagan

—AAG

*"Tell me and I forget. Teach me and I remember.
Involve me and I learn."*

—Benjamin Franklin

Pharmacology Is a Language You Can Learn

—Building the Introduction Together—

My first language is not English. While I did learn English at a young age, I recognized the barrier that not having an understanding of language can have on one's future. In teaching pharmacology and talking one-on-one with my students, I was able to earn their trust and they told me what was really hard for them—remembering these incredibly unfamiliar terms. It was a clear case of The Curse of Knowledge—I, the instructor, had been speaking the language of pharmacology for so long that I could not appreciate the struggle students had from the beginning. I realized that there was a "missing book," one that keeps health professions students engaged from the start while teaching them the ins and outs of the language of pharmacology.

But looking at the many health professions, one will find many dialects of pharmacology for each of those health care professionals. This book is meant to serve as the base of the tree, the introduction that allows students to move on to their own dialect and branches of expertise. There is a place where pharmacology intersects with the many health professions—this book serves as a foundation. Get the pharmacology language right and the student becomes a genuine part of the health care team – so the mission was on and goal clear.

What got me was how students would greet me after the semester was over. They would tell me what they remembered, the short little mnemonics that were meant to be a bit of dressing. As this happened over and over, I realized that maybe the mnemonics sit at the foundation and it's the rest that follows. Making a good mnemonic is like solving a puzzle or riddle—the brain catches it as a means to solve a problem. How do I remember this, this, and that?

As we answered the question together, we taught each other what worked and what did not. I tried to teach the students and they tried to teach their patients, forming a learning waterfall. With patient health literacy sometimes at a very low level, we realized that we needed to be clever and that mnemonics needed to be engaging and fun. Pharmacology flowed in a telephone game version with very serious consequences if we got it wrong. We needed to keep asking questions throughout. And we needed to have great analogies and images. I think we got it right because we all worked together on a memorable introduction where the reader becomes the teacher, confident in one's conversations with the patient. I hope you do also.

Tony Guerra, MHCI, PHARMD
Spring 2021

Contents

Acknowledgements

A very special thanks to the editor of this book, Jeannine Carrado, who kept a watchful eye on the many moving parts. She kept encouraging me as the pages came fast and furious.

Tony Guerra, MHCI, PHARMD

Pharmacology Made Simple

1

Introduction to Pharmacology

LEARNING OBJECTIVES

1. Define pharmacology and pathophysiology.
2. Describe over-the-counter, behind-the-counter, and prescription drugs.
3. Contrast chemical, generic, and brand names.
4. Explain DEA schedules for controlled substances.
5. Explain how to pronounce drug names.

Pharmacology and Pathophysiology

Why is pharmacology hard? How can we make it much easier?

There are a number of ways to approach **pharmacology**, the study of drugs and their actions. One way is to take a series of inorganic and organic chemistry classes and then move on to pharmacology using the various chemical structures one learns. This way is very hard, lengthy, and not necessarily appropriate for everyone taking pharmacology. There is another way, which is to study the language of pharmacology and the physiology of disease in living organisms, **pathophysiology**.

In pharmacology, we look at those parts of the drug names that have meaning and associate them to other medication names. For example, the "–cillin" in penicillin is also in amoxicillin and ampicillin. Then, we consider the diseases these medications treat, such as otitis media, or a middle ear infection—the pathophysiology.

In this book, we will marry the language of pharmacology with common pathophysiology to make pharmacology much more accessible. We cannot get away from chemistry altogether, but when we use chemistry, we will approach it more as a helpful part of learning the language.

SCENARIO 1.1. ABSORPTION

A student had heard of anatomy and physiology courses but did not recognize the word *pathophysiology*. How does pathophysiology relate to pharmacology?

Answer: Pathophysiology is a combination of "patho," which means disease, and "physiology," the study of living organisms. Pharmacology, then, is how drugs can help treat or cure a patient's pathophysiology.

* Brand discontinued, now available only as generic
† Naming conventions can vary between prescription and OTC formulations

Over-the-Counter, Behind-the-Counter, and Prescription Drugs

When we talk about medications or drugs, where we find them matters. Over-the-counter (OTC), behind-the-counter (BTC), and prescription drugs (RX) are located in different areas of the pharmacy.

If a drug is **over-the-counter (OTC)**, then the United States Food and Drug Administration (FDA) believes it is safe for most people to take the drug (medication) on their own. They do not require a prescription from a prescriber. These drugs are especially convenient to purchase in grocery stores, pharmacies, and even airports and gas stations. They tend to be less expensive and may be an option for those without prescription insurance. For example, if a patient has a fever and an infection, the prescriber might give a prescription for amoxicillin, a penicillin antibiotic, or azithromycin (Zithromax), a macrolide antibiotic, and recommend the patient pick up OTC ibuprofen (Advil, Motrin).

However, the medication might be safe if the patient has no other health conditions. Generally, patients *do* have other prescription medications and might have other health conditions. For example, if the above patient had a history of ulceration, the physician might recommend OTC acetaminophen (Tylenol) instead of ibuprofen. Acetaminophen has less of an effect on the stomach. With a pharmacist nearby, it always makes sense to consult the pharmacist or family prescriber before taking on any new OTC medications.

Behind-the-counter (BTC) medicine such as pseudoephedrine (Sudafed), a medicine for nasal congestion, is literally behind the counter. One can find these drugs usually closer to the cash register rather than on the shelf with OTC medicines. Getting this medicine requires that patients present identification to the pharmacy staff to make sure that they have not exceeded limits of use. Someone making illegal methamphetamine can use pseudoephedrine to synthesize it; limiting the purchases can help to reduce the manufacture of these illicit drugs. There is an OTC product phenylephrine that is sometimes found in combination products, but its effectiveness is inferior to pseudoephedrine.

Prescription drugs (Rx) are those that require a prescriber—such as a nurse practitioner, physician assistant, or physician—to prescribe them. Some of these medications can have multiple refills throughout a year whereas others classified under the Drug Enforcement Administration (DEA) schedules have restrictions. Often, when a provider is prescribing a drug, the medicine has to be in the provider's "scope of practice." For example, dentists limit what they prescribe to drugs for dental procedures. While a dentist could technically write a prescription for albuterol (ProAir HFA) for asthma or methotrexate (Rheumatrex*) for arthritis, these conditions are generally out of the dentist's scope of practice.

SCENARIO 1.2. NONSTEROIDAL ANTIINFLAMMATORY DRUG (NSAID) ANALGESICS

A patient has been roaming the aisles of a grocery store looking for a decongestant, but all he can find are antihistamines. Where is the medicine he is looking for?

Answer: Often, decongestants such as pseudoephedrine (Sudafed) are behind-the-counter drugs and are physically placed behind the pharmacy counter. Some stores place empty boxes or signs telling the patient to go to the pharmacy for these drugs; others do not.

Chemical, Generic, and Brand Names

Whether the prescription drug is scheduled or not, it will generally have three names: a chemical name, a generic or nonproprietary name, and a brand or trade name. It is much easier to use a few examples to make this clear.

The **chemical name** of ibuprofen (Advil, Motrin) is (RS)-2-(4-(2-methylpropyl) phenyl) propanoic acid. This long name can help a chemist draw the structure and better understand other properties about it. However, the chemical name is too cumbersome.

Instead, we use a **generic** or **nonproprietary** name, such as ibuprofen. *Nonproprietary* literally means not owned by anyone. Just as a proprietor owns a store, a nonproprietary entity has no ownership. Other nonproprietary names include acetaminophen and aspirin.

Examples of the opposite of this, a **brand name** or **trade name**, would be Advil and Motrin. Advil is ibuprofen, which the drug manufacturer Pfizer produces. Motrin comes from the Johnson & Johnson Company. To use food as an analogy, a hamburger is the generic name, whereas Big Mac or Whopper are brand names.

There are a few exceptions. For example, the OTC antacids calcium carbonate (Tums) and magnesium hydroxide (Milk of Magnesia) are such simple chemical compounds,

the chemical and generic names are the same. In writing names of medicines, the proper way is to write the generic name in lower case (unless it starts a sentence) and then capitalize the brand name in parentheses after it, like this: I use loratadine (Claritin), an antihistamine, for my seasonal allergies.

Using the generic name is especially important in making sure that the medicine a person wants is the medication a patient gets, as there is only one generic name. However, as we saw earlier, there are many brand names for the same generic entity. For example, asking someone to get Tylenol can cause problems, as there are many single and combination products that have "Tylenol" in the brand name. It is better to say, "Please buy acetaminophen liquid for an 8-year-old child" rather than "Buy some Tylenol for Jane." The first example specifies that the liquid should contain only one ingredient, acetaminophen, and it should be in a dosage form that an 8-year-old can take. The second expression does not clarify whether acetaminophen should be the only ingredient, nor does it have any information about the dosage form.

SCENARIO 1.3. CHEMICAL, GENERIC, AND BRAND NAMES

A parent has an 8-year-old daughter with a fever and the spouse instructs them to buy Advil. What would have been a better way to specify the correct medication to buy?

Answer: By specifying the purchase of ibuprofen for an 8-year-old, the spouse might avoid the parent accidentally purchasing a combination medicine or an incorrect dosage form.

DEA Drug Schedules for Controlled Substances

With narcotics, we have to be very careful because of a medicine's addictive potential. To make clear the danger, the DEA created five schedules—I, II, III, IV, and V—under the Controlled Substance Act (CSA). The numbers are the Roman numerals from I to V (1 to 5) and move from those substances that are most addictive (Schedule I) to those that are least addictive (Schedule V). The following are definitions that can help further classify these drug schedules.

A patient can have no refills on a Schedule II medication, up to 5 refills in 6 months on a Schedule III, IV, or V medication, and unlimited refills on a prescription that is not scheduled, for up to 1 year.

Schedule I

There is currently no accepted medical use for medications in Schedule I, and possession of the drug can be illegal. There is a very good chance a person could become addicted to drugs in this schedule. Examples include lysergic acid diethylamide (LSD), heroin, and marijuana. The ability to get marijuana, however, varies based on individual state laws.

Schedule II

Medications in Schedule II have a high potential for abuse because of physical or psychological dependence. Examples include fentanyl (Duragesic*, Sublimaze*), hydrocodone/acetaminophen (Vicodin*, Lortab), and oxycodone (Oxycontin).

Schedule III

The DEA schedules are relative; a Schedule III drug is more dangerous than a Schedule IV drug, but less so than those in Schedule II. Drugs in this class might include buprenorphine (Suboxone) and acetaminophen with codeine (Tylenol with codeine*).

Schedule IV

Some muscle relaxers and antianxiety medications are in Schedule IV. They might include carisoprodol (Soma), diazepam (Valium), and alprazolam (Xanax).

Schedule V

Schedule V medications have a low potential for abuse. This schedule includes liquid cough medicines that have fewer than 200 mg of codeine per 100 mL, such as Robitussin AC* and Phenergan with Codeine*.

SCENARIO 1.4. DEA DRUG SCHEDULES

A patient worries that he is going to get addicted to the medicine the provider gave him. What are the chances of his DEA Schedule V cough medicine causing him to become addicted?

Answer: While there is addictive potential in a DEA Schedule V cough medicine, it is relatively low as compared with the other DEA schedules.

How to Pronounce Drug Names

A point of frustration is that often *how* we pronounce drug names does not correspond to how we would pronounce the same letters in plain English. For example, penicillin has the letters from the word pencil in it, making it relatively easy to pronounce. We have a similar word in plain English that matches. However, with metoprolol, a word many mispronounce, we think we see full words and word parts "me," "to," "pro" from professional, and "lol" from lollipop. However, the correct pronunciation is nowhere near the word "me" as in talking about "you and me" and "to," as in "to and fro." One properly pronounces metoprolol as follows: the "me" from men, the "to" from tow, the "pro" from apron, and the "lol" from lollipop, with the stress or accented syllable as "to."

In this section, we will look over some of the origins of the pronunciations that do not fit in with what we expect so that we can better know how to pronounce drug names properly. A patient hearing a mispronunciation from a health provider might lose some trust in that provider.

The parts in italics are not classification stems like "–cillin" for penicillins; we will tackle that in the next chapter. Rather, they are word parts that might cause pronunciation problems in the future. In this first group, we see many of the elements from the Periodic Table of Elements: hydrogen, chlorine, fluorine, and sulfur.

In the first example, we see part of the element's name, "hydro-" from hydrogen.

Hydro (hydrogen)—*Hydro*codone, *HIGH-droe*

In this example, we see the hydrochlorothiazide medication (part of the thiazide drug class) takes a part of the element chlorine plus "o."

Chloro (chlorine)—Hydro*chloro*thiazide "hydrochlorothiazide", *KLOR-oh*

In this example, we see the fluoroquinolone drug class takes a part of the element fluorine plus "o."

Fluoro (fluorine)—Cipro*flo*xacin, a *fluoro*quinolone antibiotic "ciprofloxacin" *FLOR-oh*

Sometimes, the root signifies an element is very different, as in "thio" for "sulfur."

Thio (sulfur)—Hydrochloro*thia*zide "hydrochlorothiazide", *THIGH-oh*

To a chemist, these word parts indicate the number of carbon atoms that attach to a molecule made up of only carbon and hydrogen atoms. We will use these word parts to help us get the tricky part of the pronunciation right.

Methyl—*Methyl*phenidate "methylphenidate", *METH-ill*

Ethyl—Fentan*yl* "fentanyl", *ETH-ill*

Propyl—Meto*prolol*, *PROP-ill*

Butyl—Al*but*erol "albuterol", *BYOOT-ill*

Levo and dextro mean left and right in Latin, respectively:

Levo—*Levo*thyroxine "levothyroxine", *LEE-vo*

Dextro—*Dex*methylphenidate "dexmethylphenidate", *DEX-trow*

These words are chemical branches that attach to the central molecule. You may recognize part of alcohol in tramadol or the amine, from amino acid in diphenhydramine (Benadryl). We will add some more examples to help you with the pronunciation.

Acetyl—Levetir*acet*am "**levetiracetam**", *Uh-SEAT-ill*

Alcohol—Tramad*ol* "tramadol", *AL-kuh-haul*

Amide—Loper*amide* "loperamide", *UH-myde*

Amine—Diphenhydr*amine* "diphenhydramine", *UH-mean*

Disulfide—Disulfiram, *DIE-sulf-eyed*

Furan—*Fur*osemide "furosemide", *FYOOR-an*

Guanidine—Cimetidine, *GWAN-eh-dean*

Hydroxide—Magnesium *Hydroxide* "Magnesium Hydroxide", *HI-drox-eyed*

Imidazole—Omepr*azole*, "omeprazole", *im-id-AZ-ole*

Ketone—Spironolac*tone* "spironolactone", *KEY-tone*

Phenol—Acetamino*phen* "acetaminophen", *FEN-ole*

Sulfa—*Sulfa*methoxazole, *SULL-fuh*

SCENARIO 1.5. PRONOUNCING DRUG NAMES

An elderly asthmatic gets her first rescue inhaler and is having trouble pronouncing *albuterol*. As you listen, you hear the name "Al," short for Albert, butter as in "butter on toast," and "all," as in "all done." How would a person properly pronounce the "buter" in this medicine?

Answer: A person would properly pronounce albuterol with the "buter" as BYOO-ter; so Al, BYOO-ter, all is how you pronounce albuterol. The pronunciation comes from the butyl chemical group, similar to when one pronounces "butane lighter."

Summary

- Pharmacology is the study of drugs and their actions. Pathophysiology is the study of disease in living organisms. One uses pharmacology to treat or cure a pathophysiologic condition.
- OTC drugs do not require a prescription but may need the review of a health professional if a patient takes other medications or has other disease states. BTC medicines, such as pseudoephedrine (Sudafed), a medicine for nasal congestion, are physically behind the prescription counter. A patient will need to show identification to purchase a BTC medication. Prescription drugs (Rx) are those that require a prescriber to provide a prescription.
- The chemical name can help a chemist draw the structure and better understand other properties of a drug. A generic or nonproprietary name is unique to a drug

entity; the generic name is the best choice when speaking about a medication to make sure that the medicine one asks for is the drug one receives. A brand name or trade name is one created by a manufacturer and may represent different, or a combination of, generic names.
- The DEA created five schedules (I, II, III, IV, and V) under the CSA to help providers know the relative addictive potential of medicines. The lower the schedule number, the more addictive the medication can be.
- Some medications, such as penicillin, have word parts that resemble other words in plain English, such as pencil. Other medicines, like metoprolol, do not. Knowing how to pronounce a few chemical names can help with the proper drug pronunciation.

Review Questions

1. Pharmacology can best be described as the:
   a. Study of drugs and their actions
   b. A physical place
   c. A discipline that can only be understood through chemistry
   d. The study of disease in living organisms
2. When looking for a behind-the-counter decongestant, we expect that the active ingredient's generic name will be:
   a. Ibuprofen
   b. Pseudoephedrine
   c. Acetaminophen
   d. Phenylephrine
3. _____ is an example of an over-the-counter medicine that someone might use for pain or fever, which does not hurt the stomach.
   a. Amoxicillin (Amoxil*)
   b. Azithromycin (Zithromax)
   c. Ibuprofen (Advil, Motrin*)
   d. Acetaminophen (Tylenol)
4. All of the following are prescription medicines except:
   a. Albuterol (ProAir HFA)
   b. Methotrexate (Rheumatrex*)
   c. Calcium carbonate (Tums)
   d. Amoxicillin
5. All of the following are chemical names except:
   a. Calcium carbonate
   b. (RS)-2-(4-(2-methylpropyl) phenyl) propanoic acid
   c. Azithromycin
   d. Magnesium hydroxide
6. An example of the proper way to write a generic and brand name at the beginning of a sentence would look like:
   a. Albuterol (ProAir HFA)
   b. Amoxicillin, amoxil
   c. Azithromycin: Zithromax
   d. Tums, Calcium carbonate
7. The DEA schedule least likely to cause dependence and abuse, which is often given to cough medicines with limited amounts of codeine, is:
   a. Schedule II
   b. Schedule III
   c. Schedule IV
   d. Schedule V

8. Which of the following would fall into the DEA Schedule II as a high risk for addiction?
   a. Heroin
   b. Fentanyl (Duragesic*)
   c. Buprenorphine (Suboxone)
   d. Diazepam (Valium)
9. One of the following drugs is incorrectly matched to the element on the Periodic Table of Elements that it is tied to. Which is it?
   a. Thio, thorium
   b. Hydro, hydrogen
   c. Chloro, chlorine
   d. Fluoro, fluorine
10. How many months of refills could someone who has a DEA Schedule III prescription for acetaminophen/codeine be allowed?
    a. Zero
    b. Three
    c. Six
    d. Twelve

2

Drug Actions
(Pharmacodynamics)

LEARNING OBJECTIVES

1. Identify the five sources of drugs.
2. Define drug, pharmacodynamics, therapeutic effect, and adverse effect.
3. Contrast receptor affinity, agonist, and antagonist.
4. Describe a narrow and wide and high and low therapeutic index.

The Five Sources of Drugs

When we think about medications and where they came from, often we look to the local pharmacy. However, having medications premade into tablets and other dosage forms is relatively new. Traditionally, we looked to plants and recipes passed down from others to treat many illnesses (Fig. 2.1).

Almost 7000 years ago, the Sumerians put their medicinal recipes in tablets to pass them on and reduce the risk that this knowledge might fade in passing the information down orally. Over 4500 years ago, Emperor Shen Nung wrote the "Pen T'Sao" referencing hundreds of dried plants and their effects. Over 2000 years ago, Hippocrates classified many hundreds of plants and documented their effects.

Relative to these long timelines, acetylsalicylic acid (ASA), commonly known as aspirin, was a relatively recent discovery, with Germany synthesizing the active ingredient from the bark of a willow tree in the mid-1800s. The takeaway is that we are fortunate to live when we do and have the convenience of ready-made pharmaceuticals.

While plants represent an important source of drugs, there are many others (Fig. 2.2). For example, we find minerals in many common medications. Iron supplements to prevent anemia, potassium chloride to avoid potassium loss with a diuretic, and magnesium in magnesium hydroxide represent a few. Only recently did we learn to synthesize insulin. Previously, we would have insulin from cows (bovine) and pigs (porcine).

Many drugs are now the product of laboratory work, in which scientists can better control the quality and precision of drug components and active ingredients, especially as

they relate to synthetic opioids and many new antibiotics. Sometimes nature's kitchen does not have a solution and genetic engineering works to synthesize important vaccines, insulins, and monoclonal antibodies for conditions such as rheumatoid arthritis and Crohn disease. Ultimately, the more we can control the sourcing of drugs, the better we can ensure the safety of our patients.

Drug Effects and Dosing Levels

The same medication can be toxic in one dosage form and immensely helpful in another. For example, some antibiotics are too dangerous to ingest, but often we can put them into creams or topical products that will prevent bacterial infection on our skin. That is an example of a **local effect**, in which the therapeutic or toxic effect limits itself to a single site. In taking oral medications or accepting an injectable, we risk **systemic effects** (Fig. 2.3).

For example, a patient with back pain may apply a cream to relieve pain. If the cream does not work, the patient might have to take an oral medication such as **ibuprofen (Advil, Motrin)** to alleviate that pain systemically. Another example is that we can treat a condition in both ways. We can put a local anesthetic such as **lidocaine (Solarcaine*)** on a sunburn and provide ibuprofen to help with the pain systemically.

The danger in those medications, especially those that work systemically, can come from the dose itself. Safe nonprescription dosages from ibuprofen, for example, can range from 200 to 400 milligrams (mg) every 6 hours. At lower doses, ibuprofen effectively staves off pain and inflammation; at higher doses over extended periods, however, it can lead to stomach ulcers. The dosage needed to keep pain and inflammation at bay is the **maintenance dose**, or that dose required to keep the therapeutic level.

---

* Brand discontinued, now available only as generic
† Naming conventions can vary between prescription and OTC formulations

With antibiotics, **azithromycin (Zithromax)**, for example, we need a **loading dose**. A patient on azithromycin will usually take a double dose the first day, then a single dose each day thereafter for 4 more days. That initial double dose is a loading dose, a higher dose to raise drug levels quickly.

When we talk about antidepressants later, we will learn about certain classes that need only a few pills to reach a **toxic dose**, a dose that causes significant adverse effects. One such antidepressant is amitriptyline (Elavil*), a tricyclic antidepressant. Taking just a few weeks' worth of pills at once can lead to a **lethal dose**, one that kills the patient (Fig. 2.4).

Pharmacodynamics

A **drug** is a substance, other than food, intended to affect the body's function or structure. Some may talk about food as medicine; for our purposes, we will exclude that definition. From the drug prefix pharmaco-, we can create many different terms to describe the effects of drugs. For example, **pharmacodynamics** is the study of drug actions or, in a literal translation, the force of the drug on the body (Fig. 2.5).

We can also think about pharmacodynamics as the reaction between a drug and an individual (Fig. 2.6). For example, one drug might provide excellent pain relief for one patient and completely miss the mark with another. Often, this has to do with differences in patients—a certain dosage can help one patient but not another. In the next section, we will look at the difference between a drug as therapeutic, or helping a patient, and a drug as causing adverse effects. Often, the decision to use a drug is a trade-off between these two factors.

Therapeutic Drug Use

One thing that many patients take for granted is that we have a dosage chart on every medication we take. When people pick up an antihistamine from the local pharmacy, they can access a chart listing age ranges and the appropriate amount of medicine to give for each age range. However, when drugs first came to the fore, physicians had to use trial and error to determine safe dosages. Therefore, drugs can be both therapeutic and cause adverse effects at the same time (Fig. 2.7). By knowing the safe dosage forms through animal—then human—testing, researchers increased our ability to use the drugs safely.

Adverse Drug Reactions

At normal doses, a patient can experience an adverse drug reaction—a side effect we know is likely to happen is based on the dosage and duration of the medication regimen (Fig. 2.8). The classic adverse drug reaction with nonsteroidal antiinflammatory drugs (NSAIDs) is the ulcer. Many patients with arthritis depend on these antiinflammatories to help them move around better or alleviate their pain. However, needing to take an NSAID over extended periods increases the risk of an ulcer. As such, we can give another medication, an acid reducer, to avoid the possible adverse effect. Ironically, that second medicine might also have its own adverse drug effects. This prescribing cascade, a series of drugs to treat or prevent adverse drug reactions from subsequent medications, is all too common in situations in which patients have to take many medicines.

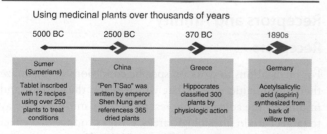

• **Fig. 2.1** History of Plants as Drugs

SCENARIO 2.1. PHARMACODYNAMICS

When a dentist prescribes an antibiotic to prevent infection after a procedure, the patient questions the dose. The prescription asks the patient to take four tablets initially, then two tablets daily thereafter. What kind of dose do the four tablets represent? What kind of dose do the two tablets daily thereafter represent?

Answer: The initial four tablets represent a loading dose while the two tablets thereafter represent a maintenance dose.

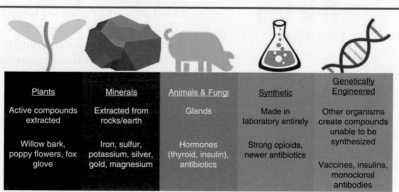

• **Fig. 2.2** Sources of Drugs

Drug effects

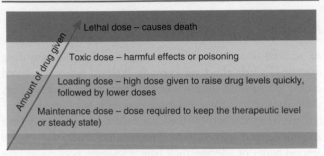

Local effects	Systemic effects
Limited to administration site	Widespread through the body
Example: Benzocaine (Solarcaine) sprayed onto sunburn	Example: Ibuprofen (Motrin) tablets ingested for sunburn relief

• **Fig. 2.3** Drug Effects

Dosing levels

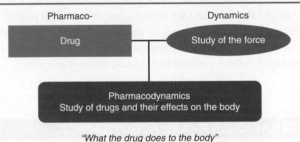

Amount of drug given

Lethal dose – causes death

Toxic dose – harmful effects or poisoning

Loading dose – high dose given to raise drug levels quickly, followed by lower doses

Maintenance dose – dose required to keep the therapeutic level or steady state)

• **Fig. 2.4** Dosing Levels

Definition – pharmacodynamics

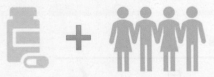

Pharmaco-
Drug

Dynamics
Study of the force

Pharmacodynamics
Study of drugs and their effects on the body

"What the drug does to the body"

• **Fig. 2.5** Definition of Pharmacodynamics

Pharmacodynamics

• Reactions between the drug and living systems

• **Fig. 2.6** Pharmacodynamics as a Reaction

Pharmacodynamics

Therapeutic: drug use treats disease

Adverse: drug use causes harm/unwanted effects

These effects often based on the drug's dose

• **Fig. 2.7** Therapeutic Use Versus Adverse Use

Adverse drug reactions (ADR)

An unintended response at normal doses

Example: A peptic ulcer forms when taking non-steroidal antiinflammatory drugs (NSAIDs) like ibuprofen

• **Fig. 2.8** Adverse Drug Reactions

Receptors

• Drugs produce their effect by attaching to <u>receptors</u>

Receptors: a protein drugs attach to in the body

• These can be best explained by the lock-and-key model

• When a drug attaches to the receptor, an action happens

• **Fig. 2.9** Receptors

Affinity

• The chance that a drug will act at a receptor is considered <u>affinity</u>

• Affinity: how attracted/sticky a drug is to the target receptor

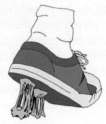

• **Fig. 2.10** Affinity

Receptors and Affinity

Receptors

For medications to work on specific conditions to maximize their therapeutic effect, that which helps the patient and minimizes the adverse drug reactions, they must have a way to target certain physiologic areas. Drugs produce that effect by attaching to a **receptor**. A receptor is often a protein that the drug can attach to that will relay the message to make a physiologic change, such as decreasing heart rate to lower blood pressure or open the bronchioles to help an asthmatic (Fig. 2.9). We will discuss a lock and key analogy a little bit further down, but for anything to happen there must be an attraction between the receptor and the drug, something we call **affinity**.

Affinity

Affinity is the attraction between a receptor, which receives the message from a drug, and the medication itself. Another way to think of affinity is how "sticky" a drug will be, just as gum can stick to person's shoe sole if they step on it (Fig. 2.10). If the drug does not have an attraction for the receptor,

Receptors

High affinity: will stick and stay at receptor for a while

Low affinity: will attach to receptor but can switch quickly

• **Fig. 2.11** High Affinity Versus Low Affinity

or affinity, then it is unlikely the pharmacologic response we want, such as lowering blood pressure, will happen.

We can often separate receptors into two classes, those that have a high affinity and those that have a low affinity for the receptor (Fig. 2.11). One specific example comes from two different classes of NSAIDs. Drugs such as ibuprofen (Advil, Motrin) or naproxen (Aleve, Naprosyn) have affinity for cyclooxygenase-1 (COX-1) and cyclooxygenase-2 (COX-2). One of these enzymes is responsible for mostly helpful effects and another for mostly harmful effects. However, celecoxib (Celebrex) has a much higher affinity for COX-2, which can help to prevent ulcers common with NSAIDs. In this way, we can use affinity to produce a better result for a patient.

Another example is that of affecting beta-receptors. Often, we use Greek letters such as alpha, beta, and mu [MYOO] to describe which receptor the drug will affect. We find many beta-1 receptors in the heart and many beta-2 receptors in the lungs. By selecting for beta-1 receptors with a second-generation beta-blocker such as metoprolol (Toprol XL), we can reduce heart rate and blood pressure. However, a first-generation beta-blocker such as propranolol (Inderal) will block both beta-1 and beta-2 receptors, lowering heart rate and blood pressure. Unfortunately, it will also close up the lungs' bronchioles to some degree. By paying attention to receptor affinity, we can create medications such as the second-generation metoprolol that are safer for certain populations such as asthmatics.

SCENARIO 2.2. RECEPTORS AND AFFINITY

Albuterol is an asthma medication that opens bronchioles in the lungs by activating beta-2 receptors. However, albuterol can also increase heart rate by activating beta-1 adrenergic receptors at very high doses. Does albuterol have a greater affinity for beta-2 or beta-1 receptors?

Answer: Because albuterol activates beta-2 receptors at normal doses, we expect albuterol to have a greater affinity for beta-2 receptors.

Agonists and Antagonists

Agonists

We might affect a receptor with an agonist or antagonist. We will cover **antagonists**, or those molecules that block receptors, in the next section. An **agonist** is a substance

Pharmacodynamics – Endogenous agonists

Endogenous agonist
Substance found naturally in the body that activates receptor

Receptor
Usually located on the cellular membrane and causes effects when activated or antagonized

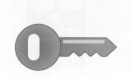
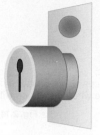

• **Fig. 2.12** Endogenous Agonist

Pharmacodynamics – Agonists

Drug agonist
Substance not found In the body that binds activates receptor

Receptor
Usually located on the cellular membrane and causes effects when activated or antagonized

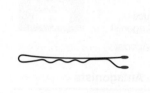
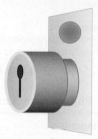

• **Fig. 2.13** Agonists

that activates a receptor; in our analogy, we will call this the key. A receptor is a protein, usually on the cell membrane, that will cause an effect when the key turns in the lock (Fig. 2.12).

We can, in some ways, "trick" the body into releasing agonists by using drugs that activate the receptors. We can think of this as not having the original key but instead using something like a bobby pin, a sprung hairpin, to "pick" the lock and still open the door to a therapeutic effect (Fig. 2.13). However, we may see **full agonists** that cause a maximal response. For example, if maintenance managers in apartment buildings had to have one key for each of 100 different apartments, that would make it very difficult for them to find and keep that many keys with them. It would be much easier to use a skeleton key, a key that opens all of the locks with a single key. Think of a full agonist as a skeleton key, one that opens all of the locks to create a maximal effect (Fig. 2.14). On the other hand, we can have a **partial agonist**, which we can think of as a single apartment key. While the key might open all the doors in a single apartment, the response is not as great as the skeleton key, which can open all the doors in the complex. The response is lower in this case (Fig. 2.15).

Agonists

- Different drugs may attach to the same receptor, and have the same response. These are <u>agonists</u>

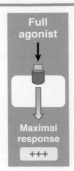

Full agonist

↓

Maximal response

+++

Agonists:
Substances which initiate a physiological response when combined with receptors

• **Fig. 2.14** Full Agonist

Agonists

- If a drug sticks to a receptor and produces a positive response, but a response less than the original substance, this is considered a <u>partial agonist</u>

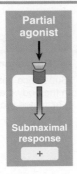

Partial agonist

↓

Submaximal response

+

Partial agonists:
Drugs that bind to the receptor to produce submaximal reponse relative to the full agonist

• **Fig. 2.15** Partial Agonist

Pharmacodynamics – Antagonists

Drug antagonist	Receptor
Substance that binds and blocks receptor to prevent activation	Usually located on the cellular membrane and causes effects when activated or antagonized

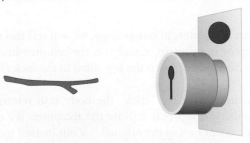

• **Fig. 2.16** Antagonists

Antagonists

Another important aspect of drug pharmacodynamics is the receptor **antagonist**. While a drug may not activate the receptor, it can prevent the receptor's activation. Any time you read that a drug is an inhibitor or blocker, this might be a clue the drug is an antagonist. An antagonist could work like a stick in a keyhole (Fig. 2.16). Two things happen. First, the stick does not open the door; it has no effect on the door opening. Second, the stick blocks a key from working at all. It antagonizes, or prevents, the physiologic effect. For example, a beta-1 blocker will block beta-1 receptors. Normally, when beta-1 receptors activate, heart rate

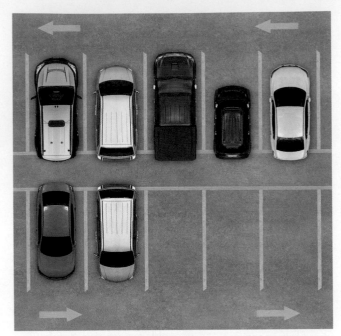

• **Fig. 2.17** Competitive Agonists (©istock #915375802)

goes up. By blocking that receptor, heart rate goes down or stays at a certain level.

When talking about antagonists, we talk about those that are competitive or noncompetitive. Each of these can divide into irreversible or reversible. A **competitive antagonist** binds to the same site as an agonist but does not activate it. A **noncompetitive antagonist** binds to what we call an **allosteric** or nonagonist site to prevent receptor activation.

Imagine a parking lot. If someone parks in the spot you wanted, that person is acting as a competitive antagonist. However, if a green car two spaces over is parked over the yellow line, forcing the black car next to it to be parked over the white line, blocking the parking spot you wanted, the green car acts as a noncompetitive antagonist (Fig. 2.17).

The antagonist can also fall into reversible or irreversible categories. A **reversible antagonist** will move away, that is, the car will not stay parked there forever. This drug will move away and allow the agonist to act later.

An **irreversible antagonist** is like a broken-down car in a parking spot—it is not going anywhere. This drug will stay on the receptor forever, never again allowing an agonist to act there.

SCENARIO 2.3. AGONISTS AND ANTAGONISTS

Allopurinol (Zyloprim) inhibits uric acid through noncompetitive inhibition. Is allopurinol working at the same or different site than the agonists?

Answer: As a noncompetitive inhibitor, allopurinol acts on a different site.

Therapeutic index

- A narrow therapeutic index means they have a small window of safe doses

- A wide therapeutic index is the opposite in that they have a larger window of safe doses

- Drugs with a narrow therapeutic index need to be dosed carefully and monitored frequently by pharmacists and doctors

- **Fig. 2.18** Therapeutic Index

Therapeutic index

- Therapeutic index is the window of drug doses that can be used in patients that are both efficacious and non-lethal
- You can calculate the therapeutic index yourself!

$$\text{Therapeutic index} = \frac{TD_{50}}{ED_{50}}$$

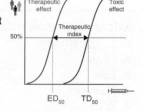

- **Fig. 2.19** Calculating the Therapeutic Index

Therapeutic index

You can have a narrow therapeutic index...

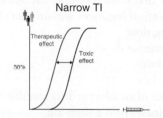

- **Fig. 2.20** Narrow Therapeutic Index

Therapeutic index

...or a wide index!

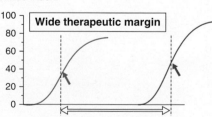

- **Fig. 2.21** Wide Therapeutic Index

Therapeutic Index

Therapeutic Index Generally

We always want to know how safe a drug is, especially when we give it to children. However, safety often comes from the dosages that we need to give and how easy or hard it is to miss the mark with that dosage. A **therapeutic index** is the difference between at what points a drug will help the patient (therapeutic effect) or hurt the patient (toxic effect). We can express the therapeutic index visually and mathematically (Fig. 2.18).

We calculate the therapeutic index mathematically by placing the range between the ED50 and the TD50. The ED50 is the effective dose for half, or 50%, of the population taking the drug. Similarly, the TD50 is that dose which will cause toxicity in 50% of the population who take the drug. The safest medicines have an ED50, or effective dose in half the population, that is much lower than the toxic dose (Fig. 2.19).

Narrow Therapeutic Index

We say the therapeutic index for a drug such as the antiepileptic phenytoin (Dilantin), which has a small gap between a safe and dangerous dose, is a **narrow therapeutic index**. Because mathematically a narrow therapeutic index is a lower number than a wide therapeutic index, we can use the expression "low therapeutic index" as a synonym (Fig. 2.20).

Wide Therapeutic Index

We call the therapeutic index for a drug such as ibuprofen, which has a larger gap between a safe and dangerous dose, a **wide therapeutic index**. Because mathematically a wide therapeutic index is a higher number than a narrow therapeutic index, we can use the expression "high therapeutic index" as a synonym (Fig. 2.21).

SCENARIO 2.4. THERAPEUTIC INDEX

Drug A has a therapeutic index of 3. Drug B has a therapeutic index of 6. Which medication is safer?

Answer: A larger number indicates a wider index or that the toxic dose in 50% of the population (TD50) is much higher than the effective dose in half the population (ED50). Drug B would be the safer of the two.

Summary

- We may want to use drugs that exert a local effect if the medication would be toxic to ingest. Alternatively, we can pair a medication such as ibuprofen with systemic effects to relieve pain further with another local-effect medication such as lidocaine to treat a sunburn better.
- Affinity is the attraction of a molecule to a receptor, a protein that drugs can readily bind. Molecules can have a high affinity (or significant attraction) for the receptor or a low affinity (or weak attraction) for the molecule.
- Agonists activate a receptor while antagonists block an agonist's action. Full agonists create a maximal effect while partial agonists create a less than maximal effect. Antagonists can block a receptor directly (competitive antagonist) or indirectly (noncompetitive antagonist). We can classify an antagonist's action as reversible (it will not permanently attach to the receptor) or irreversible (a permanent binding).
- Therapeutic indices can be wide or narrow. A wide therapeutic index indicates a safer drug while a narrow therapeutic index points to a drug that is less safe.

Review Questions

1. A drug with significant attraction to a receptor would have a _____ affinity.
   a. High
   b. Low
   c. Narrow
   d. Wide
2. The ED50 mainly reflects a drug's _____ at a certain dosage.
   a. Weakness
   b. Effectiveness
   c. Strength
   d. Toxicity
3. Which of the following represents the most recent sources of drugs?
   a. Genetically engineered
   b. Plants
   c. Minerals
   d. Animals
4. The mathematical expression for a "therapeutic index" is the:
   a. TD50/ED50
   b. ED50 alone
   c. TD50 alone
   d. ED50/TD50
5. Phenytoin (Dilantin), an antiepileptic, has a _____ therapeutic index.
   a. Strong
   b. Weak
   c. Narrow
   d. Wide
6. A drug with a weak attraction to a receptor would have a _____ affinity.
   a. High
   b. Low
   c. Narrow
   d. Wide
7. An agonist is a drug that:
   a. Reversibly blocks a receptor
   b. Irreversibly blocks a receptor
   c. Activates a receptor
   d. Inactivates a receptor
8. When the first dose is double the subsequent dosages in a medication regimen, we consider this a:
   a. Loading dose
   b. Maintenance dose
   c. Toxic dose
   d. Lethal dose
9. An example of an adverse drug reaction would include:
   a. Drowsiness from a sleep aid
   b. An ulcer from an antiinflammatory
   c. Acid reduction from an acid reducer
   d. Pain relief from an analgesic
10. A drug has a TD50 of 40 and an ED50 of 10. What is the therapeutic index?
    a. 4
    b. 30
    c. 50
    d. 400

3

Drug Movement (Pharmacokinetics)

LEARNING OBJECTIVES

1. Identify the four major components of pharmacokinetics.
2. Define normal and abnormal absorption.
3. Discuss how adipose tissues and hemodynamics affect distribution.
4. Demonstrate how the liver affects metabolism.
5. Contrast a healthy versus an injured kidney and excretion.

Introduction

In this chapter, we will visit the cousin of pharmacodynamics, pharmacokinetics. While we need to know how drugs will interact with the body, we also need to know the effects the body has on those drugs. The "kinetics" part of pharmacokinetics is similar to the kinetics prefix in kinesiology. A student who studies kinesiology is studying movement or motion. A pharmacology student studying pharmacokinetics studies drug movement (Fig. 3.1).

Pharmacokinetics Versus Pharmacodynamics

We want to contrast these two fundamental principles so that we do not confuse them. In pharmacokinetics, we are studying how the drug moves through the body; often, we shorten this to "what the body does to the drug." In pharmacodynamics, we study the drug's effect on the body; we can say pharmacodynamics is "what the drug does to the body" (Fig. 3.2). By understanding both pharmacokinetics and pharmacodynamics, we have a much better picture of how we can use medications safely and effectively by knowing both the drug effects and drug movement.

Kinetics and ADME

To remember the four major components of pharmacokinetics, we use the mnemonic ADME, pronounced "add me." In this chapter, we will look closely at each component (Fig. 3.3). The **A** represents **absorption** that takes into account what the body does, whether a patient swallows a dose or receives an injection. **D** is for **distribution**; it is how the body moves that drug to various areas of the patient's physiology, inside as well as outside the cells.

We can best describe the word **metabolism**, the **M** in ADME, by comparing it to two other words: anabolism and catabolism. **Anabolism** is the synthesis or creation of molecules, sometimes called *constructive* metabolism or to build. **Catabolism** is the breakdown of molecules into smaller parts, sometimes called *destructive* metabolism. Metabolism itself is not necessarily construction or destruction of molecules; rather it is the changing of a molecule from one thing to another, and it is the altering of a drug chemically. Finally, **E** is for **excretion**, how the body removes chemicals. While urine output is certainly one of the more common means, there are many others.

Absorption

Site of Action

Our first step with absorption is to look at the site of action. Where would the body best take in our medication? A tablet is the most convenient way for a patient to take medicine; the small intestine helps us by absorbing the bulk of the medication. However, it is often better to have a local rather than a systemic effect (Fig. 3.4). While a systemic drug could reach the site, we might expect adverse systemic reactions. By creating a local site for absorption, we might avoid those extraneous effects.

For example, an asthmatic who needs to reduce inflammation and narrowing of the airways could benefit from an inhaler that sprays medicine directly into the lungs. A patient with a small cut could use a local antibiotic that could be spread on rather than an oral, or even intravenous, antibiotic. Sometimes, the stomach destroys a medicine and it is better for absorption when a patient has a direct intramuscular (IM) injection into the arm muscle,

Definition – pharmacokinetics

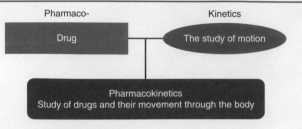

"What the body does to the drug"

- **Fig. 3.1** Definition of Pharmacokinetics

Pharmacokinetics vs Pharmacodynamics

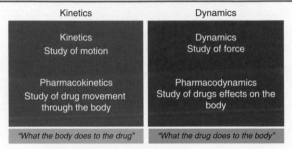

- **Fig. 3.2** Pharmacokinetics Versus Pharmacodynamics

Kinetics and ADME

Movement of the drug through the body can be split into 4 steps (ADME)			
Absorption	**Distribution**	**Metabolism**	**Excretion**
Drug absorbed into body via route of administration	Drug moved into intra- and extracellular spaces	Drug altered chemically within body	Drug removed from body

- **Fig. 3.3** Phamacokinetics and ADME

Absorption

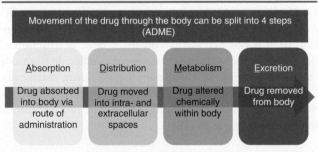

- **Fig. 3.4** Absorption

as with the influenza vaccine. By paying attention to the body's effect on the drug, we can hope for a better therapeutic outcome.

Stomach or Small Intestine?

A common misconception is that absorption happens mostly in the stomach, but that is *not* the case (Fig. 3.5).

Stomach absorption?

Most oral medications are absorbed in the small intestine, not the stomach

Role of the stomach is to break down medication
- Break tablet into smaller and smaller pieces
- Eventually, put the medication into solution, like salt in water

Medications can't be absorbed by small intestine unless they are in solution

- **Fig. 3.5** Stomach Absorption

Absorption Blood flow

Food	Gastrointestinal illness	Blood flow	Age
Delays stomach emptying	Passage through GI tract speeds up (loose stools, diarrhea)	Less blood moving around small intestine allows less drug absorption	Slower stomach emptying, less breaking down of medications (dissolution)
Levothyroxine needs empty stomach	Birth control is less effective with antibiotics and illness	All drugs become less effective	Enteric-coated aspirin is released sooner, causing more GI adverse drug reactions

- **Fig. 3.6** Absorption Changes

Most absorption happens in the small intestine where tiny villi, fingerlike projections, help increase the surface area of the intestine and contain specialized cells that transport substances into the bloodstream. The stomach's role is not absorption; rather, it is to break down materials well enough to help the small intestine do its work.

Aspirin, which the stomach easily absorbs, is acidic, but other drugs are not. We do not want to confuse the two terms dissolution and dissolving. **Dissolution** is how fast a drug comes out of a vehicle, like a capsule. **Dissolving** is how fast or slow the body breaks a drug down into smaller parts.

Absorption Changes

Just as we need to pay attention to the way the body absorbs drugs, we also need to respond to changes that might occur (Fig. 3.6). If a patient takes medicine with food, it delays stomach emptying, which can affect levothyroxine (Synthroid), a synthetic thyroid replacement hormone. If gastrointestinal emptying speeds up, as with diarrhea, it may not give the body enough time to absorb the medication, as with birth control medicine. If there is poor blood flow to an area, we might see less absorption as well. The drug is simply not around the target site long enough. Finally, as patients age, they experience slower stomach emptying, which can affect an enteric-coated aspirin (Ecotrin). The coating would not last long enough to reach the small intestine; thus, the aspirin would be released in the stomach.

Distribution

- Movement of drug into tissues throughout the body after absorption
- Blood moves drugs around body, but drugs don't always stay in blood – based on drug properties

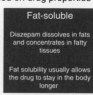
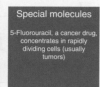

Water-soluble	Fat-soluble	Special molecules
Atenolol dissolves in water and stays in the blood and space between cells	Diazepam dissolves in fats and concentrates in fatty tissues Fat solubility usually allows the drug to stay in the body longer	5-Fluorouracil, a cancer drug, concentrates in rapidly dividing cells (usually tumors)

• **Fig. 3.7** Distribution

Distribution changes

Adipose tissue

Drug can be pushed into adipose tissue and release into blood over time, leading to increased drug levels

Hemodynamic status

Decreased heart function – less movement of blood around the body

Kidney impairment – may lead to high drug levels because it is not being filtered out of blood

• **Fig. 3.8** Distribution Changes

SCENARIO 3.1. ABSORPTION

An asthmatic had significant side effects from an oral medication taken to help reduce the inflammation from a severe asthma attack. What site of action might be a better choice for ensuing treatment?

Answer: Prednisone, an oral steroid for inflammation, can often cause significant side effects—even in short bursts. A better choice might be to provide a daily inhaled steroid to keep the asthma inflammation at bay and to prevent a recurrence of an asthma attack.

Distribution

Water Versus Lipid-Soluble Drugs

Distribution, the second component of our ADME mnemonic, represents how the body will move a drug around (Fig. 3.7). This distribution often depends on certain drug properties. If the drug is **water soluble**, that is it readily dissolves in water, then it will likely stay in the blood and spaces between the cells. Atenolol (Tenormin), a beta-blocker for cardiovascular issues, is an example. However, a drug might be **fat soluble**, such as the benzodiazepine diazepam (Valium). Its ability to dissolve in fats can allow it to remain in the body longer. Certain **special molecules** such as 5-fluorouracil, an antineoplastic (anticancer drug), concentrate its levels in rapidly dividing cells, which are prevalent in tumors.

Distribution Changes

We can target fat tissue (adipose tissue) as a way to keep the drug in the body longer. However, there are often other factors to assess. In patients with poor hemodynamic status, for example, their hearts are not working optimally; we have to consider the consequences in that case. Decreased heart function means that the drugs will take longer to reach target areas since there is less movement in the body. Another potential distribution issue comes from the kidney. Patients with kidney disease cannot clear the medication as quickly, leading to possibly toxic levels (Fig. 3.8).

SCENARIO 3.2. DISTRIBUTION

A patient receives an injection every 4 weeks versus taking a tablet once daily. Is this drug form likely water soluble or fat soluble?

Answer: It is more likely fat soluble because those medications can remain in the body longer.

Metabolism

Metabolism is the chemical change of a drug in the body (Figs. 3.9 and 3.10). The liver is often the center of metabolism, though drug changes can happen in other ways. A metabolite is the substance that comes after metabolism. Some of these metabolites are helpful and initiate the therapeutic effect; others are harmful and can lead to adverse drug reactions. Knowing how the body will change drugs into these metabolites is critical for safely administering medicines. One such drug is tramadol (Ultram), a weak opioid pain reliever that works as an analgesic. After entering the liver, there are many metabolites; some are helpful, some are harmful, and some do nothing at all (inert).

It is also important to know how long a drug will last in the body before being eliminated. We use the term **half-life** to describe the time it takes for a drug to decrease by half. For example, if we begin with 100 milligrams (mg) of a drug, one half-life will reduce that amount to 50 mg. Two half-lives will further reduce the drug to 25 mg, three half-lives to 12.5 mg, four half-lives to 6.25 mg, and five half-lives to 3.125 mg. We consider a drug to have been eliminated once we reach five half-lives.

We can use our knowledge of metabolism, or the lack of metabolism, to treat issues in the bladder. For example, if a patient takes nitrofurantoin (Macrobid), an antibiotic for urinary tract infections, it will pass to the kidneys without any change in the liver. Thus, it can exert its effect on the bacteria in the bladder.

One concern is liver function. If a patient has poor liver function because of illness or disease, the liver may lack the capacity to clear toxic metabolites successfully (Fig. 3.11). Knowing where the body metabolizes the medicine is critical to patient safety. Toxic metabolites can build up, harming this patient.

Metabolism

- Chemical changes to the drug by the body
- Most drugs metabolized in liver
- Some are metabolized extensively

Tramadol
Weak opioid, used
for moderate pain

Lots of chemical
changes by liver
(extensive metabolism)

Some metabolites are active and cause side effects,
others are inert

• **Fig. 3.9** Metabolism (Part 1)

Metabolism

- Chemical changes to the drug by the body
- Most drugs metabolized in liver
- Some aren't metabolized at all

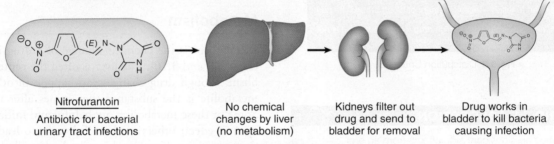

Nitrofurantoin
Antibiotic for bacterial
urinary tract infections

No chemical
changes by liver
(no metabolism)

Kidneys filter out
drug and send to
bladder for removal

Drug works in
bladder to kill bacteria
causing infection

• **Fig. 3.10** Metabolism (Part 2)

Metabolism changes

- Liver damage or disease decreases metabolism
- Some drugs require hepatic metabolism to work
- Others need the liver to remove toxic metabolites

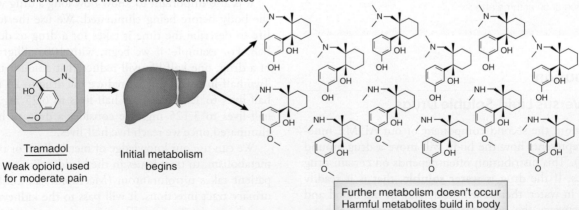

Tramadol
Weak opioid, used
for moderate pain

Initial metabolism
begins

Further metabolism doesn't occur
Harmful metabolites build in body

• **Fig. 3.11** Metabolism Changes

Other factors that can affect metabolism include race. Some races produce less renin, an enzyme important in blood pressure control. Others have different genetics, which can affect enzyme activity. A disease can affect the rate of metabolism, as shown with liver disease, discussed earlier. Protein binding is another concern. A drug that is highly protein bound can make it difficult to get to a target. The drug has to be able to separate from the protein, such as albumin, to reach its target.

SCENARIO 3.3. METABOLISM

A patient takes a medication that the liver does not metabolize at all. Where might the site of infection be if this is the case?

Answer: Some drugs for bladder infection rely on the liver ignoring them as they pass through the body.

Excretion

While we think of excretion as the kidneys creating urine to remove harmful chemicals, other sites of excretion are available. For example, the lungs excrete air, pores excrete sweat, and the breasts excrete breast milk. Other avenues of excretion include the feces, bile, tears, and saliva. However, in this section, we will focus primarily on the kidneys and their filtering of chemicals through their nephrons, the functional units of the kidney (Fig. 3.12).

There are many reasons for excretion changes. Three primary reasons are chronic kidney disease (CKD), hypotension, and dehydration (Fig. 3.13). Kidney damage may impair the body's ability to filter chemicals. Hypotension, or decreased blood pressure, can result in a slowing of the filtration rate. Dehydration can cause less fluid to enter the nephron, reducing filtration.

One specific change to excretion can come from direct damage to the kidney (Fig. 3.14). In a car accident, for example, the kidney might incur a blockage or significant damage. Or, the cause might come from CKD, reduced activity of the kidney over time.

Healthy Kidneys

In healthy kidneys, the body can readily excrete the drug in the urine. The drug levels decrease over time and eventually the drug is eliminated from the body (Fig. 3.15).

Injured Kidneys

When the kidneys sustain damage, they cannot keep up with the amount of drug in the body. The drug remains to exert toxic or sustained effects beyond that which the clinician wants. We can often avoid this drug buildup by detecting the lower rate of excretion and lowering the dosage or increasing the time interval between doses (Fig. 3.16).

SCENARIO 3.4. EXCRETION

What are the three scenarios in which the filtration rate in the kidney may decrease, keeping drug levels elevated?

Answer: CKD, hypotension, and dehydration can all contribute to a slower filtering rate.

Excretion

- Removal of waste products from the body produced during metabolism
- Most done by the kidneys, acting as the body's filters
- Nephron - site of filtration inside the kidney

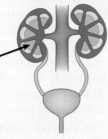

• **Fig. 3.12** Excretion

Causes for excretion changes

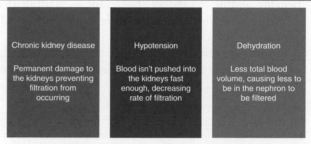

Chronic kidney disease	Hypotension	Dehydration
Permanent damage to the kidneys preventing filtration from occurring	Blood isn't pushed into the kidneys fast enough, decreasing rate of filtration	Less total blood volume, causing less to be in the nephron to be filtered

• **Fig. 3.13** Causes for Excretion Changes

Excretion blood flow

- Injury
  - Blunt trauma, like car crash
  - Acute kidney injury (AKI) - decreased blood flow to kidneys, blockage to bladder
- Disease
  - Chronic kidney disease (CKD)

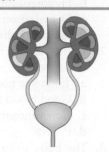

• **Fig. 3.14** More Causes for Excretion Changes

Healthy kidneys

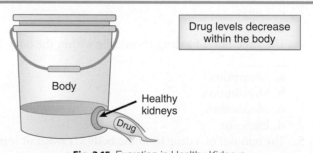

Drug levels decrease within the body

Body

Healthy kidneys

Drug

• **Fig. 3.15** Excretion in Healthy Kidneys

Injured kidneys

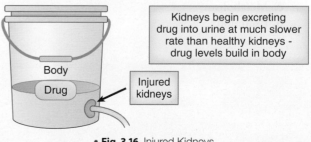

Kidneys begin excreting drug into urine at much slower rate than healthy kidneys - drug levels build in body

Body

Drug

Injured kidneys

• **Fig. 3.16** Injured Kidneys

Summary

- We can summarize pharmacokinetics as what the body does to the drug and pharmacodynamics as what the drug does to the body. Knowing the pharmacokinetics and pharmacodynamics of a drug makes it much easier to provide safe and effective administration. We use the ADME mnemonic, taking the first letters of absorption, distribution, metabolism, and excretion to remember the four primary components of pharmacokinetics.
- With absorption, we are especially concerned with the site of action. Whether the drug absorbs in the small intestine, lungs, skin, or muscle, each area comes with benefits and/or drawbacks. For example, a drug that directly reaches the lungs might have fewer systemic side effects.
- Most drugs are either water soluble or fat soluble. If the prescriber wants to provide a medication that will last longer, we expect the drug to more likely be fat soluble. However, changes in distribution, such as with heart conditions or kidney disease, can alter our approach and dosages.
- Metabolism represents the change of one chemical into one or many others. If the body extensively metabolizes a drug and illness prevents this metabolism, it is critical that the prescriber change the dose accordingly. A metabolite is one product of metabolism. A drug that does not metabolize at all could end up as a treatment for a bladder infection.
- Excretion is the removal of products from the body. While the urine is the primary site of excretion, the lungs, sweat glands, and intestines can also play an important role. Three causes of excretion changes are CKD, hypotension, and dehydration.

Review Questions

1. Which of the following factors does not affect a body's ability to excrete drugs?
   a. Chronic kidney disease
   b. Hypotension
   c. Dehydration
   d. Healthy kidney function
2. Which of the following is not a concern regarding absorption?
   a. Taking or not taking food
   b. Good blood flow
   c. Gastrointestinal illness
   d. Patient's age
3. The body primarily absorbs oral medications in the _____.
   a. Small intestine
   b. Stomach
   c. Lungs
   d. Skin
4. The alteration of a drug chemically within the body is _____.
   a. Absorption
   b. Distribution
   c. Metabolism
   d. Excretion
5. The removal of a drug from the body via sweat or tears is a result of _____.
   a. Absorption
   b. Distribution
   c. Metabolism
   d. Excretion
6. The movement of a drug throughout the body into spaces inside and outside the cell is:
   a. Absorption
   b. Distribution
   c. Metabolism
   d. Excretion
7. A metabolite is the result of which pharmacokinetic path?
   a. Absorption
   b. Distribution
   c. Metabolism
   d. Excretion
8. Which of the following is the primary organ for excretion?
   a. Liver
   b. Bile
   c. Kidney
   d. Feces
9. Which of the following is the primary organ for metabolism?
   a. Liver
   b. Bile
   c. Kidney
   d. Feces
10. How many half-lives must pass for a body to excrete a drug fully?
    a. 2
    b. 3
    c. 4
    d. 5

4

Drug Laws and Preventing Medication Errors

LEARNING OBJECTIVES

1. Identify federal regulatory agencies.
2. Understand federal versus state laws.
3. Outline the progression of drug laws.
4. Identify look-alike sound-alike drugs.
5. Understand the use of tall man letters.

Federal Regulatory Agencies—Food and Drug Administration, Drug Enforcement Administration, and Centers for Disease Control and Prevention

The Food and Drug Administration (FDA), Drug Enforcement Administration (DEA), and Centers for Disease Control and Prevention (CDC) are all federal regulatory agencies critical to the safe use of medications.

Food and Drug Administration

The FDA is a branch of the United States Department of Health and Human Services. The FDA was formed in 1906 after the passing of the Pure Food and Drug Act. The agency's responsibility has grown over time as the number of available medications has increased. Currently, FDA responsibilities include the management of cosmetics, medicines, medical devices, radiation-emitting products, food and drugs used for farm animals, domestic and imported food, bottled water, and wine beverages that have less than a 7% alcohol by volume ratio. As such, approvals may take time, and there is often pressure on the FDA to make approvals quickly if there is a specific need for medicine more urgently.

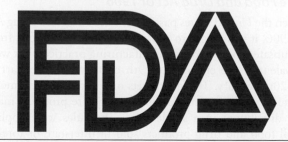

Drug Enforcement Administration

The DEA was created after the passing of the Controlled Substances Act in 1970. It enforces controlled substance laws and regulations and prosecutes those who grow, manufacture, or distribute illegal substances. The DEA keeps a close watch on the number of controlled medications that pharmacies distribute, as one of the most significant paths to addiction includes prescribed opioid analgesics.

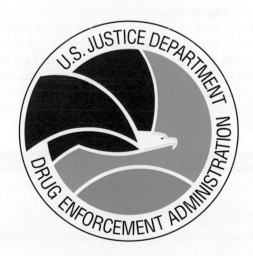

Centers for Disease Control and Prevention

The CDC began in 1946. Its role is to investigate, prevent, and help control diseases. This role allows the agency to protect the United States from health, safety, and security threats. It also provides statistics and information to health professionals about the treatment of a wide variety of common and rare diseases. It is a collaborative entity working with many others to create a much healthier and safer country.

* Brand discontinued, now available only as generic
† Naming conventions can vary between prescription and OTC formulations

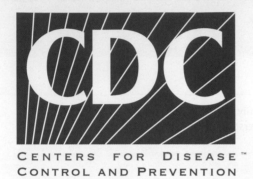

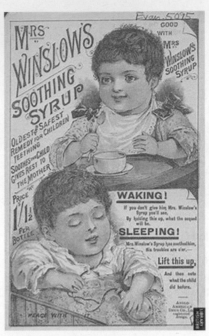

• **Fig. 4.1** Advertisement for Mrs. Winslow's Soothing Syrup circa 1883 from http://www.bl.uk/onlinegallery/onlineex/evancoll/a/014eva00000 0000u05095000.html © British Library Board

Federal Versus State Laws

The federal and state governments are in charge of different parts of practice. The federal government primarily regulates interstate commerce, patient privacy laws, and regulations around drug manufacturing, approval, and safety. State governments are the primary regulators of practice and licensing. State law sets the minimum qualifications for individuals involved with a practice, including setting requirements, if any, for licenses or credentials to be registered with the state board.

Typically, state laws are stricter than federal regulations. For example, the maximum amount of pseudoephedrine that a person can purchase in a month is 7.5 grams (g) in Iowa compared with 9 g in the federal law. When state and federal laws disagree, the stricter laws prevail. This leads to variations in what a practitioner and patient can and cannot do regionally.

Progression of Drug Laws

Patent Drugs

Before 1906, there were not many regulations for medications. There were no prescription drugs, as all the medicines were made by physicians or pharmacists and sold directly to consumers. Some drugs were patented, but many were just trademarked. These drugs are known as patent drugs. Many of the medicines contained ingredients that were minimally efficacious and were sometimes harmful.

One example of a patent drug was Clark Stanley's Snake Oil Liniment, a lotion or cream that claimed to give immediate relief for many ailments, including rheumatism, sore throats, and animal bites, and contracted muscles. No ingredients were listed on the label, but the U.S. Bureau of Chemistry tested it and found it to contain mineral oil, fatty oil, capsaicin, turpentine, and camphor.

Another patent drug was Mrs. Winslow's Soothing Syrup, which was marketed for constipation and pain relief for teething babies (Fig. 4.1) The drug contained alcohol, but 65 mg of morphine per ounce was not listed on the label. It is estimated that thousands of children needlessly died from using this drug.

Milestones in Progression of Drug Laws
Pure Food and Drug Act of 1906

When the United States passed the Pure Food and Drug Act of 1906, it was meant to protect the American public from the unsafe food and drug manufacturing practices that were prevalent at the end of the 19th century and the start of the 20th century. The law targets only interstate commerce because it was unconstitutional to regulate products made and distributed in a single state. The rules were applied to all food and drug products sold in interstate or foreign commerce.

The Pure Food and Drug Act sought to eliminate misbranding or adulteration of patent drugs by requiring labels that listed all drugs, including habit-forming medications. Also, expected side effects were to be listed as well. The labels could not contain false therapeutic claims, and the government could seize products that did not comply. The drugs also had a purity standard established by the United States Pharmacopeia (USP).

A list of 10 problematic drugs with addictive or dangerous properties was created to ensure reporting on the product label. This list included alcohol, morphine, opium, cocaine, heroin, alpha or beta eucaine, chloroform, cannabis indica, chloral hydrate, and acetanilide. Coca-Cola changed its formula after this law passed, as the cocaine ingredient turned to caffeine.

The Pure Food and Drug Act also created the FDA. The FDA had the responsibility of testing all drugs and food made for human consumption.

Major Outcomes

I. Products needed labeling that included drugs and side effects.
II. The government could seize products sold across state lines that did not comply.

Sulfanilamide Disaster of 1937

Sulfanilamide is the active ingredient in an antibiotic that was commonly used for streptococcal infections. Safe tablet and powder forms existed; however, in 1937, the S. E. Massengill Company created an elixir form meant to help with sore throats. Diethylene glycol, a popular active ingredient in antifreeze, was used as the solvent to get the product into the liquid form. Over 100 people died in less than a year from ingesting the sulfanilamide elixir.

As no safety tests were required before bringing drugs to the market, the manufacturer did not have to ensure that it was safe for consumption. While the Pure Food and Drug Act of 1906 required an authentic ingredients label, the lay public might not have been able to determine that the chemicals were not indeed safe for consumption. It was up to the FDA to find the products and their shipments. The company did have to pay a fine because the end product was not a genuine elixir made with alcohol as the solvent.

Major Outcome

I. The FDA could approve or deny new drug applications through the Food, Drug, and Cosmetic Act of 1938.

Food, Drug, and Cosmetic Act of 1938

The Food, Drug, and Cosmetic Act (FDCA) of 1938 was a result of the sulfanilamide elixir tragedy and replaced the Pure Food and Drug Act of 1906. The earlier act was most concerned with the product's purity rather than its safety. The FDCA of 1938 allowed the FDA to require manufacturers to prove that a drug was safe as part of a new drug application before marketing and sale. Under this law, the drugs also had to be labeled with adequate directions so that the patient could use it correctly.

Major Outcomes

I. Required drugs are labeled with adequate directions.
II. Manufacturers had to prove that a drug was safe before the sale.

SCENARIO 4.4. MILESTONE LAWS

Which law states that medications must have directions for use and appropriate safety warnings?
Answer: The Food, Drug, and Cosmetic Act of 1938

Durham-Humphrey Amendment of 1951

Even with the enactment of the FDCA, there were still gaps in the safety of medications sold to the general public. The Durham-Humphrey Amendment of 1951 amended the FDCA, giving the FDA the authority to determine whether medicines are safe to use without a prescription, over the counter (OTC), or if they should require a prescription. The amendment also laid out specific requirements for the safe and appropriate dispensing of prescription medications (Fig. 4.2).

The Durham-Humphrey Act specifically creates two categories of drugs: prescription (also known as legend) and OTC. Medications that cannot be safely used OTC from that time onward could only be legally dispensed based on the prescriber's authority. Medications designated as prescription must also have "Caution: Federal law prohibits dispensing without prescription" on the label.

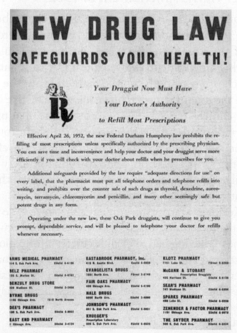

• **Fig. 4.2** Durham-Humphry Act. Notice from http://oprfmuseum.org/this-month-in-history/health-care-reform-1952

Major Outcomes

I. Prescription medications can be dispensed only with a valid prescription and must include a specific statement.

II. OTC medications do not need a prescription.

SCENARIO 4.5. MILESTONE LAWS

Which amendment to the Food, Drug, and Cosmetic Act gave the FDA the authority to determine whether a medication is OTC or will require a prescription?

Answer: The Durham-Humphrey Amendment of 1951

Thalidomide Disaster of 1962

Back in 1962, thalidomide, a medication now used for skin lesions caused by leprosy and multiple myeloma, was in the process of being approved in the United States. Europeans often used the drug for pregnancy-induced nausea. Before its approval in the United States, physicians began using it off-label for morning sickness. Many of these patients gave birth to children with particular congenital disabilities, including deafness, severe underdevelopment or absence of arms (known as phocomelia), and defects in the leg bones. Fortunately, the FDA discovered the severe side effects and did not approve thalidomide for use in the United States. Unfortunately, the drug had already been distributed to over 20,000 patients in the United States during the clinical trial phase.

Major Outcome

I. The Kefauver Harris Amendment to the FDCA, which increased regulation of which drugs can be on the market.

Kefauver-Harris Amendment of 1962

The Kefauver-Harris Amendment of 1962 came about as a response to the thalidomide tragedy, when dangerous side effects of the drug were discovered during the clinical trial phase. This amendment allowed the FDA to regulate further which drugs could be on the market. It put the onus of proof on the manufacturer that a drug was effective and safe through clinical trials before approval. The manufacturer needs to report side effects that occurred after approval. This amendment also required the FDA to evaluate the effectiveness of drugs approved from 1938 to 1962 for safety but not necessarily effectiveness. There is no use for a drug that lacks therapeutic efficacy as compared with placebo.

The Kefauver-Harris Amendment also allowed the FDA to set good manufacturing practices as well as control drug advertising. The marketing had to include correct information about side effects and control generic drug marketing to make sure that generic medications, which are supposed to be less expensive, were not sold at higher prices with new brand names.

Major Outcomes

I. Drug manufacturers had to prove drug effectiveness and safety.

II. Drug advertising needed to be accurate regarding side effects.

Comprehensive Drug Abuse Prevention and Control Act of 1970

Congress passed the Comprehensive Drug Abuse Prevention and Control Act of 1970 to combat illegal drug use that had increased during the 1960s. The first part of the law created what we now know as the drug schedules. A Latin number would be assigned to each schedule: Schedule I (one) was the most dangerous and Schedule V (five) was the least dangerous.

Schedule I drugs have a high potential for abuse and no accepted medical use. Examples include heroin, LSD, and ecstasy.

Schedule II drugs have a high potential for abuse and have an accepted medical use. Examples include morphine, cocaine, and amphetamines.

Schedule III drugs have a lower potential for abuse compared with Schedule I and Schedule II drugs. Examples include acetaminophen with codeine, ketamine, and testosterone.

Schedule IV drugs have a low potential for abuse or dependence. Examples include benzodiazepines and zolpidem.

Schedule V drugs have the lowest potential for abuse or dependence. Examples include pregabalin, diphenoxylate/atropine, and cough syrups with limited amounts of codeine.

The other part of the law provided penalties for controlled substance importation, exportation, and criminal forfeiture, allowing the agency to combat the drug trade better.

Major Outcome

I. Created drug schedules to manage potentially addictive medications.

SCENARIO 4.6. MILESTONE LAWS

The Comprehensive Drug Abuse Prevention and Control Act of 1970 has allowed for the management of potentially addictive medications. Which DEA schedule has the highest abuse potential but still has medical use?

Answer: Schedule II medications have high abuse potential but still have medical use associated.

Poison Prevention Packaging Act of 1970

The Poison Prevention Packaging Act of 1970 was passed to prevent accidental childhood poisonings. It addressed the problem of children trying to get into medication bottles and/or taking pills because some pills look like candy. This law gave the Consumer Product Safety Commission the power to establish standards for packaging of drugs and other household products to prevent poisoning. How do we determine whether a package is child resistant (Fig. 4.3)? Upon testing, a package is considered to be child resistant if:

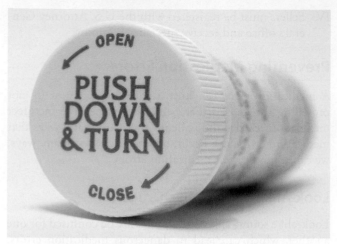

• **Fig. 4.3** Child Resistant Bottle (© istock #147665766)

(a) 80% of children under 5 years old cannot open the package
(b) 90% of adults can open the package

Child-resistant packaging is the default for most drugs that a pharmacy dispenses unless the patient specifically asks for non–child-resistant packaging. Older adults often request nonsafety packaging because of conditions such as arthritis. The law provides other exceptions, but a patient must provide a signature to receive nonsafety packaging to assert that there are no small children in the home who could be in danger from the medication.

Major Outcomes

I. Requires special packaging to protect children from injury.
II. The package is considered child resistant if 80% of kids under 5 years old cannot open the package but 90% of adults can.

SCENARIO 4.7. MILESTONE LAWS

When a child gets into a medication, it can lead to unintentional poisoning. As a way to prevent this, medication bottles can come with child-resistant lids. What is the maximum percentage of children that should be able to open these specific lids?
  Answer: Less than 20% of children under 5 years old

Orphan Drug Act of 1983

Moving a drug from a chemical to a therapeutically approved medication is a long and expensive process. As such, pharmaceutical companies are more likely to create medicines that can benefit from more significant sales in more common conditions, such as hypertension and diabetes. However, this leaves patients who have rare diseases with fewer treatment options since companies do not devote as many resources to developing medications for those diseases.

The Orphan Drug Act of 1983 aimed to increase the treatment options for rare diseases. A "rare disease" is one that affects fewer than 200,000 people. These include Tourette syndrome and Huntington disease. It allows the FDA to provide financial incentives to drug companies to develop and market drugs to treat rare diseases and provide options for patients and providers. These incentives include 7 years of market exclusivity, tax credits for up to 50% of research and development, and grants for clinical testing of orphan drugs. In 2019, the FDA approved 21 orphan drugs versus 27 nonorphan drugs.

Major Outcomes

I. Companies earn federal incentives to develop and market drugs for rare diseases.
II. A 7-year exclusive patent on drug sales and tax breaks come with making an orphan drug.

SCENARIO 4.8. MILESTONE LAWS

How does one define a rare disease eligible for an orphan drug mathematically?
  Answer: An orphan drug is a medication to treat a rare disease that affects less than 200,000 patients.

Omnibus Budget Reconciliation Act of 1990

The Omnibus Budget Reconciliation Act of 1990 (OBRA 90) was the most extensive deficit reduction package ever passed and included many important parts that affect medications. First, pharmacists are required to complete a prospective drug use review before filling every prescription to determine whether the medication is appropriate and necessary. Second, the pharmacists must offer to counsel Medicare and Medicaid patients about the relevant drug information and potential adverse effects. Finally, the pharmacy must keep accurate and up-to-date patient profiles with this information. Just as discussed earlier with respect to other laws, states are able to enact more stringent rules than those required under OBRA 90. One-third of states require pharmacists to counsel on *all* medications, including new prescriptions and refills, while two-thirds of states require pharmacists to counsel only on *new* medicines. Most states have applied OBRA 90 rules to all patients, not just Medicare and Medicaid patients.

Major Outcomes

I. Pharmacists must offer to counsel Medicare and Medicaid patients about drug information and possible adverse effects.
II. Requires state Medicaid provider pharmacists to review Medicaid recipients' drug profiles before filling their prescription(s).

Health Insurance Portability and Accountability Act of 1996

The value of digital information exponentially changed as the Internet expanded. The Health Insurance Portability and Accountability Act (HIPAA) of 1996 was created to protect patient-specific health information from being disclosed without the patient's knowledge, especially electronically. HIPAA restricts those situations in which health care providers can disclose protected health information for treatment and/or payment. It also grants patients the right to access their records and see who else has accessed their records.

HIPAA also sets standards for improved electronic security of protected health information (PHI). It created a standardized set of codes that hospitals share for health transactions and requires unique identifiers. Finally, it sets standards for the security of PHI and electronic signatures, including storage, transmission, and access. The only people who can or should access a patient's PHI are those who need the information to treat the patient properly.

Major Outcomes

I. Standardizes codes among hospitals for health transactions.
II. Requires unique identifiers to reduce errors and costs.
III. Specifies requirements for security, physical storage, and transmission of PHI.
IV. Limits nonconsensual PHI use and release of PHI.
V. Allows patients the right to access their record and see who else accessed it.

Combat Methamphetamine Epidemic Act of 2005

The Combat Methamphetamine Epidemic Act of 2005 regulates products sold OTC that contain ephedrine, pseudoephedrine, and phenylpropanolamine. Each of these substances can be used in the manufacture of methamphetamine, often known as "meth." These drugs must be kept behind the pharmacy counter away from easy access or held in locked cases. The law limits how much can be sold to 3.6 g in one day and 9 g per month. To buy these drugs, patients must provide identification and sign a sales log. Sellers of these drugs must also be registered with the U.S. Attorney General's office and receive specialized training. Currently, many states have connected networks; thus, patients cannot go to multiple pharmacies and exceed the legal limits.

Major Outcomes

I. Ephedrine, pseudoephedrine, and phenylpropanolamine must be kept behind pharmacy counters or in locked cases.
II. Limits sales of these drugs to 3.6 g per day and 9 g per month.
III. Patients must provide identification and sign a sales log.

IV. Sellers must be registered with the U.S. Attorney General's office and receive specialized training.

Preventing Medication Errors

A medication error can hurt a patient directly or by not providing the needed therapeutic help when the incorrect medication reaches the patient. There are many ways that medication errors can occur, but there are also many ways, we can try to prevent medication errors.

Look-Alike Sound-Alike Drugs

Look-alike sound-alike drugs can easily be confused for one another, which can lead to dangerous medication errors. The Institute for Safe Medication Practices maintains a list of look-alike sound-alike drugs. Examples include:
- clonidine and Klonopin
- amlodipine and amiloride
- misoprostol and mifepristone
- oxcarbazepine and carbamazepine

It is essential to have ways to keep these drugs separated. Some ways to do this include:
- using tall man letters
- using the brand and generic names on labels
- providing the indication of the medication on the prescription label
- distinguishing the medication bottles
- keeping the medication in separate areas

Tall Man Letters

One commonly used method to decrease medication errors from look-alike sound-alike drugs is using tall man letters to help differentiate drug names. Each drug's unique portion is capitalized and sometimes bolded, italicized, or sometimes in a different color. While these letters can be in the beginning, middle, and end of the medication, they are not drug class prefixes, infixes, or suffixes, such as the cef- from cefepime, -pred- in methylprednisolone, and -cillin in amoxicillin.

Some examples of tall man letters include:
- rif**AMP**in and rif**AXIM**in
- **SAX**agliptin and **SIT**agliptin
- diaze**PAM** and diltiazem

SCENARIO 4.9. PREVENTING MEDICATION ERRORS

What is one way to prevent medication errors due to look-alike sound-alike drugs?
Answer: Tall man letters

Summary

- The FDA, DEA, and CDC are federal agencies that regulate different aspects of medication development, safety, and use. The FDA regulates drug approvals and safety, the DEA regulates controlled substances, and the CDC manages data and statistics for diseases.
- When federal laws and state laws conflict, the stricter regulation must be followed.
- Laws have been changed over time to increase patient safety. Notable federal drug laws include the Pure Food and Drug Act of 1906, the Federal Food, Drug, and Cosmetic Act of 1938, the Durham-Humphrey Amendment of 1951, the Kefauver-Harris Amendment of 1962, the Comprehensive Drug Abuse Prevention and Control Act of 1970, the Poison Prevention Packaging Act of 1970, the Orphan Drug Act of 1983, the Omnibus Budget Reconciliation Act of 1990 (OBRA 90), the Health Insurance Portability and Accountability Act of 1996 (HIPAA), and the Combat Methamphetamine Epidemic Act of 2005.
- Medication errors can be dangerous. It is essential to utilize ways to distinguish look-alike sound-alike drugs from one another, such as using tall man letters.

Review Questions

1. Which federal regulatory agency enforces controlled substance laws and regulations?
   a. State organizations
   b. Drug Enforcement Administration
   c. Food and Drug Administration
   d. Centers for Disease Control and Prevention
2. When a state pharmacy law and the federal pharmacy law conflict, which law should be followed?
   a. The state law
   b. The federal law
   c. The more strict law
   d. The less strict law
3. Which act was created due to the events of the elixir sulfanilamide incident?
   a. 1938 Federal Food, Drug, and Cosmetic Act
   b. Durham-Humphry Amendment of 1951
   c. Kefauver-Harris Amendment of 1962
   d. Comprehensive Drug Abuse Prevention and Control Act of 1970
4. Which act was created due to the events of the thalidomide disaster and led to drug manufacturers needing to prove the effectiveness and safety of their drugs before approval?
   a. 1938 Federal Food, Drug, and Cosmetic Act
   b. Durham-Humphrey Amendment of 1951
   c. Kefauver-Harris Amendment of 1962
   d. Comprehensive Drug Abuse Prevention and Control Act of 1970
5. According to the Controlled Substance Act, in what class of controlled medication is heroin?
   a. I
   b. II
   c. III
   d. IV

6. According to the Controlled Substance Act, what class of controlled medication is acetaminophen/codeine (Tylenol #3*)?
   a. I
   b. II
   c. III
   d. IV
7. According to the Controlled Substance Act, in what class of controlled medication is zolpidem (Ambien)?
   a. I
   b. II
   c. III
   d. IV
8. What is required to fulfill a request to use a non–child-resistant prescription vial?
   a. Prescriber's signature
   b. A patient saying he doesn't want a lid
   c. Patient's signature
   d. The prescriber saying it is OK
9. Which act gave tax incentives to manufacturers to encourage them to develop medications for rare diseases?
   a. 1938 Federal Food, Drug, and Cosmetic Act
   b. Orphan Drug Act of 1983
   c. Omnibus Budget Reconciliation Act of 1990
   d. Comprehensive Drug Abuse Prevention and Control Act of 1970
10. Under *federal law*, what is the maximum amount of pseudoephedrine that can be bought in a month?
    a. 3.6 g
    b. 4 g
    c. 7.5 g
    d. 9 g

5

Drug Administration

1. Compare and contrast the enteral versus parenteral routes.
2. Discuss enteral administration.
3. Discuss parenteral administration.
4. Provide examples of other administration routes.

Enteral Versus Parenteral

Enteral means that something is passing through the intestines—whether in a natural opening, such as the mouth, or an artificial opening. Often, people see the word "parent" in **parenteral**, but the prefix is really "para" + enteral. **Para** can mean beside, as in parathyroid, abnormal, as in paranormal, or beyond, as in para-enteral. Over time, the second "a" dropped, making the word simply parenteral, or beyond enteral. So, an enteral medication goes through the gastrointestinal (GI) tract and a parenteral medication is outside the GI tract, as in using a needle for an intramuscular flu shot.

Advantages and Disadvantages

As with deciding which medication to give, a prescriber must also weigh the differences in the routes. While both enteral and parenteral routes have advantages and disadvantages, usually patient-specific factors make the choice readily apparent (Table 5.1). When a patient has a stomachache from excess acid, an antacid tablet might be enough. However, if a patient needs a preventative vaccination, and the medicine would be otherwise damaged by the stomach, then an intramuscular injection makes more sense.

Usually, with each enteral advantage, we can find a parenteral administration disadvantage and vice versa. It is much less expensive to give an ibuprofen (Motrin) tablet for analgesic pain relief than a ketorolac (Toradol) injection. However, the ibuprofen tablet would take longer to work. Table 5.1 outlines some of the situations in which enteral and parenteral dosage forms have opposite advantages and disadvantages.

How to Choose the Best Route

Generally, there is a standard of practice, a certain dosage administration form that prescribers use more commonly. For example, a patient self-treating a headache might grab an over-the-counter (OTC) oral pain reliever. If this headache progresses to a migraine and the patient starts vomiting, then the oral medication might not make it into the GI tract for absorption. In this case, the standard of care might progress to using a parenteral injection such as migraine-specific sumatriptan (Imitrex). While experience dictates the choice many times, these decisions often come from a common-sense cascade.

Enteral

Enteral forms include oral, nasogastric, gastrostomy, sublingual, buccal, vaginal, and rectal. As with deciding between enteral and parenteral dosage forms, the best administration type often has to do with the patient's individual conditions. In this section, we will dive deeper into each form, giving examples of when one would or would not use them.

Oral

The most common route is oral, often abbreviated PO, which is Latin for *per os* or, literally, through the opening. It is often the most practical route because it is relatively easy to take or give an oral dose, the pills can be inexpensive, and a patient might be able to take the medicine without help. The complexity comes from the various oral dosage forms, which are often a solid or liquid.

Solid dosage forms include **capsules** that encase the medicine. When drugs first come on the market, we will often see a capsule form because it is much easier to manufacture a capsule and put something in it than to get the tablet form perfectly right. It is not that tablets cannot be manufactured, it is that the tablet must dissolve at a certain rate as it goes through the stomach and GI tract. A **tablet** is simply an amount of medication compressed into a pellet with certain fillers to keep it stable. Patients are not meant to swallow a **lozenge**; rather, unlike a capsule or tablet, they should allow the medicine to dissolve slowly. We often see lozenges in medicines for sore throats (Fig. 5.1).

TABLE 5.1	Advantages and Disadvantages of Enteral Versus Parenteral Administration	
Enteral Advantages	**Parenteral Disadvantages**	
Less expensive	More expensive	
Easier to make (nonsterile)	Harder to make (sterile)	
Self-administration	Needs professional administration	
Enteral Disadvantages	**Parenteral Advantages**	
Slower onset of action	Rapid action	
Poor/bitter taste	Taste is not a consideration with an injection	
Patient must be conscious	Patient can be unconscious	

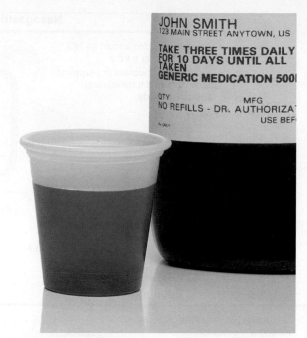

• **Fig. 5.2** Liquid Dosage Forms (© istock #92261289)

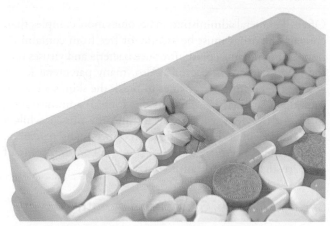

• **Fig. 5.1** Solid Dosage Forms (© istock #528907589)

Liquid dosage forms include five major types: solutions, syrups, suspensions, emulsions, and elixirs (Fig. 5.2). A **solution** is clear, with the drug completely dissolved. By contrast, a **suspension** includes a medicine that is not completely dissolved. Often, we store drugs such as amoxicillin as a powder. When the patient is ready, we will add water and create a suspension. To keep the medicine relatively uniform, the patient must shake the container before taking it. A **syrup** simply contains significant sugar as part of its composition. Two forms we might see less often are an **emulsion**, in which one liquid is not an equal mixture with another, such as oil in water, or an **elixir**, which has 5% to 40% alcohol in it.

Nasogastric and Gastrostomy

There are times when the patient's GI system works but the patient cannot take medicine by mouth. An underweight neonate, for example, might have to have a tube put through the nose that goes through the throat and feeds directly into the stomach. This is the route for nasogastric administration. We call this an NG tube for short. If the tube went directly into the stomach, bypassing the throat entirely, we would call that a gastrostomy (Fig. 5.3).

Sublingual

Just as a *sub*marine is *below* the ocean and a *lingu*ist uses the *tongue* to speak, a *sublingual* dose dissolves under the tongue (Fig. 5.4). The term **hypoglossal** is a synonym for sublingual. An advantage of a sublingual dose is that it absorbs directly into the circulation and avoids the first-pass effect. The liver often metabolizes or changes drugs that come into the body. A sublingual dose avoids this effect, keeping the medicine intact. While the medicine might cause a little bit of mouth irritation, the advantages far outweigh the disadvantages. Two drugs that use sublingual dosage forms include the antinausea medicine ondansetron (Zofran) and nitroglycerin (Nitrostat) for angina or chest pain (Fig. 5.5).

Buccal

Another route that can bypass the first-pass effect is the buccal route. This involves placing the medicine between the teeth and the cheek, where it dissolves (Fig. 5.6). In this case, we have a much slower dosage form meant for longer administrations. The classic example of a buccal route medicine is the nicotine lozenge for smoking cessation.

Vaginal/Rectal

If a patient cannot take an oral medicine because of vomiting or being unconscious, two routes we can use are the vaginal or rectal routes. Instead of a tablet, we will likely use a suppository, a dosage meant to dissolve over a short period of time and melt from the increase in temperature

Nasogastric and Gastrostomy

- Nasogastric, also known as NG, involves placing a tube
- Gastrostomy involves the surgical placement of a tube leading outside the body

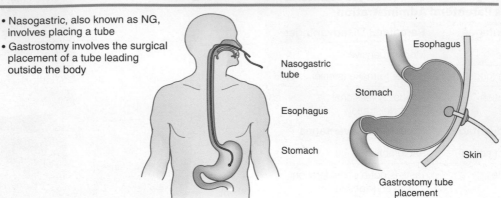

- **Fig. 5.3** Nasogastric and Gastrostomy

Sublingual

- Sublingual (SL) involves holding a medication to dissolve under the tongue
- Sublingual is quick and easy as it is absorbed directly into the circulation

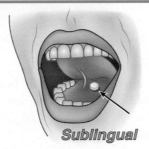

- **Fig. 5.4** Sublingual Route (Part 1)

Sublingual

- An advantage of the sublingual route is that the onset is quick and avoids the stomach and first-pass effect
- Great for nauseous patients as well
- May cause some irritation of the mouth
- Medication examples include:
  - Ondansetron for nausea
  - Nitroglycerin for chest pain

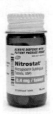

- **Fig. 5.5** Sublingual Route (Part 2)

that the body produces. One common rectal medication is the promethazine (Phenadoz) suppository for nausea and vomiting (Fig. 5.7).

SCENARIO 5.1. ENTERAL DOSAGE FORMS

A patient holds the chest and complains of chest pain. The patient opens a small amber vial labeled nitroglycerin (Nitrostat). How would this patient likely take this dosage form?

Answer: Nitroglycerin (Nitrostat) goes under the tongue. It is a sublingual dose meant to work rapidly to counter the chest pain or angina.

Parenteral

Often, parenteral administration becomes more complex than enteral. The drugs must be aseptic, or free from contamination. Contaminants could introduce bacteria and viruses into the bloodstream, for example. Also, many parenteral forms require the health care provider to break the skin, such as an intramuscular (IM) or subcutaneous (SubQ) administration form. An IM dose will go directly into the muscle while a SubQ dose will go beneath the skin. Since many parenteral forms require a syringe and needle, we will go over some of the parts that are important to our study.

Syringe, Needle, Gauge, and Length

A **syringe** has three parts: plunger, barrel, and tip. The **plunger** pushes the contents from inside the barrel. The **barrel** is that part of the outside of the syringe with measurement lines. The **tip** connects to the needle.

A **needle** also has three parts: the hub, shaft, and bevel (Fig. 5.8). The **hub** connects the needle to the tip of the syringe. The **shaft** is the metal part of the needle. The **bevel** is the needle tip's slanted part. The lumen is the hole in the needle itself.

To describe a needle's size, we use the terms gauge and length.

A needle's **gauge** is the shaft's diameter, which generally varies from #18 to #28. A large gauge indicates a smaller diameter; a small gauge indicates a larger diameter.

The shaft **length** varies, but generally falls between ½ to 2 inches. We assess a patient's muscle development and weight when deciding which length to use.

Parenteral Administration Types

In this section, we will review five parenteral administration methods: intravenous, intradermal, subcutaneous, intramuscular, and intrathecal (Fig. 5.9).

- Intravenous—into the vein
- Intradermal—into the skin

Buccal

- Another route that involves the oral cavity and bypasses the first-pass effect is **buccal**
  - Buccal: Med placed between cheek and gum and left there until it dissolves
- This route is slower than sublingual, but allows for sustained administration of medications
  - Example: Nicotine lozenges for smoking cessation

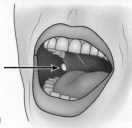
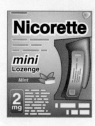

• **Fig. 5.6** Buccal Route

Vaginal / rectal

- If a patient is unconscious or vomiting, we can use the vaginal canal or rectal route to administer medications
- The process involves inserting a suppository or liquid into the areas for absorption
- Examples of common medications include the promethazine suppository for nausea

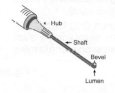

• **Fig. 5.7** Vaginal/Rectal Route

Parenteral adminstration – equipment

- Needles are made up of three parts: <u>bevel</u>, <u>cannula</u>, and <u>hub</u>
  - Bevel: slanted part at the needle's tip
  - Cannula: actual metal part of needle
  - Hub: part of the needle that connects into the syringe

• **Fig. 5.8** Parts of a Needle

Parenteral administration types

- There are various ways to "avoid the gut"
  - Intravenous
  - Intradermal
  - Subcutaneous
  - Intramuscular
  - Intrathecal

• **Fig. 5.9** Parenteral Administration Types

- Subcutaneous—below the skin
- Intramuscular—into the muscle
- Intrathecal—into the spinal canal

Intravenous

To get medicine directly into the circulation, providers will often use the **intravenous** (**IV**) route. This injection goes directly into the vein at an angle of 25 degrees. The IV route is a common parenteral route in the hospital (Fig. 5.10).

Intradermal

Intradermal injections, by contrast, go directly into the upper skin layers (Fig. 5.11). The angle for an intradermal

Intravenous

- The intravenous route involves administering medications into the veins
  - This provides direct access to the circulation
- Injecting intravenously uses an angle of 25 degrees
- The intravenous route is the most common administration route, and the majority of medications are given this way in the hospital

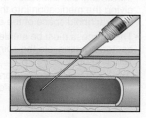

• **Fig. 5.10** Intravenous Method

Intradermal

- Intradermal administration involves administering medication into the top layers of the skin
- To inject intradermally, you need to angle your needle at 10-15 degrees
- This route is mostly used for diagnostic use

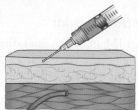

• **Fig. 5.11** Intradermal Method

Subcutaneous

- The subcutaneous route requires injecting the medication into the fatty tissue under the skin
- The angle for subcutaneous injection is 45 degrees
- A common medication given subcutaneously is insulin

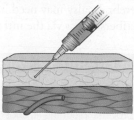

• **Fig. 5.12** Subcutaneous Method

injection varies between 10 and 15 degrees. Some diagnostic measures require an intradermal injection.

Subcutaneous

Under the skin, or dermis, we find fatty tissue. By injecting at a 45-degree angle, we can get into the subcutaneous tissue (Fig. 5.12). Insulin is a medicine we often see injected via the subcutaneous route.

Intramuscular

- An intramuscular injection is just how it sounds—you inject medications into the skeletal muscle
- The angle for intramuscular administration is 90 degrees
- A common medication given intramuscularly is the flu shot, given every fall

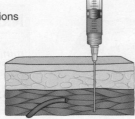

• **Fig. 5.13** Intramuscular Method

Intrathecal

- Intrathecal administration involves giving the medication into the subarachnoid space of the spine
- This process must be sterile as bacteria getting into the spinal fluid can be deadly
- An example of a medication given intrathecally is baclofen for cerebral palsy

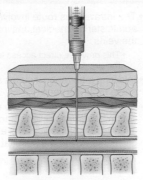

• **Fig. 5.14** Intrathecal Method

Transdermal route

- The transdermal route achieves effects by application of drugs to the skin
- The rate of effect varies by the drug and person
- Patches and topical ointments can be used for transdermal delivery
- Transdermal is great for sustained delivery of drugs, such as fentanyl for chronic pain

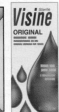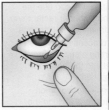

• **Fig. 5.15** Transdermal Route

Ophthalmic route

- Ophthalmic delivery involves giving the medication onto the eyes
- Common medications given this route are eye drops such as Visine

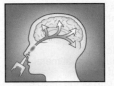

• **Fig. 5.16** Ophthalmic Route

Nasal route

- The nasal route involves giving medications through the nose canal
- Common drug forms include nasal sprays, such as fluticasone for allergies

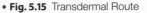

• **Fig. 5.17** Nasal Route

Intramuscular

An IM injection goes directly into the muscle (Fig. 5.13). The needle goes in at a 90-degree angle. A provider gives a flu shot via the IM route.

Intrathecal Method

An intrathecal injection goes directly into the subarachnoid space of the spine (Fig. 5.14). It is especially important that the medicine be sterile and free from bacteria, as treating spinal fluid infections can be very difficult. Patients with cerebral palsy may need baclofen, a muscle relaxer that prescribers inject via the intrathecal route.

SCENARIO 5.2. PARENTERAL DOSAGE FORMS

A patient is a diabetic and is coming in to get a flu shot. At what angle does a diabetic inject insulin? At what angle will a provider inject the flu shot?

Answer: The diabetic injects insulin subcutaneously, at an angle of 45 degrees. A flu shot is an intramuscular injection given at a 90-degree angle.

Other Administration Routes

While enteral and parenteral administration forms cover most of the ways that health professionals use medicines, there are a few more, including the transdermal, ophthalmic, nasal, otic, and inhalation routes.

Transdermal Route

Transdermal literally means across the skin (Fig. 5.15). When we use patches and other transdermal dosage forms, such as topical ointments, we are able to allow drugs to continuously work on a patient. Nicotine patches for smoking cessation and fentanyl (Duragesic), a strong opioid for pain, are two common drugs that work via this route.

Ophthalmic Route

When a patient has an eye infection, irritation, or allergy, it is often easier to directly place drops on the affected area (Fig. 5.16). These drops, however, must be free of bacteria so as not to infect the eye. Sometimes you will see an ophthalmic drop prescribed for someone's ear infection or other condition. That is acceptable. What is not acceptable is to use an ear drop in the eye.

Nasal Route

When a condition is in the sinuses or nose, it may make sense to send medicine directly to those areas (Fig. 5.17).

For example, when someone has temporary nasal congestion, using a nasal decongestant in the short term avoids most systemic effects. However, if the patient needs chronic treatment, an oral dosage form might make more sense. Manufacturers often make allergy sprays that work via the nasal route.

Otic Route

Ear infections are sometimes easier to treat via an otic antibiotic, one that goes directly into the ear canal (Fig. 5.18). Again, it is okay for ophthalmic (eye) drops to be prescribed for the ear, but we cannot use ear drops in the eye.

Inhalation Route

While we will discuss this route in more detail in the respiratory chapter, avoiding side effects by directly spraying medicine into the lungs is a common practice (Fig. 5.19). The dosage can be a gas, vapor, or powder. Asthma medicines such as albuterol (ProAir), a rescue inhaler, work via the respiratory route.

SCENARIO 5.3. OTHER DOSAGE FORMS

A patient reports having antibiotic medicine from a prior ear infection and not wanting to waste money on a new medicine for the eye. Can the patient use the old medicine?

Answer: First, antibiotics vary and sometimes a patient considers all antibiotics to work equally, which is not true. Second, a patient cannot use an ear medicine in the eye; the sterility of eye medicine is much higher than that of an ear medicine.

Otic route

- Otic route involves giving medication through the ear canal
- Medications that are given in the ear canal include antibiotics for ear infections

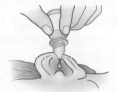

• **Fig. 5.18** Otic Route

Inhalation route

- The inhalation route introduces medications through the respiratory system in the form of a gas, vapor, or powder
- Examples of this medication include albuterol, an inhaler for asthma

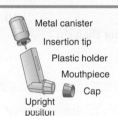 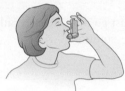

Metal canister
Insertion tip
Plastic holder
Mouthpiece
Cap
Upright position

• **Fig. 5.19** Inhalation Route

Summary

- An enteral medicine passes through the intestines and a parenteral medicine goes via another route. Enteral medicines have advantages, such as low cost and ease of use, but also disadvantages, such as their speed of onset, and the patient must be conscious to take them. While parenteral medicines enjoy advantages, such as a faster onset and that taste is not an issue, they can be expensive and require significant skill to administer.
- Enteral dosage forms include solid dosage forms, such as capsules and tablets, and liquid dosage forms, such as solutions and suspensions. While capsules and tablets can be convenient and inexpensive, the patient's circumstances often dictate which to use. A suspension would be a better choice for a child who cannot swallow pills,

for example. Other enteral forms include oral, nasogastric, gastrostomy, sublingual, buccal, vaginal, and rectal.
- Parenteral administration can be more complex, as it must often be aseptic, free of bacteria. We often need to determine the proper syringe, needle, gauge, and length to properly use a parenteral form. Parenteral forms include intravenous—into the vein, intradermal—into the skin, subcutaneous—below the skin, intramuscular—into the muscle, and intrathecal—into the spinal canal.
- Other administration forms include transdermal—across the skin, ophthalmic—in the eye, nasal—in the nose, otic—in the ear, and inhalation routes to the lungs.

Review Questions

1. Which of the following is an example of an abbreviation for an enteral dosage form route?
   a. IM
   b. IV
   c. SubQ
   d. PO

2. When administering a medicine via the transdermal route, we expect to see a:
   a. Tablet
   b. Patch
   c. Capsule
   d. Solution

3. A liquid dosage form in which all of the medicine completely dissolves is a:
   a. Solution
   b. Suspension
   c. Elixir
   d. Syrup

4. When looking to reach the lungs directly, the _____ administration form is the best.
   a. Oral
   b. Nasal
   c. Respiratory
   d. Otic

5. A medicine that must go into the eyes rather than the ears is a(n) _____ solution.
   a. Otic
   b. Ophthalmic
   c. Transdermal
   d. Subcutaneous

6. We expect a ninety-degree angle from an _____ injection.
   a. Intravenous
   b. Intramuscular
   c. Intrathecal
   d. Intradermal

7. When a diabetic injects insulin, the _____ route is appropriate.
   a. Intramuscular
   b. Intravenous
   c. Subcutaneous
   d. Intradermal

8. The _____ is the slanted part of the needle's tip.
   a. Bevel
   b. Cannula
   c. Hub
   d. Plunger

9. If a patient is actively vomiting, which enteral dosage form allows the patient to still receive medicine?
   a. Oral
   b. Sublingual
   c. Rectal
   d. Buccal

10. When treating chest pain with nitroglycerin, which enteral dosage form is most appropriate?
    a. Oral
    b. Rectal
    c. Vaginal
    d. Sublingual

6

Dosage Calculations

1. Identify four measures of weight used in dosage calculations.
2. Identify three common measures of volume used in dosage calculations.
3. Describe tools to administer the proper dosages.
4. Demonstrate dosage calculations with the ratio/proportion method.
5. Demonstrate dosage calculations with the formula method.
6. Use dimensional analysis to solve dosage calculations.

Measures of Weight

While a person can measure weight in pounds or kilograms, generally we dose a patient in kilograms. This requires us to perform a basic conversion from one measure to the other. There are other measures of weight as well. However, it is much easier to use examples in actual drug forms. A drug package will often display an abbreviation of the weight or volume form (Table 6.1).

Pound (lb)—a unit of weight equal to 0.4536 kilograms

Kilogram (kg)—the base mass unit in the metric system also known as the International System of Units (SI). Also might be abbreviated in common speech as a "kilo" (short for kilogram) or "kig" pronouncing the abbreviation letter "k" and "g" together. Generally, 1 kilogram = 2.2 pounds.

Gram (g)—1/1000 of a kilogram

Milligram (mg)—1/1000 of a gram, sometimes pronounced as "mig." A provider might say the patient needs 10 migs per kig per day, meaning they need 10 milligrams per kilogram of body weight daily.

Microgram (mcg or μg)—1/1000 of a milligram. Sometimes shortened to "mic," which should be pronounced like the name "Mike." The patient needs 50 mics/hour, for example. The letter that looks like a "u" in μg is actually a Greek letter mu (pronounced "myoo").

MilliEquivalent (mEq)—a milliEquivalent is a special case in which a milligram equivalent is listed next to the number of milliEquivalents. For example, 10 mEq of potassium is 750 mg of potassium.

Measures of Volume

Milliliter (mL)—1/1000 of a liter.

Cubic centimeter (cc)—is equal to 1 milliliter, thus, 10 cc = 10 mL.

Teaspoon (tsp)—a measure equal to 5 milliliters (5 mL)

Tablespoon (tbsp)—a measure equal to 15 milliliters (15 mL)

Fluid ounce (fl oz)—a measure equal to 30 milliliters (30 mL)

Liter (L)—1 kilogram of water in standard conditions

Tools to Administer Proper Dosages

Hearing that a patient needs two teaspoonfuls of a medication can be misleading, because one should never use a kitchen utensil to measure medicine—they vary too much in volume. Unfortunately, the image of a bottle pouring into a metal teaspoon is all too common and should be avoided (Fig. 6.1).

The proper method to measure liquid medicine is to use either the plastic measuring cup that comes with the medicine or a plastic syringe that the pharmacy or prescriber provides (Fig. 6.2). Both devices will have markings in milliliters to help with measurement. We may need to convert instructions, such as 1 teaspoonful to 5 mL or 2 teaspoonfuls to 10 mL.

The data show that it is better to use a plastic syringe for accuracy if the patient will allow it. Children sometimes equate plastic syringes to those syringes they had to endure for immunizations and may refuse it. Either way, these devices are the correct method of providing the proper dose.

SCENARIO 6.1. MEASUREMENT AND DEVICES

A parent calls asking whether it is necessary to use the plastic cup that came with the medicine to measure 2 teaspoonfuls, as it seems to have been misplaced. The parent says that there are plenty of teaspoons lying around the house, and it's a 20-minute drive each way to the pharmacy.

Answer: Yes, either the parent needs to find the lost cup or find a measuring device that can be used to measure 10 mL exactly for the child to get the proper dose.

TABLE 6.1	Examples of Dosages	
Drug	**Sample Abbreviation**	**Extended Dosage Explanation**
Omeprazole	20-mg tabs	Milligrams per tablet
Amoxicillin	200 mg/5 mL	Milligrams per milliliter
Azithromycin	1 g/packet	Grams per packet
Fentanyl transdermal system	50 mcg/h	Micrograms per hour
Potassium	20 mEq K (1500 mg)	20 milliEquivalents potassium (milligrams)

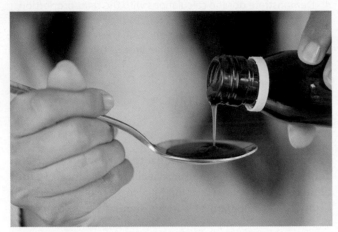

• **Fig. 6.1** Household teaspoons and tablespoons should not be used because of variability in size (© istock #1013348316)

Methods of Calculation

Ratio and Proportion Method

A ratio is a comparison in fraction form, such as miles per hour. A proportion is an equation that says that two fractions across from each other are equivalent. We show ratios and proportions by putting two fractions across from each other and cancel them by multiplying or dividing. Often, a person uses this method without even thinking about it. For example, in a math class, you may remember that 1/2 = 2/4. The 1/2 and 2/4 are the ratios and putting an equal sign between them is a proportion.

What if, however, you had that 1/2 = 2/x? How would you determine what x represents?

From before, it is clear that the question mark is a 4, but how did we get there?

We cross-multiply the bottom and opposite top numbers to get (x) * (1) = (2) * (2), then divide the (2) (2) / (1) = (x), which gives us the 4 answer from before.

Comparing Solid Medication

If a patient needs 500 mg of medication and there are 250 mg in each tablet, how many tablets do we need for the patient?

We can set this up as a ratio and proportion by putting x tablets/500 mg = 1 tablet/250 mg, which becomes

$$x \text{ tablets} = (500 \text{ mg}) * (1 \text{ tablet}) / (250 \text{ mg})$$

After completing the calculation, the solution ends up as 2 tablets.

If we think about this intuitively, we realize this must be true. If you have a dosage that's twice as big, we would need twice as many tablets.

Comparing Liquid Medication

If a patient needs 2 mL of medication to achieve a 25-mg dose, how much liquid does the patient need to achieve a 100-mg dose?

$$100 \text{ mg}/x \text{ mL} = 25 \text{ mg}/2 \text{ mL}$$

$$x \text{ mL}/100 \text{ mg} = 2 \text{ mL}/25 \text{ mg}$$

$$x \text{ mL} = (100 \text{ mg}) (2 \text{ mL}) / (25 \text{ mg})$$

$$x \text{ mL} = 8 \text{ mL}$$

We notice here that just as 100 mg is four times as big as 25 mg, the answer, 8 mL, is four times as big as 2 mL.

The Formula Method

The formula method is also known as the desired-over-have method. It allows a person to convert factors by knowing the (1) ordered DOSE amount (D), (2) the amount on HAND (H), and the (3) QUANTITY of medicine (Q). These three fit into the formula D/H x Q = Amount to Give. For example, if the prescriber orders a dose of 800 mg, but only 200 mg per 1 tablet are on hand, then the D = 800 mg, H = 200 mg, and Q = 1 tablet. Inputting the variables into the formula D/H x Q = 800 mg/200 mg * 1 tablet = 4 tablets.

This method works with liquids as well. If the prescriber orders a dose of 1000 mg of amoxicillin but the liquid on hand is 250 mg per 5 mL, we set up the equation in this way: D = 1000 mg, H = 250 mg, Q = 5 mL.

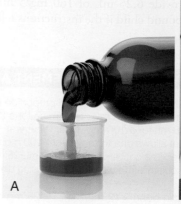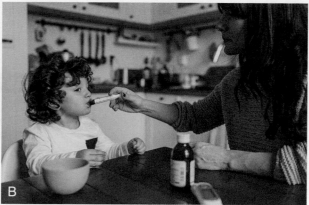

• **Fig. 6.2** Using a measuring cup (A) or measuring syringe (B) provides a more accurate dose (© istock #186604633 and #1088379538)

$$D/H * Q = 1000 \text{ mg}/250 \text{ mg} * 5 \text{ mL} = 20 \text{ mL}$$

The Dimensional Analysis Method

The dimensional analysis method also has other names, such as the unit-factor method or factor-label method. In this method, we use conversion factors that can change one quantity to another. Students often encounter this method in algebra or introductory chemistry classes.

A common conversion that travelers need to use is from miles per hour to kilometers per hour. There are 1.61 kilometers in a single mile. How do we use this information to make the conversion?

If a driver finds the distance between two cities as 161 kilometers and drives 50 miles per hour, how long will it take the driver to get there? First, we can determine the number of miles to travel by converting the kilometers to miles with the 1.61 kilometers per mile conversion factor. Notice that when we have the kilometers on the bottom and the kilometers on top, we cross out those factors and replace them with the new one, miles.

$$161 \text{ km} \times (1 \text{ mile}/1.61 \text{ km}) = 100 \text{ miles}$$

Second, we use the conversion factor of 50 miles per hour to convert 100 miles into a number of hours.

$$100 \text{ miles} \times (1 \text{ hour}/50 \text{ miles}) = 2 \text{ hours}$$

In the same way as above, we cross out miles and allow for the conversion to hours. In taking care of patients, we complete similar conversions.

If a 5-year-old child needs acetaminophen for a fever and there are 160 mg in each 5 mL of medicine, how many milligrams of medicine does the child receive with a 7.5-mL dose?

Our conversion factor is 160 mg/5 mL. We already know that there is a 7.5-mL dose in a volume, but we are unsure what the milligram dosage turns out to be. As such, we set up the problem in this way:

$$7.5 \text{ mL} \times (160 \text{ mg}/5 \text{ mL}) = 240 \text{ mg}$$

While students consider the dimensional analysis method the most complex way to solve problems, they often like that all problems solvable with the ratio and proportion or formula method can also be solved through the dimensional analysis method. For example, we solved this equation with the ratio and proportion method to find that the patient needed 2 tablets.

If a patient needs 500 mg of medication and there are 250 mg in each tablet, how many tablets do we need for the patient? Answer: 2 tablets. In the same way, we can set up the dimensional analysis method to solve this problem as well.

$$500 \text{ mg} \times (1 \text{ tablet}/250 \text{ mg}) = 2 \text{ tablets}$$

We can also use dimensional analysis to solve any problems that we would solve with the formula method such as the one above.

If the prescriber orders a dose of 1000 mg of amoxicillin but the liquid on hand is 250 mg per 5 mL, how many mL will we need? Answer: 20 mL.

$$1000 \text{ mg} * (5 \text{ ml}/250 \text{ mg}) = 20 \text{ mL}$$

The advantage of this method is that we can solve more complex problems with more than one factor. For example, if we have to dose acetaminophen for a 44-pound child but the instructions tell us to use 10 mg/kg * dose (might be described as 10 "migs" per "kig" per dose), how do we solve this?

We begin with the conversion from pounds to kilograms using our 2.2 pounds = 1 kilogram conversion factor.

$$44 \text{ pounds} * (1 \text{ kg}/2.2 \text{ pounds}) = 20 \text{ kg}$$

We then multiply the number of kilograms to determine the milligram.s per dose in this way.

$$20 \text{ kg} \times (10 \text{ mg/kg} \times \text{dose}) = 200 \text{ mg dose}$$

However, the parent of that 44-pound child will need to give dosages in a certain liquid measure. Thus, if we have 160 mg/5 mL, how many milliliters do we give to the patient?

$$200 \text{ mg} \times (5 \text{ mL}/160 \text{ mg}) = 6.25 \text{ mL dose}$$

We provide 6.25 mL of 160 mg/5 mL acetaminophen for a 44-pound child if the instructions tell us to use 10 mg/kg * dose.

SCENARIO 6.2. MEASUREMENT AND DEVICES

Previously, we used the ratio and proportion method to determine that, with 2 mL of medicine for a 25-mg dose, we needed 8 mL for a 100-mg dose. What was the conversion factor that allows one to move from 100 mg to 8 mL?
Answer: The conversion factor is 2 mL/25 mg. We would set up the problem in this way if we were using dimensional analysis.

$$100 \text{ mg dose} \times (2 \text{ mL}/8 \text{ mL}) = 25 \text{ mg dose}$$

Summary

- The most common weights we use in the metric system include the kilogram, gram, milligram, and microgram. Each weight is 1/1000 of the other such that 1 gram is 1/1000 of a kilogram.
- The most common measures of volume in the metric system are the liter and milliliter. In general, we want to convert household measures such as teaspoonfuls to milliliters such that 1 teaspoonful is 5 milliliters and 1 tablespoonful is 15 milliliters.

- When measuring out a dosage, it is better to use a plastic syringe or measuring cup than a household measure, which might vary in its volume.
- The three primary methods for calculating dosages are ratio and proportion, formula, and dimensional analysis. Using dimensional analysis, one can perform any calculation that can be done by the ratio and proportion or formula method.

Review Questions

1. Which of the following is the smallest unit of measure?
   a. Kilogram
   b. Gram
   c. Milligram
   d. Microgram
2. The abbreviation for mcg stands for which measure?
   a. Kilogram
   b. Microgram
   c. Gram
   d. Pound
3. If a patient needs 440 mg of medication per dose but the only available tablets are 220 mg per tablet, how many tablets does the patient need?
   a. 2 tablets
   b. 3 tablets
   c. 4 tablets
   d. 5 tablets
4. To determine the number of pounds in a certain number of kilograms we use that 1 kilogram equals _____ pounds.
   a. 2.0
   b. 1.61
   c. 2.2
   d. 5

5. A dosage calls for 8 cc; how many mL of medicine is in the dosage?
   a. 2 mL
   b. 4 mL
   c. 6 mL
   d. 8 mL
6. A patient needs 10 mg of medication, but the medicine comes in a 2 mg/1 mL dosage form. How many milliliters are required?
   a. 2 mL
   b. 5 mL
   c. 7 mL
   d. 10 mL
7. Given a medicine that has 500 mg per capsule, how many grams would 6 capsules contain?
   a. 3000
   b. 6000
   c. 3
   d. 6
8. If a microgram is 1/1000 of a milligram, what is a microgram to a gram?
   a. 1/100
   b. 1/10,000
   c. 1/1,000,000
   d. 1/1,000,000,000

9. In the formula method, what does the "Q" stand for?
   a. Quantity of medicine
   b. Ordered dose amount
   c. Amount on hand
   d. Amount to give

10. The factor-label method is the same as:
   a. The ratio and proportion method
   b. The desired/have method
   c. The formula method
   d. The dimensional analysis method

7

Drug Classifications

LEARNING OBJECTIVES

1. Discuss the methods of drug classification.
2. Recognize common stem positions.
3. Review the placement and importance of common stems of gastrointestinal, musculoskeletal, and respiratory medications.

4. Review the placement and importance of common stems of immune, neuropsychology, cardiology, and endocrine medications.

Methods of Drug Classification

There are many ways to classify drugs. However, brand names do not lend to easy classification, though often they hint at the drug's function. For example, the nasal steroid fluticasone brand name Flonase helps improve nasal flow. The brand name takes "Flo" from flow and "nas" from nasal. However, generic names often readily fit into classifications because those names were created in a systematic way. A drug similar to penicillin must have -cillin at the end, and nonsteroidal antiinflammatory drugs (NSAIDs) such as ibuprofen and ketoprofen, for example, will share the same -profen ending.

The more we can learn about where certain drug names come from, the more likely we are to avoid potential mistakes. This chapter will not cover all of the medicines but will provide a preview of what you will see in future chapters. Think of this section as a primer to get you ready to tackle seven pathophysiologic classes: gastrointestinal, musculoskeletal, respiratory, immune, neuropsychology, cardiology, and endocrine.

Where Do Generic Names Come From?

While a brand name is a proprietary name, one that comes from the drug manufacturer, the generic medication names, sometimes called INNs (International Nonproprietary Names), generally have a systematic classification. This classification might have a stem in the prefix, infix, or suffix position that has meaning. This meaning can allude to a classification by:
1. Chemical structure (e.g., tetracycline alludes to a four-membered chemical ring)
2. Neurotransmitter that they affect (e.g., fluoxetine (Prozac) is a selective serotonin reuptake inhibitor that works on one neurotransmitter)

3. Receptor that they affect (e.g., angiotensin II receptor blockers [ARBs] such as losartan (Cozaar) and valsartan (Diovan))
4. Therapeutic class (e.g., amoxicillin (Amoxil) is a penicillin antibiotic)

Not all generic names have these clues, but many do. In this chapter, we will examine the United States Adopted Names Council (USANC). This group works to standardize medication names to classify new drugs that resemble old ones. We will look at medication classifications in the same order as they appear at the end of this book. We need to start with drugs for the gastrointestinal, musculoskeletal, respiratory, immune, nervous, cardiovascular, and endocrine systems. Let us first better understand what stems in the prefix, infix, and suffix positions mean.

Note: Trademark does not protect generics. Most generics, unless they begin a sentence, start with a lowercase letter. We always capitalize brand names. Usually, the convention works like this: acetaminophen (Tylenol), where acetaminophen is the generic name and Tylenol is the brand name.

Recognizing Stem Positions

Prefix—A prefix is a part of a word that comes at the beginning or before the other letters. Just as a pre-med student takes classes before medical school, a prefix signals an important commonality at the start of a generic drug name. Meaningful prefixes are in *pred*nisone, a steroid, and *cef*epime, a cephalosporin antibiotic. These letters, common to the group, provide us with a hint at the drug classification at the beginning of the drug name. We will then recognize when we see *pred*nisolone and *cef*dinir that these drugs are a steroid and cephalosporin antibiotic, respectively.

Suffix—Suffix resembles the word affix, and you affix these letters to the end of the generic drug name. Generic drugs with meaningful suffixes, such as doxy*cycline*, a

---

* Brand discontinued, now available only as generic
† Naming conventions can vary between prescription and OTC formulations

tetracycline antibiotic, or metopro*lol*, a beta-blocker, help us recognize other drugs when they come along. For example, when we see mino*cycline* and aten*olol*, we know they are a tetracycline antibiotic and beta-blocker, respectively.

Infix—Think of an infix as *in* the middle. Rarely, we see these in the middle of a drug name. Just as pred- can indicate that a drug is a steroid by being at the beginning of the drug name, it can do the same in the middle, as in methyl*pred*nisolone.

By reviewing common prefixes, suffixes, and infixes, we can learn to see quickly what the drug's purpose might be before we even see the whole word. These will be covered by chapter order starting with the gastrointestinal system. Note that many medication stems in this chapter are in italics for emphasis but, normally, we would not italicize them. Finally, there are many drugs without stems and it is just as important to know when a little extra memorization might be required.

SCENARIO 7.1. DRUG CLASSIFICATION

When a patient takes many medications and has many prescribers, sometimes we see what is called a therapeutic duplication. A patient gets two drugs that do essentially the same thing when the patient is supposed to have only one. How can we identify prednisone and methylprednisolone as a therapeutic duplication?

Answer: In both cases, the "pred" stem indicates that prednisone and methylprednisolone are steroids. The pred-stem is in the prefix position in prednisone and the -pred-stem is in the infix position in methylprednisolone.

Stems by Physiologic Class

Gastrointestinal Medications (See Chapter 8)
H2RAs Histamine-2 Antagonists

Much of what health professionals do is serve as translators. While a patient might speak about having an acid reducer, it is important to know the proper medication classification. For example, famotidine is a histamine-2 (H2) receptor antagonist H2RAs that binds to H2 receptor sites. It can reduce acid in the stomach and treat heartburn or even ulcers. We see the -tidine ending in famotidine (Pepcid), nizatidine (Axid), and cimetidine (Tagamet*).

Note: in the Respiratory chapter, we will see loratadine, which has the —atadine ending for certain H1 blockers. Those histamine-1 blockers are for seasonal allergies.

Proton Pump Inhibitors

Another gastrointestinal medication we can see over-the-counter (OTC) or by prescription (Rx) is the proton pump inhibitor (PPI) omeprazole (Prilosec OTC). These PPIs also work for excess acid and ulcers, though the dose for an ulcer is often twice that for heartburn. Other examples include esomeprazole (Nexium 24HR) and lansoprazole (Prevacid 24HR). It is very rare, but sometimes we will see another stem with the same letters as -prazole for PPIs in

the antipsychotic medications aripiprazole (Aricept) and brexpiprazole (Rexulti). The actual stem for the antipsychotics is —piprazole. Watch out for these look-alikes.

Monoclonal Antibodies

While -tidine for H2RAs and -prazole for PPIs readily define a drug and its function, sometimes the stem is not that useful. For example, the -mab ending in infliximab (Remicade), a medicine for Crohn disease and ulcerative colitis, simply lets us know how it was made. However, there are many drugs that end with -mab for many different therapeutic indications.

SCENARIO 7.2. GASTROINTESTINAL STEMS

A patient has generic loratadine and famotidine in his hands. However, he has excess acid that is causing severe heartburn. Does the -atadine stem in loratadine or the -tidine stem in famotidine indicate that it is a medicine for this condition?

Answer: The -tidine stem in the suffix position indicates a medicine for excess acid and heartburn. The -atadine stem in loratadine would refer to a histamine-1 blocker for seasonal allergies.

Musculoskeletal Medications (See Chapter 9)
Nonnarcotic Analgesic

Just as nonfiction books cover real events but we name them as not-fiction instead of real books, we name pain medicines that are not narcotics as nonnarcotics. Many people rely on OTC acetaminophen (Tylenol) for pain and fever relief. It is a relatively old medication and has no identifying stem. The name comes from parts of the chemical name N-*acetyl*-p-*amino*-*phen*ol. The abbreviation APAP also comes from letters in the chemical name.

Nonsteroidal Antiinflammatory Drugs

Ibu*profen* (Advil, Motrin) has the —profen stem, indicating its relationship to the NSAID class. Thus, if we see keto*profen*, we recognize it as similar to ibuprofen. Although naproxen (Aleve, Naprosyn) does not have the same stem, it is a long-acting NSAID and has similar ending letters in -proxen to help with recognition. A prescription NSAID that can sometimes avoid the gastrointestinal side effects common to NSAIDs is celecoxib (Celebrex) with the —coxib stem.

Narcotic (Opioid) Analgesics

Most opioid analgesics have similar spellings and are related to morphine. For example, both hydrocodone with acetaminophen (Vicodin*) and oxycodone with acetaminophen (Percocet) have -codone at the end. While this is not a stem, it is a way to tie them together. The hydro- is for a hydrogen element and the oxy- is for an oxygen element.

Bisphosphonates

Bisphosphonates are drugs for osteoporosis and end with -dronate. Both alen*dronate* (Fosamax) and iban*dronate* (Boniva) help someone who has weakening bones, generally due to age.

SCENARIO 7.3. MUSCULOSKELETAL STEMS

A patient goes to the hospital and leaves with ketoprofen for minor pain after a procedure. However, he is soon running out of that medicine and wants to know if ibuprofen is similar to ketoprofen. Is it?

Answer: While ibuprofen is similar to ketoprofen, it would take a health professional to properly assess the pain and make the transition from the prescription ketoprofen to the OTC ibuprofen.

Respiratory Medications (See Chapter 10)

Allergic Rhinitis

Sometimes, on electronic notecards, someone might post that -sone and -lone are both suffixes for steroids. Neither is an official stem, but it is good to see where these come from. One medicine for allergic rhinitis, a nasal inflammation, is triamcinolone (Nasacort Allergy 24HR). Another is fluticasone (Flonase Allergy Relief). Both end in either -sone and -lone respectively. Clobetasol, a topical steroid, and budesonide, another nasal steroid, do not end in either -sone or -lone. While this can be useful as a clue, be wary when you hear something like all steroids end in -sone or -lone.

Allergy, Cold, and Cough

Among the hundreds of medications for allergy, cold, and cough, there are actually very few different active ingredients.

Antihistamines might or might not end in a stem. For example, loratadine (Claritin) has the -atadine stem, but cetirizine (Zyrtec) does not.

Decongestants such as pseudoephedrine (Sudafed) have the -drine suffix for sympathomimetics (drugs that mimic the fight-or-flight effect), but oxymetazoline (Afrin) and phenylephrine (Neo-Synephrine) do not have that stem.

Antitussives, drugs that prevent a cough, include dextromethorphan, the DM in Robitussin Adult Cough and Congestion DM and Mucinex DM, which has the -orphan stem.

Expectorants, those medicines that help bring up and break up mucus, like guaifenesin, the active ingredient in plain Robitussin and Mucinex, lack a recognizable stem. Nonetheless, these medicines, along with the analgesics ibuprofen and acetaminophen, comprise the bulk of ingredients in allergy, cold, and cough medicines.

Bronchodilators and Antiinflammatory Drugs for Asthma

Asthma has two parts: bronchoconstriction, a narrowing of the bronchioles, and inflammation. As such, we have medicines for each of these two aspects of the disease. To open bronchioles, we use a bronchodilator such as albuterol (ProAir HFA) or ipratropium (Atrovent HFA) with the -terol and -tropium stems, respectively. To reduce inflammation,

we use an inhaled steroid, much like we would for a nasal steroid. Fluticasone in Advair HFA and budesonide in Symbicort have similar -sone or -son- parts to them. These, again, are not true stems, although they can hint at steroids for the lung inflammation that comes along with asthma. The important lesson is that asthma medicines can have very consistent stems and suffixes.

SCENARIO 7.4. RESPIRATORY STEMS

A patient has a combination medicine with salmeterol/fluticasone (Advair) to prevent asthma attacks. Based on the endings of the two generic names, what is each component for?

Answer: Salmeterol, like albuterol (ProAir HFA), has the -terol ending indicating that it is a bronchodilator to open up the lungs. Salmeterol is longer acting and not meant as a rescue inhaler like albuterol for a severe attack. Fluticasone has the -sone ending and is a steroid.

Immune System Medications (See Chapter 11)

Antibacterials can have drug prefixes or suffixes that can either make them easier to classify or cause someone to mistake that there is a relationship between two drugs.

Amoxicillin is a penicillin-type antibiotic. We can see the -cillin ending that makes it easy to recognize. Another example includes the tetracycline antibiotics ending in -cycline. This makes it easy to recognize doxycycline (Doryx) or minocycline (Minocin) as tetracycline antibiotics.

However, drugs that end in -mycin can be many different types of antibiotics. The -mycin indicates that the antibiotic came from the *Streptomyces* strain of bacteria but does not tell someone which kind of antibiotic class it is. For example, azithromycin (Zithromax) is a macrolide antibiotic and vancomycin (Vancocin) is a glycopeptide antibiotic; these are from two different classes.

In antifungals, we might see an ending such as -conazole, as in fluconazole (Diflucan). In antivirals, non-HIV drugs, such as acyclovir (Zovirax) or valacyclovir (Valtrex), have the –cyclovir stem. The –vir suffix indicates an antiviral, but additional letters may further classify it. For example, the –cyclovir in its entirety tells us that these drugs help treat herpes virus. Similarly, we also see the –vir stem in antivirals for influenza, HIV, or hepatitis. There are too many -vir stems to put in this chapter, but we will visit more in the Immune chapter.

Most of the antibiotics, antifungals, and antivirals treat an active infection. However, it is much better to prevent infection in the first place. Vaccines protect against bacteria, fungi, and viruses. Often, we will separate these into three groups: those that are preventative against *bacteria*, such as the pneumococcal vaccine (Prevnar 13); those that are preventative against *fungi*, such as fluconazole (Diflucan) mentioned earlier; and those that are preventative against viruses, such as the human papillomavirus (HPV) vaccine (Gardasil).

A patient sees that his antibiotic, azithromycin (Zithromax), has the same ending as a drug the doctor prescribed when he had a severe skin infection in the hospital—vancomycin (Vancocin). Does the patient necessarily have that same skin infection?

Answer: The -mycin stem can mislead more than help. Azithromycin is a macrolide antibiotic; a prescriber might use it for a sinus or upper respiratory infection, not a life-threatening skin infection.

Neuropsychology Medications (See Chapter 12)

There are many medications that affect the nervous system and work for psychological disorders. This section is a preview of the different conditions and stems that can help connect the drug name to that condition.

Anxiety

The CALM mnemonic can help you remember that the generic clonazepam (Klonopin), alprazolam (Xanax), lorazepam (Ativan), and midazolam (Versed*) are benzodiazepines. The –azepam and –azolam stems confirm these as benzodiazepines. Benzodiazepines are important in reducing anxiety, inducing sleep, and relaxing muscles.

Epilepsy

Sometimes stems do not help as much with a therapeutic purpose. With generic carbamazepine (Tegretol), the –pine stem relates to the drug structure having a three-ring backbone. However, in phenytoin, there is a specific stem, –toin, that lets us know this drug is an antiepileptic.

Parkinson Disease

Parkinson disease is a condition of too little **dopamine**, an important neurotransmitter, in the brain. With carbidopa/levodopa (Sinemet) the –dopa stem refers to dopamine receptor agonists, those drugs that activate dopamine. Technically, only levodopa actually acts as a dopamine agonist; carbidopa helps reduce the breakdown of levodopa.

Migraine

Both eletriptan (Relpax) and sumatriptan (Imitrex) help with migraines. Health professionals often call the group triptans as a way to name the drug class. That is much easier to say than serotonin receptor agonist, the drug's mechanism of action.

Depression

Three of the major antidepressive classes are the selective serotonin reuptake inhibitors (SSRIs), serotonin norepinephrine reuptake inhibitors (SNRIs), and tricyclic antidepressants (TCAs). An example of an SSRI is sertraline (Zoloft), with the -traline stem. Another SSRI is venlafaxine (Effexor XR), with the –faxine stem. The –triptyline stem in amitriptyline (Elavil*) relates to its three-ring structure, a tricyclic antidepressant.

There is a point of possible confusion. Duloxetine (Cymbalta), an SNRI, has the –oxetine stem. This can also be found in fluoxetine (Prozac), an SSRI for depression and anxiety, and atomoxetine (Strattera), a nonstimulant for attention deficit/hyperactivity disorder (ADHD).

Schizophrenia

Drugs for schizophrenia span two generations. The older medicines, such as haloperidol (Haldol) and chlorpromazine (Thorazine*), represent the first generation. They have adverse effects, such as sedation and movement disorders, that are different from those drugs in the second generation. The second-generation drugs for schizophrenia—such as olanzapine (Zyprexa) and clozapine (Clozaril), and aripiprazole (Abilify) and brexpiprazole (Rexulti)—do have similar endings and stems.

A drug class usually has only a single drug ending. However, a patient had clonazepam (Klonopin) and then the prescriber switched to alprazolam (Xanax). Is this patient still on a medication in the same drug class?

Answer: Benzodiazepines can have two stems: -azepam, as in clonazepam and lorazepam, and -azolam, as in alprazolam and midazolam.

Cardiovascular Medications (See Chapter 13)

Many of the medicines in the cardiovascular system are newer and follow a very logical classification system.

Diuretics

Patients who have heart failure or other conditions often retain too much fluid. Diuretics help release this fluid. A thiazide diuretic works at the distal convoluted tubule (DCT), farther from the high-pressure glomerulus capillary bed. We can recognize hydrochlorothiazide (Hydrodiuril*) by the –thiazide ending. We often use this as the drug for someone recently diagnosed with hypertension. One very important loop diuretic, especially for congestive heart failure, is furosemide (Lasix), and we can recognize the -semide stem.

Angiotensin-Converting Enzyme Inhibitors

Generic lisinopril is a drug that blocks an important enzyme in the renin-angiotensin-aldosterone system (RAAS). In blocking this enzyme, the blood vessels cannot constrict as well, leading to decreased blood pressure. We call these angiotensin-converting enzyme (ACE) inhibitors (ACEIs)—such as lisinopril (Zestril, Prinivil) and benazepril (Lotensin)—prils.

Angiotensin II Receptor Blockers

Angiotensin II normally helps cause blood vessels to constrict. However, drugs such as losartan (Cozaar) and valsartan (Diovan) can block the receptor to lower blood pressure. As with the prils, we sometimes call these drugs sartans by their endings, or by the acronym ARBs.

Beta-Blockers

The heart contains many beta-1 receptors. Both propranolol (Inderal) and metoprolol (Toprol XL) can block those receptors, thus lowering the heart rate. Although these are no longer the drugs of choice for hypertension, they are in an important drug class. They have the -olol beta-blocker stem. The stem does not have all the information, however. Beta-blockers come in generations and the stem does not differentiate between propranolol, a first-generation beta-blocker that affects both beta-1 and beta-2 receptors affecting the heart and lungs, and metoprolol which affects only beta-1 receptors. Because metoprolol would not affect the lungs, it is the preferred choice with asthmatics, for example.

Statins

Often, we have many names for a drug in a class. Drugs like lovastatin (Mevacor*) and atorvastatin (Lipitor) are 3-hydroxy-3-methylglutaryl-coenzyme A (HMG-CoA) reductase inhibitors, cholesterol-lowering drugs, antihyperlipidemic agents, or simply statins after their -statin stem. These drugs lower bad cholesterol, low-density lipoproteins (LDLs). They also include the substem -va to separate them from a drug such as nystatin (Mycostatin*), an antifungal.

SCENARIO 7.7. CARDIO STEMS

A cardiac patient is switched from hydrochlorothiazide to furosemide. Is his condition likely worsening or getting better?

Answer: A patient on hydrochlorothiazide might have only a little bit of excess fluid; however, furosemide, a much stronger diuretic, would indicate a worsening condition.

Endocrine Medications (See Chapter 14)

Diabetes

Although there are many facets to diabetes care, the most important therapeutic goal is to lower blood sugar. In oral diabetic medications, we often see the prefix gli- or gly- in the generic name. The g-l intentionally recalls the first letters of glucose, the sugar we are trying to reduce in a diabetic. In the medication name metformin (Glucophage), the —formin stem lacks gli or gly, but from the brand name Glucophage, it is possible to see that this biguanide medicine is meant to eat (phage) excess glucose. The thiazolidinedione, pioglitazone (Actos), has the —glitazone stem with gli in it, but a longer total stem. Nateglinide (Starlix) and repaglinide (Prandin) have the -glinide stem, indicating meglitinide antidiabetics. Finally, the dipeptidyl peptidase-4 (DPP-4) inhibitors sitagliptin (Januvia) and saxagliptin (Onglyza) both have a -gliptin stem.

Progestins and Estrogens

Oral contraceptives are either progestin only or an estrogen-progestin combination. A drug such as etonogestrel (NuvaRing) works like a traditional oral contraceptive, but the patient uses it as a vaginal ring. Norelgestromin (Xulane) is a contraceptive patch. Notice the -gest- stem for progesterone. When we see an oral combination contraceptive with estrogen *and* progestin, we might also include ethinyl estradiol, the estr- indicating that there is an estrogen component.

Benign Prostatic Hyperplasia

Benign prostatic hyperplasia translates to an enlarged prostate. Finasteride (Proscar) and dutasteride (Avodart) block the conversion of testosterone to active androgen dihydrotestosterone (DHT) that will cause the enlargement and extra cell growth. The -steride stem helps us classify the drugs as a 5-alpha reductase inhibitor.

SCENARIO 7.8. ENDOCRINE STEMS

A patient notices that all of his diabetes generic-named medication except metformin has gl- in the name. Is metformin for diabetes?

Answer: Metformin is a biguanide diabetes medicine. Sometimes, the patient will see only the generic name, but if the medication has the same the brand name, he would recognize Glucophage as having part of the word glucose in it.

Summary

- Generic medication names, International Nonproprietary Names (INNs), have a systematic classification with a stem in the prefix, infix, or suffix position. We might classify the meaning by chemical structure, neurotransmitter that they affect, receptor that they affect, or therapeutic class.
- Acid reducers such as famotidine (Pepcid+) that are histamine-2 (H2) receptor antagonists have the -tidine suffix, while proton pump inhibitors such as omeprazole have the -prazole ending.
- While nonnarcotic analgesics such as acetaminophen may not have a stem, they come from parts of the chemical name N-*acetyl*-p-*amino-phen*ol. The APAP abbreviation also comes from letters in the chemical name. NSAIDs such as ibu*profen* (Advil, Motrin) and ketoprofen (Orudis*) have the —profen stem. A prescription NSAID that can reduce gastrointestinal distress common to NSAIDs is celecoxib (Celebrex) with the -coxib stem.
- Asthma is a condition of bronchoconstriction and inflammation. To open bronchioles, we use bronchodilators such as albuterol (ProAir HFA) and ipratropium (Atrovent HFA) with the -terol and -tropium stems, respectively. To reduce inflammation, we use inhaled steroids such as fluti*ca*s*one* in Advair HFA and bude*son*ide in Symbicort with the -sone or -son- parts.
- Antibacterials have drug prefixes or suffixes that can either make them easier to classify or possibly cause a mistaken classification. Tetracycline antibiotics end in -cycline, making it easy to recognize doxycycline (Doryx) and minocycline

(Minocin) as being in the same drug class. Drugs that end in -mycin can fall into many different antibiotic classifications. Examples include azithromycin (Zithromax) as a macrolide antibiotic and vancomycin (Vancocin) as a glycopeptide antibiotic, from two different classes.

- Benzodiazepines are important in reducing anxiety, inducing sleep, and relaxing muscles. The CALM mnemonic—taking the first letter of the generics clonazepam (Klonopin), alprazolam (Xanax), lorazepam (Ativan), and midazolam (Versed*)—can help one remember four benzodiazepines. The -azepam and -azolam stems confirm the drug class. Drugs for schizophrenia span two generations. The first generation causes adverse effects such as sedation and movement disorders. Second-generation drugs for schizophrenia—such as olanzapine (Zyprexa)

and clozapine (Clozaril) or aripiprazole (Abilify) and brexpiprazole (Rexulti)—have similar endings. Second-generation drugs often cause metabolic effects such as diabetes, hyperlipidemia, and weight gain.

- Beta-blockers span generations. The stem does not differentiate between propranolol, a first-generation beta-blocker that affects both beta-1 and beta-2 receptors affecting the heart and lungs, and metoprolol, which affects only beta-1 receptors. Because metoprolol does not affect the lungs, it is the preferred choice with asthmatics, for example.

- In oral diabetic medications, we see the prefix gli- or gly- in many generic names. The gl recalls the first letters of glucose. Pioglitazone (Actos), nateglinide (Starlix), and sitagliptin (Januvia) exemplify this fact.

Review Questions

1. A(n) _____ is a meaningful stem in the middle of a generic medication name.
   a. Prefix
   b. Suffix
   c. Infix
   d. Substem
2. The acronym for a medication that has the -pril stem is _____.
   a. NSAID
   b. DMARD
   c. ARB
   d. ACEI
3. At the end of a diuretics generic name, we might see the suffix:
   a. -pril
   b. -olol
   c. -sartan
   d. -thiazide
4. Which medication would best lower high cholesterol?
   a. Angiotensin-converting enzyme inhibitors
   b. HMG CoA reductase inhibitors for cholesterol
   c. Alpha-blockers
   d. Beta-blockers
5. What is the brand name for the antidiabetic metformin?
   a. Nateglinide
   b. Actos
   c. Glucophage
   d. Lasix
6. Which medication is approved for the treatment of benign prostatic hyperplasia?
   a. Ibuprofen
   b. Naproxen
   c. Valsartan
   d. Finasteride
7. Which medication(s) is (are) associated with bronchodilation?
   a. Albuterol
   b. Atenolol
   c. Atorvastatin
   d. Budesonide
8. If a patient is on sumatriptan, what is the prescriber treating?
   a. Diabetes
   b. Hypertension
   c. Edema
   d. Migraines
9. Which drug ending would indicate the drug works on the renin-angiotensin-aldosterone system (RAAS) to lower blood pressure?
   a. -glitazone
   b. -olol
   c. -sartan
   d. -statin
10. Which drug stem can represent up to three drug classes?
    a. -triptyline
    b. -traline
    c. -faxine
    d. -oxetine

8

Gastrointestinal

LEARNING OBJECTIVES

1. Discuss the stepwise management of gastrointestinal conditions of peptic ulcer disease, constipation, diarrhea, emesis, irritable bowel syndrome, and inflammatory bowel disease.
2. Describe the pathophysiology of common gastrointestinal conditions.
3. Identify various medication classifications in the therapeutic treatment of gastrointestinal diseases.

4. Compare and contrast medicines within a given medication class as they relate to the Periodic Table of Elements, chemical receptors, and dosage types.
5. Discuss the mechanisms of action, indications, drug interactions, and adverse effects of common gastrointestinal medications.

Peptic Ulcer Disease

Peptic ulcer disease (PUD) happens when the gastrointestinal (GI) tract experiences an abnormal state (Fig. 8.1). For example, the acidic stomach environment is aggressive. The pH, or measure of acidity, is 2, which defines hydrochloric acid as very strong. When the stomach's protection fails, the acidic environment can lead to ulcers in the stomach or first part of the small intestine, the duodenum (from the Latin *duodeni* twelve each, from *duodecim* twelve; from its length, about 12 fingers' width). A patient with an ulcer often presents with burning pain 1 to 3 hours after eating. Depending on the location of the ulcer, this pain may worsen when lying down at night.

PUD has many causes but the most common is *Helicobacter pylori* infection. *H. pylori* is a Gram-negative, helicopter-shaped bacterium that digs its way in between the mucus and epithelium stomach layers. We find *H. pylori* in 60% to 70% of PUD patients. Those without *H. pylori* might suffer from a nonsteroidal antiinflammatory drug (NSAID)–induced ulcer. Ibuprofen and naproxen are examples of NSAIDs. A side effect of NSAIDs is blocking prostaglandin synthesis. Prostaglandins help create good blood flow, protective mucus, and bicarbonate to neutralize acid. Without these three protections, ulcers may develop over time. In addition, increased acid levels and pepsin, an enzyme, can cause PUD (Fig. 8.2). Cigarette smoking can delay ulcer healing.

The body can normally defend itself against developing ulcers (Fig. 8.3). The stomach secretes a mucus layer, which blocks acid and pepsin. The production of bicarbonate should neutralize stomach acid as food moves to the duodenum. Adequate blood flow allows for better healing when there are ulcers.

---

*Brand discontinued, now available only as generic

†Naming conventions can vary between prescription and OTC formulations

Acid Reducers

Treatments for PUD include acid reducers such as (1) antacids, (2) histamine-2 receptor antagonists, and (3) proton pump inhibitors, as well as antibiotic treatment of *H. pylori* infection (Table 8.1).

Antacids

Antacids directly neutralize stomach acid; patients should take them after a meal. Antacids raise the stomach pH. The acidity of the stomach is based on a range called the pH scale. A measure of acidity or alkalinity of water-soluble substances (pH stands for potential of hydrogen). The pH scale ranges from 0 to 14. A zero sits left on the scale for the very acidic compounds and a 14 sits right for the basic ones. A 7, which is in the middle of the scale, is neutral. Stomach acid has a pH of 2; neutral is 7 and blood is 7.35. There are, however, some side effects from antacids.

Calcium carbonate (Tums, Children's Pepto), like magnesium hydroxide, are uncommon in that their chemical name is their generic name. One can remember the Tums with the word tummy to remember the drug's antacid effect.

Magnesium hydroxide (Milk of Magnesia) looks like milk, which can work similarly to an antacid in calming an acidic stomach. Milk has a pH of around 6, which is higher than stomach acid, making it more alkaline. Put together the "milky texture" and the diarrhea of lactose sugar intolerance to remember magnesium hydroxide's laxative effect.

Indications: Acid indigestion, heartburn, and hyperacidity.

Adverse effects: Calcium carbonate (Tums), a chewable tablet, can be constipating. Magnesium hydroxide (Milk of Magnesia) is a liquid suspension, but it can have a laxative

PUD – Pathology

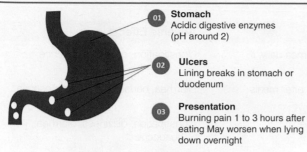

01 Stomach
Acidic digestive enzymes
(pH around 2)

02 Ulcers
Lining breaks in stomach or
duodenum

03 Presentation
Burning pain 1 to 3 hours after
eating May worsen when lying
down overnight

• **Fig. 8.1** PUD Pathology

PUD Causes (Invaders)

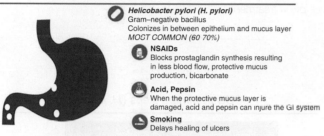

Helicobacter pylori (H. pylori)
Gram–negative bacillus
Colonizes in between epithelium and mucus layer
MOST COMMON (60 70%)

NSAIDs
Blocks prostaglandin synthesis resulting
in less blood flow, protective mucus
production, bicarbonate

Acid, Pepsin
When the protective mucus layer is
damaged, acid and pepsin can injure the GI system

Smoking
Delays healing of ulcers

• **Fig. 8.2** PUD Causes (Invaders)

PUD Defenses (Castle)

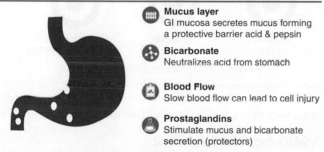

Mucus layer
GI mucosa secretes mucus forming
a protective barrier acid & pepsin

Bicarbonate
Neutralizes acid from stomach

Blood Flow
Slow blood flow can lead to cell injury

Prostaglandins
Stimulate mucus and bicarbonate
secretion (protectors)

• **Fig. 8.3** PUD Defenses (Castle)

effect (Fig. 8.4). Antacids do not prevent ulcers. Antacids are no less effective than other options but are inconvenient to take many times throughout the day.

Patient education and care: Antacids interact with tetracycline and fluoroquinolone antibiotics. The multivalent cations calcium and magnesium bind to these antibiotics, decreasing their effectiveness. **Calcium carbonate (Children's Pepto)** and **bismuth subsalicylate (Adult Pepto Bismol)** both have Pepto in the brand name but have different ingredients and should not be interchanged as the subsalicylate can harm children.

Histamine-2 Receptor Antagonists

A patient asking for antihistamine likely means a medication that will help relieve allergic symptoms such as sneezing and runny nose. The allergy antihistamine affects histamine-1 (H_1) receptors. When the body activates histamine-2 receptors in the stomach, it induces gastric acid secretion, lowering stomach pH (making it more acidic). Histamine-2 receptor antagonists (H2RAs) such as famotidine (Pepcid+)

and ranitidine (Zantac) block these receptors, preventing an increase in gastric-acid secretion (Fig. 8.5). Remember the H2RA medications with the -tidine stem.

Famo*tidine* (Pepcid+) has the -tidine stem, indicating that it is an H_2 blocker. The brand name **Pepcid** contains pep from peptic, which relates to digestion, and cid from acid.

Proton Pump Inhibitors

Proton pump inhibitors (PPIs) such as omeprazole (Prilosec+) and esomeprazole (Nexium) act by shutting off the stomach's proton pumps (Fig. 8.6). PPIs reduce acid and cause a rise in the gastric pH. Many drugs have chemical structures that have mirror images. We call them enantiomers. Instead of saying they are right- and left-handed mirror images, we call them "R" and "S" from the Latin words *rectus* (right) and *sinister* (left). In the case of esomeprazole, the drug includes only the "S" isomer form, which is more active biologically.

Esome*prazole* (Nexium+) has the PPI -prazole ending. Think of **Nexium+** (coming after **Prilosec+**) as the next PPI drug to affect hydron*ium* ions.

Ome*prazole* (Prilosec+) also has the -prazole ending. The brand name combines Pr for hydrogen *pro*tons and *lo* and *sec* for *lo*w *sec*retion of those ions.

Indications: Gastric and duodenal ulcers or hypersecretory conditions such as Zollinger-Ellison syndrome.

Adverse effects: Like H2RAs, PPIs are not recommended for long-term use because of the risks of osteoporosis, fractures, and hypomagnesemia. Because it is possible the body will try to compensate for a lack of acid, the discontinuance of PPIs must be tapered to avoid gastric acid–rebound hypersecretion.

Patient education and care: It is best to take PPIs around 30 minutes before breakfast, or the first meal of the day. Unlike antacids, which work immediately, it can take up to a week to see full effects. Both H2RAs and PPIs are for preventing heartburn and not for immediate treatment. This is because PPIs have a long onset of action.

SCENARIO 8.1. PEPTIC ULCER DISEASE

A patient has acid reflux after large meals and finds the aisle for stomach acid relief. She chooses calcium carbonate (Tums). When would she take the medicine?

Answer: Antacids act by neutralizing stomach acid. Thus, the patient would take the calcium carbonate 1 to 3 hours after a meal.

Treatment—*H. pylori* Versus NSAIDs Versus Nondrug

H. pylori Treatment

Treatment for *H. pylori* infection includes treating with at least two antibiotics and an antisecretory agent that is usually a PPI. By using two antibiotics, we reduce the chance

TABLE 8.1   Acid Reducers, Classes, Dosages, and Adverse Effects

Generic (Brand)	Drug class	Common dosage	Adverse Effects
Calcium carbonate (Tums)	Antacid	500–2000 mg 4–6 times daily, if needed	Constipation, nausea, flatulence
Magnesium hydroxide (Milk of Magnesia)	Antacid	5–10 mL, 1–3 hours after meals	Diarrhea, nausea, hypermagnesemia
Famotidine (Pepcid+)	Histamine-2 receptor antagonist (H2RA)	20–40 mg at bedtime	Constipation, dizziness, diarrhea, headache
Omeprazole (Prilosec+)	Proton pump inhibitor (PPI)	20 mg once daily with a meal (twice daily as part of *H. pylori* treatment)	Hypomagnesemia, osteoporosis, fractures
Esomeprazole (Nexium+)	PPI	40 mg once daily with a meal (twice daily as part of *H. pylori* treatment)	Hypomagnesemia, osteoporosis, fractures

PUD treatment – antacids

Calcium carbonate (tums)

Neutralize stomach acid (raise pH)
Chewable tablets
Constipating

Magnesium hydroxide (Milk of Magnesia)

Neutralize stomach acid (raise pH)
Liquid suspension
Laxative effect

Notes:
Take 1-3 hours after a meal
No less effective than H₂RAs, PPIs but more inconvenient
Not for preventing dyspepsia, only treating
Both can bind to tetracyclines and fluoroquinolone antibiotics, decreasing effectiveness

• **Fig. 8.4** Antacids

PUD treatment – histamine-2 receptor antagonist

Histamine-2 receptors line the stomach helping secrete gastric acid

Famotidine (Pepcid+)

Block H₂ receptors and prevent acid secretion
Don't use for more than 14 days

Notes:
Taken 1 hour before meal
Best for nighttime GERD caused more by histamine
Cimetidine (Tagamet) H2RA causes adverse effects and many drug interactions
Long-term use puts patients at pneumonia risk

• **Fig. 8.5** Histamine-2 Receptor Antagonist

PUD treatment – proton pump inhibitors (PPIs)

Omeprazole (Prilosec+)

Shuts off stomach proton pumps raises gastric pH

Esomeprazole (Nexium+)

Shuts off stomach proton pumps raises gastric pH
S-isomer of omeprazole

Notes:
Usually take 30 minutes before the first meal of the day
Can take up to 7 days to work
Taper when stopping to avoid rebound hypersecretion
Long term use can increase osteoporosis, fractures, and hypomagnesemia risk (only use short term)

• **Fig. 8.6** Proton Pump Inhibitors (PPIs)

PUD treatment steps (*H. pylori*)

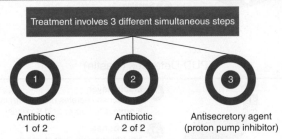

Treatment involves 3 different simultaneous steps

1 — Antibiotic 1 of 2
2 — Antibiotic 2 of 2
3 — Antisecretory agent (proton pump inhibitor)

• **Fig. 8.7** PUD Treatment Steps (Antibiotics)

of resistance and, instead of raising the dose of one medicine, we can use lower doses of two medications (Fig 8.7).

NSAID-Induced Treatment

Treatment for NSAID-induced PUD involves NSAID discontinuation (Fig 8.8). Sometimes this is possible if there is another medication for the patient's pain or if the condition is acute. However, for patients with chronic arthritis, for example, this is not possible. We also treat with an H2RA or a PPI to create the best healing environment.

Patient education and care: In addition to medicines, lifestyle changes might improve PUD issues (Fig. 8.9). For example, a larger meal can often trigger more acid; if a patient eats 5 to 6 small meals per day instead, this might help the condition. PUD patients should also avoid smoking, stop NSAIDs if possible, and avoid alcohol and caffeine. Finally, some reports show that PUD can be induced by stress. Thus, patients should reduce their stress load whenever possible.

Constipation

We can divide constipation into two categories: primary and secondary. Primary constipation comes from intrinsic bowel issues. These can include slowed or delayed bowel transit, or bowel obstruction. Secondary constipation comes from

PUD treatment steps *(NSAIDs)*

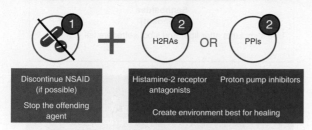

• **Fig. 8.8** PUD Treatment Steps (NSAIDs)

PUD treatment - *nondrug*

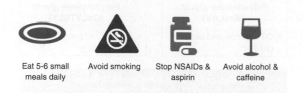

Eat 5-6 small meals daily   Avoid smoking   Stop NSAIDs & aspirin   Avoid alcohol & caffeine

Last: reduce stress as much as possible

• **Fig. 8.9** PUD Treatment—Nondrug

Constipation Pathology

01 Primary Constipation
Caused by:
• Slowed or delayed transit
• Obstruction of bowel

02 Secondary Constipation
Caused by:
• Diet (fiber)
• Lifestyle
• Medications
• Underlying conditions

• **Fig. 8.10** Constipation Pathology

TABLE 8.2	**Laxatives**			
Generic (Brand)	**Drug class**	**Common dosage**	**Onset**
Psyllium (Metamucil)	Bulk-forming laxative	1–2 teaspoons, 1–3 times per day	0.5–3 days
Docusate sodium (Colace)	Surfactant laxative	50–200 mg per day	1–3 days
Sennosides (Senokot)	Stimulant laxative	0.5–2 g	6–12 hours
Polyethylene glycol (MiraLAX)	Osmotic laxative	17 g of powder dissolved in 4–8 oz of liquid	1–3 days
Polyethylene glycol (GoLytely)	Osmotic laxative	4 L bowel prep 8 oz every 10 minutes	1 hour or less

outside factors, such as the lack of fiber in a diet, lifestyle factors, medications, and underlying conditions (Fig. 8.10).

SCENARIO 8.2. TREATMENT—*H. PYLORI* VERSUS NSAIDS VERSUS NONDRUG

A patient has NSAID-induced PUD and asks what lifestyle changes can help lower chances of future ulcer recurrences. What would the prescriber suggest?

Answer: The prescriber would likely tell the patient to stop taking NSAIDs or aspirin, avoid alcohol, smoking, and caffeine, and try to break down big meals into 5 or 6 small meals throughout the day. This will be in addition to medical treatment with H2RAs or PPIs.

When considering laxatives, there are four main types: bulk-forming, surfactant, osmotic, and stimulant (Table 8.2). We colloquially refer to the first two as mush, as these medicines help soften the stool, and the second two as push, as these types work to move the feces from the body (Fig. 8.11).

Bulk-Forming Laxatives

Bulk forming laxatives soften the stool and allow for smooth and easy passage. We include psyllium (Metamucil) in this category. It acts like dietary fiber and swells with water to increase fecal mass as well as softness. Because of its lack of side effects and similarity to fiber in the diet, it is the preferred temporary constipation relief (Fig. 8.12).

Surfactant Laxatives

Surfactant laxatives, like bulk-forming ones, also soften the stool for easier passage (Fig. 8.13). Drugs such as docusate

sodium (Colace) will lower stool surface tension. This effect allows water to enter the feces. It is important that patients take this with plenty of water as the drug can dehydrate the patient. The medicine takes time to work but should produce a bowel movement in 1 to 3 days. We see this medicine commonly with opioids, such as morphine. The end of the words **docusate** and "penetrate" rhyme to help you remember that it works by helping water penetrate into the bowel. A mnemonic to remember **Colace** is that it improves the *col*on's p*ace*.

Stimulant Laxatives

A stimulant, just as it sounds, induces the bowel to push the feces forward (Fig. 8.14). **Sennosides (Senokot)** is one example that most use after fiber and stool softeners fail. It is common to see patients with eating disorders abuse these. A patient can expect a bowel movement (BM) in half a day.

Constipation treatment – laxatives

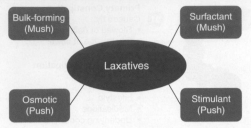

• **Fig. 8.11** Constipation Treatment—Laxatives

Laxatives – bulk-forming (mush)

> **Psyllium**
> **(Metamucil)**
>
> Acts like fiber in the diet
> Swells with water to increase fecal mass and softness
> Preferred temporary constipation treatment
> Minimal side effects
>
> Notes:
> Talk with patients about dietary fiber
> Mix well with liquids before taking
> Can take 3 days to produce a bowel movement

• **Fig. 8.12** Laxatives—Bulk Forming

Laxatives – surfactant (mush)

> **Docusate sodium**
> **(Colace)**
>
> Lowers stool surface tension and water enters the feces
>
> Notes:
> Take with water to prevent dehydration as water leaves the body with the stool produces bowel movement (BM) in 1-3 days
> *Should be given to everyone taking on opioid medication.*

• **Fig. 8.13** Laxatives—Surfactant

Osmotic Laxatives

Two osmotic forms of a laxative have two very different effects. **Polyethylene glycol (MiraLAX)** is an OTC powder for gentle constipation relief. However, **polyethylene glycol (GoLYTELY)** is a prescription form for bowel prep for a patient who must undergo a colonoscopy (Fig. 8.15). These have a high risk of dehydration; thus, plenty of fluids are necessary. MiraLAX will produce a stool in 72 hours or less. GoLYTELY's effect is immediate—patients should be near a toilet when starting this bowel prep.

Diarrhea

Diarrhea involves an abnormal consistency in bowel movements characterized by very soft or liquid stools 3 times or more in 24 hours. Diarrhea is not a disease but rather a symptom, and it often has a pathology behind it. There are

Laxatives – stimulant (push)

> **Sennosides**
> **(Senokot)**
> Use stimulants after fiber and stool softeners fail.
>
> Notes:
> Often used and abused
> Expect a bowel movement within 12 hours (overnight)
> Tablets and suppositories available

• **Fig. 8.14** Laxatives—Stimulant

Laxatives – osmotic (push)

> **Polyethylene glycol**
> **(MiraLAX)**
> • OTC gentle and okay for children
>
> **Polyethylene glycol**
> **(GoLYTELY)**
> • Rx for bowel prep before colonoscopy
>
> Miralax produces a BM within 72 hours;
> GoLYTELY's effect is immediate

• **Fig 8.15** Laxatives—Osmotic

viral, bacterial, or parasitic infections, or other drugs that might be the cause (Fig. 8.16).

SCENARIO 8.3. CONSTIPATION

A patient has acute pain from a broken arm and is on opioid treatment. She chooses docusate (Colace) to help her with a bout of recent constipation. Does this medicine work by lowering stool surface tension to soften the stool or by increasing the stool size by mimicking fiber?

Answer: Docusate works by lowering stool surface tension to soften the stool.

Antidiarrheals—Opioids

Opioid medications can cause constipation, but medications with those properties can help combat diarrhea (Table 8.3). **Loperamide (Imodium A-D)** is a weak opioid that is available as an OTC drug. Loperamide cannot cross the blood-brain barrier to a significant extent; thus, it has very little effect on the central nervous system (CNS) or pain. However, it still produces a constipating effect (Fig. 8.17).

Loperamide (Imodium A-D) has the lo for s*lo*w and per for *per*istalsis. Low peristalsis is a slow-moving bowel, the goal after treatment for diarrhea.

Diphenoxylate/atropine (Lomotil) is a Drug Enforcement Administration (DEA) controlled-substance (opioid) prescription medication that makes therapeutic sense if a less aggressive loperamide did not work.

Patient education and care: Loperamide is for diarrhea that is *not* from an infection. Another use is to reduce discharge volume in ileostomies; these are surgical openings in the abdominal wall. The atropine portion of diphenoxylate/atropine discourages abuse, but a high dose might still bring on a morphine-like response. A case of overdose can be treated with naloxone.

Antidiarrheals—Nonspecific

Bismuth subsalicylate (Pepto Bismol) is a nonspecific OTC antidiarrheal that is available as a liquid or as a chewable tablet. **Bismuth sub*sali*cylate (Pepto Bismol)** has the "b" in **bismuth subsalicylate**, which can remind you of the black tongue, and black stool that some patients experience as side effects. **Pepto** looks like peptic, which has to do with digestion (Fig. 8.18).

Patient education and care: A harmless side effect is black tongue and/or stool. Patients should know this ahead of time so that they do not mistake the dark stool for blood in the stool. Because bismuth subsalicylate is similar to aspirin, it can cause Reye syndrome in children. A parent should not mistake that this pink liquid should be given to children.

Antidiarrheal Treatment—Infectious

A major cause of diarrhea is a bacterial infection (Fig. 8.19). *Escherichia coli* (*E. coli*) infections are usually self-limiting, but a prescriber might give ciprofloxacin (Cipro), for example. There are new FDA guidelines regarding ciprofloxacin use for urinary tract infections and respiratory infections because of its ability to cause tendon rupture; thus, prescribers may give it less often.

Diarrhea – Pathology

A change in normal bowel movements characterized by unusually soft or liquid stools ≥ 3 times in 24 hours lasting < 14 days

Common causes:
- Viral, bacterial, or parasite infection
- Other drugs
- Food allergies
- GI conditions

• **Fig. 8.16** Diarrhea Pathology

Emesis

Emesis happens because the chemoreceptor trigger zone (CTZ) in the brain sends signals to the body to vomit (Figs. 8.20, 8.21). There can be more to the condition, however. For example, we can divide emesis due to chemotherapy into three types:

- **Anticipatory emesis** occurs before a patient takes the drug when a memory of severe nausea triggers the episode.
- **Acute emesis** occurs within minutes and resolves in a few hours.
- **Delayed emesis** happens more than 1 day after therapy (usually 48 to 72 hours after).

Dopamine Antagonists

One medication, **promethazine (Phenergan),** blocks the dopamine-2 receptors in the CTZ, preventing its activation. We see promethazine use with vomiting secondary to surgery, cancer, and chemotherapy. As a patient might actively vomit while needing treatment, a suppository form is available (Table 8.4)

Promethazine (Phenergan) is technically an antihistamine sometimes used as a liquid with codeine. In this chapter, we focused on its use in nausea. In addition to the suppository form, it also comes in oral, intramuscular (IM) and intravenous (IV) forms (Fig. 8.22).

5-HT₃ Receptor Antagonists

Ondansetron (Zofran) is a 5-HT_3 receptor antagonist. It has become a mainstay treatment for chemotherapy-induced nausea and vomiting (CINV). The blocking of serotonin 5-HT_3 receptors in the CTZ prevents activation of the vomiting response. It has many dosage forms,

TABLE 8.3	Antidiarrheals			
Generic (Brand)	**Drug class**	**Common dosage**	**Adverse Effects**	
Loperamide (Imodium A-D)	Antidiarrheal	4 mg at first, then 2 mg after each stool up to 8 mg/day	Abdominal pain, drowsiness, nausea	
Diphenoxylate/atropine (Lomotil)	Antidiarrheal with anticholinergic	5 mg up to 3–4 times/day	Sedation, dizziness, nausea, dry mouth, blurry vision	
Bismuth subsalicylate (Pepto Bismol)	Salicylate antidiarrheal	30 mL every 30–60 minutes, up to 8 times daily	Possible black tongue and stool	

Antidiarrheals – opioids

Loperamide (Imodium A-D)

- Weak, OTC opioid
- For diarrhea not of infectious origin
- Reduces the volume of discharge from ileostomies

Diphenoxylate/atropine (Lomotil)

- Controlled substance
- Atropine discourages abuse
- High doses can bring on morphine-like response

Notes:
Treat overdose with naloxone

- **Fig. 8.17** Antidiarrheals—Opioids

Antidiarrheals – nonspecific

Bismuth subsalicylate (Pepto Bismol)

- OTC available liquid or chewable tablets
- Causes harmless black stool and black tongue
- Children's Pepto is calcium carbonate [not bismuth subsalicylate]

Notes:
Avoid in children due to risk of Reye syndrome

- **Fig. 8.18** Antidiarrheals—Nonspecific

Antidiarrheals – infectious origin

Escherichia coli: Usually self-limiting
Ciprofloxacin **(Cipro)**

New urinary tract and respiratory infections guidelines regarding use for minor urinary tract and respiratory infections

- **Fig. 8.19** Antidiarrheals—Infectious Origin

Emesis pathology

Caused by activation of the vomiting center in the brain.

Indirect activation happens when the chemoreceptor trigger zone (CTZ) is first activated.

This goes on to activate the vomiting center.

- **Fig. 8.20** Emesis Pathology

Chemotherapy – induced nausea/vomiting

3 types of emesis to manage

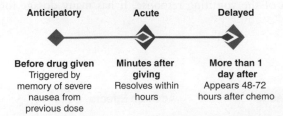

Anticipatory	Acute	Delayed
Before drug given	Minutes after giving	More than 1 day after
Triggered by memory of severe nausea from previous dose	Resolves within hours	Appears 48-72 hours after chemo

- **Fig. 8.21** Chemotherapy-Induced Nausea/Vomiting

including a tablet, an orally disintegrating tablet, and IV (see Table 8.4).

Ondan*setron* (Zofran) has a -setron suffix. Ondansetron is actually a clever word scramble; it has every letter but

Antiemetics – dopamine antagonist

Block the dopamine-2 receptors in the CTZ, preventing activation
Useful for emesis caused by surgery, cancer, chemotherapy, and toxins

Promethazine (Phenergan)

Contraindicated for children under 2
Available as suppository

Notes:
Can cause extrapyramidal side effects due to lack of dopamine

- **Fig. 8.22** Antiemetics—Dopamine Antagonist

the "i" in serotonin, the neurotransmitter that it is involved with (Fig. 8.23).

Patient education and care: With promethazine, there is the extrapyramidal side effect of uncontrolled movement disorders, which might be the result of promethazine's effect on dopamine. Ondansetron's side effects include headache, dizziness, diarrhea, and prolonged QT intervals in the heart. Prolonged QT intervals can lead to torsades de pointes, a possibly fatal ventricular dysrhythmia.

SCENARIO 8.5. EMESIS

A patient has to undergo chemotherapy and the prescriber is concerned about CINV. What receptor does ondansetron act on to prevent the CTZ from sending signals for the body to vomit?

Answer: Ondansetron (Zofran) is a serotonin 5-HT_3 receptor antagonist.

Inflammatory Bowel Disease

An abnormal and exaggerated immune response in the bowel is what we consider inflammatory bowel disease (IBD; Fig. 8.24). The major classes include ulcerative colitis (UC), which is an inflammation of the mucosa and submucosa of the colon and rectum. This can cause rectal bleeding and require hospitalization. Crohn disease is inflammation of the entire intestinal wall and, while it usually happens in the ileum, it can occur anywhere in the GI tract.

IBD Treatment

Immunomodulators such as **infliximab (Remicade)** are monoclonal antibodies that neutralize tumor necrosis factor (TNF) alpha (Fig. 8.25). Affecting this important inflammatory modulator decreases the immune response and inflammation. **Infl*iximab* (Remicade)** is a biologic agent. Conditions such as ulcerative colitis can go into remission. **Remicade** is a "remission aide."

Patient education and care: A provider must administer infliximab through IV infusion; thus, we expect infusion site reactions. Because of a possible increased risk of lymphoma, prescribers must screen patients for tuberculosis and other infections.

TABLE 8.4 Antiemetics

Generic (Brand)	Drug class	Common dosage	Adverse Effects
Promethazine (Phenergan)	Dopamine antagonist	25 mg twice daily	Extrapyramidal effects
Ondansetron (Zofran)	5-HT$_3$ antagonist	8 mg 30 minutes prior to chemotherapy	Confusion, dizziness, headache

Antiemetics – 5-HT$_3$ serotonin receptor antagonist

Ondansetron
(Zofran)

- First approved for chemotherapy Induced nausea/vomiting (CINV)
- For regular emesis and CINV
- Available as regular tablet, orally disintegrating tablet, and IV

Notes:
Can cause prolonged QT interval and potentially torsades de pointes (V-Tach)
Common side effects: headache, dizziness, diarrhea

• **Fig. 8.23** Antiemetics—5-HT$_3$ Serotonin Receptor Antagonist

GI Autoimmune Pathology (IBD)

Caused by exaggerated immune response to normal bowel flora

Ulcerative colitis
- Inflammation of the mucosa and submucosa of the colon and rectum
- Can cause rectal bleeding
- May require hospitalization

Crohn Disease
- Characterized by transmural inflammation
- Usually affects terminal ileum (can affect all parts of GI tract)

• **Fig. 8.24** Gastrointestinal Autoimmune Pathology (IBD)

IBD – Immunomodulators

Infliximab
(Remicade)

- Monoclonal antibody designed to neutralize tumor necrosis factor alpha (TNF), a key immunoinflammatory modulator
- For moderate to severe Crohn Disease
- Has to be given by IV infusion leading to infusion reactions
- Increases risk of lymphoma

Notes:
Must screen patients for tuberculosis and other infections before starting
Infusion reactions happen every time – can prevent after the first infusion

• **Fig. 8.25** Immunomodulators

SCENARIO 8.6. INFLAMMATORY BOWEL DISEASE

It is easy to recognize infliximab as a monoclonal antibody. How?

Answer: Monoclonal antibodies have the -mab suffix. While this does not relate to the drug's therapeutic purpose, it helps identify it as a biologic agent.

Summary

- The most common PUD cause is *H. pylori* infection. Those without *H. pylori* likely suffer from NSAID-induced ulcers. Treatment for *H. pylori* infection includes administering at least two antibiotics and an antisecretory agent that is usually a PPI. For NSAID-induced ulcers, just the PPI is used.
- The three major antisecretory classes include antacids, such as calcium carbonate (Tums), histamine-2 receptor antagonists, such as famotidine (Pepcid), and PPIs, such as esomeprazole (Nexium).
- When considering laxatives, there are four main types: bulk forming, such as psyllium (Metamucil), surfactant, such as docusate sodium (Colace), osmotic, such as polyethylene glycol (MiraLAX), and stimulants, such as Sennosides (Senokot).
- Treating diarrhea depends on whether it is mild or severe, infectious or not. Loperamide (Imodium A-D) is a weak

OTC opioid for mild noninfectious diarrhea. Prescribers reserve diphenoxylate/atropine (Lomotil) for more severe cases. Infectious diarrhea would warrant the use of antibiotics.
- There are three types of emesis. *Anticipatory emesis* occurs before a patient takes the drug. *Acute emesis* occurs within minutes and resolves in a few hours. *Delayed emesis* happens more than 1 day after therapy (usually 48 to 72 hours after).
- Ondansetron (Zofran) is a 5-HT$_3$ receptor antagonist, a mainstay treatment for CINV.
- Immunomodulators such as infliximab (Remicade) are monoclonal antibodies that neutralize tumor necrosis factor to reduce the immune response and inflammation in IBD.

Review Questions

1. A medication that ends in -tidine is most likely a(n):
   a. Antacid
   b. PPI
   c. H2RA
   d. Stool softener

2. A patient who needs an OTC antacid should use:
   a. Esomeprazole (Nexium 24HR)
   b. Magnesium hydroxide (Milk of Magnesia)
   c. Calcium carbonate (Tums)
   d. Omeprazole (Prilosec OTC)

3. A medication that ends in -prazole is most likely a(n):
   a. PPI
   b. Antacid
   c. Stool softener
   d. H2RA

4. Someone looking for a stimulant laxative would use which medication?
   a. Psyllium (Metamucil)
   b. Sennosides (Senokot)
   c. Loperamide (Imodium A-D)
   d. Polyethylene glycol (MiraLAX)

5. Which of the following is a stool softener that helps a patient who needs an opioid for pain?
   a. Docusate (Colace)
   b. Sennosides (Senokot)
   c. Loperamide (Imodium A-D)
   d. Polyethylene glycol (MiraLAX)

6. All of the following medicines would be appropriate for constipation except:
   a. Docusate (Colace)
   b. Sennosides (Senna)
   c. Loperamide (Imodium A-D)
   d. Polyethylene glycol (MiraLAX)

7. Patients should know that bismuth subsalicylate (Pepto Bismol) can cause a harmless side effect of:
   a. Torsades de pointes
   b. Black tongue and stools
   c. Diarrhea
   d. Heart attack

8. Which of the following is *not* a common side effect of ondansetron (Zofran)?
   a. Bradycardia
   b. Headache
   c. Dizziness
   d. Diarrhea

9. Which of the following is the correct mechanism of action for the antiemetic promethazine (Phenergan)?
   a. Histamine agonist
   b. 5-HT$_3$ antagonist
   c. Dopamine-2 antagonist
   d. Proton pump inhibitor

10. Infliximab is in which drug class?
    a. Glucocorticoid
    b. H2RA
    c. Antibiotic
    d. Immunomodulator

9

Musculoskeletal

LEARNING OBJECTIVES

1. Identify various medication classes in the therapeutic treatment of musculoskeletal diseases.
2. Compare and contrast drugs within a given medication class as they relate to the musculoskeletal medication dosages.
3. Discuss the stepwise management of musculoskeletal conditions.

4. Describe the pathophysiology of common musculoskeletal conditions.
5. Discuss the mechanisms of action, indications, drug interactions, and adverse effects of common musculoskeletal medications.

Introduction

Treatment of musculoskeletal conditions usually involves resolving pain. However, pain comes in many forms and, therefore, so does treatment. We treat a common headache differently than a migraine. We treat osteoarthritis (OA) differently than rheumatoid arthritis (RA). In this chapter, we will describe some of the common musculoskeletal conditions that cause pain and review many of the ways that patients find relief from these conditions.

Nonsteroidal Antiinflammatory Drug Analgesics

NSAID stands for a nonsteroidal antiinflammatory drug that we use to treat some of the most common forms of pain and inflammation (Table 9.1). You will likely recognize the names **ibuprofen (Motrin, Advil)** and **naproxen (Aleve)** from your pharmacy shelves. However, there are more NSAIDs that we will cover here. Most NSAIDs inhibit cyclooxygenase, abbreviated COX. This enzyme comes in two primary forms.

COX-1 is involved in the stomach lining, kidneys, and a response to bleeding. Therefore, inhibition of this enzyme leads to gastric erosion and ulcers, kidney impairment, and bleeding. We call this the "good COX" because it helps control these three factors.

COX-2 causes many of the effects involved with the inflammatory and pain process. Thus, inhibition leads to suppression of inflammation, a reduction in pain and fever, and colorectal protection. We call this the "bad COX" because it causes inflammation and pain (Fig. 9.1).

We refer to medications as COX inhibitors and classify them as selective or nonselective between COX-1 and

COX-2. Inhibition of COX-1 generally results in bad side effects, while inhibition of COX-2 improves pain, inflammation, and fever. Ideally, we would just inhibit COX-2.

Nonselective COX inhibitors such as ibuprofen (Advil, Motrin), naproxen (Aleve, Naprosyn), and meloxicam (Mobic) inhibit both COX-1 and COX-2. A specific medication, celecoxib (Celebrex), affects only COX-2 with the idea that it should reduce the risk of gastrointestinal (GI) distress.

SCENARIO 9.1. NSAID ANALGESICS

A patient needs an over-the-counter (OTC) remedy for her headache. She has a history of ulcers, however, and wants to know if taking this medicine on a regular basis could be a problem.

Answer: The patient is correct. Since ibuprofen is a nonselective COX inhibitor, its use can lead to gastric erosion and ulceration. The prescriber might consider celecoxib (Celebrex) or OTC acetaminophen (Tylenol), if it is effective.

Aspirin

Aspirin (ASA) is an old medicine and the first of the NSAID class (Fig. 9.2). It acts as an irreversible, nonselective COX inhibitor, which means that its effects on platelets, blood components critical for proper clotting, last for days. The acronym ASA comes from the chemical name: *a*cetyl*s*alicylic *a*cid. One common brand name, Ecotrin, indicates that it is an *enteric-coat*ed aspi*rin* to protect the stomach.

Indications: At first, patients used aspirin as an analgesic for pain and an antipyretic for fever. They also used it for its antiinflammatory properties. It also reduces the aggregation of platelets.

---

* Brand discontinued, now available only as generic

† Naming conventions can vary between prescription and OTC formulations

TABLE 9.1   Nonopioid Analgesics

Generic (Brand)	Drug Class	Common Dosage	Adverse Effects
Aspirin (Ecotrin)	First-generation nonsteroidal antiinflammatory drug (NSAID)	350–650 mg every 4 hours, as needed	GI bleeding, renal impairment, salicylism, Reye syndrome
Ibuprofen (Advil, Motrin)	First-generation nonaspirin NSAID	200–800 mg every 6 hours, as needed	Nausea, vomiting, bleeding
Naproxen sodium (Aleve)	First-generation nonaspirin NSAID	220 mg every 8–12 hours	Nausea, vomiting, bleeding
Meloxicam (Mobic)	First-generation nonaspirin NSAID	7.5–15 mg daily	Nausea, vomiting, bleeding
Celecoxib (Celebrex)	Second-generation nonaspirin NSAID	100–200 mg twice daily	Dyspepsia, renal impairment, cardiovascular issues, including stroke and myocardial infarction
Acetaminophen (Tylenol)	Nonnarcotic analgesic	Up to 1000 mg every 6 hours with a maximum of 3000 mg daily per the manufacturer of Tylenol	Liver toxicity in excess

Cyclooxygenase inhibitors

Enzyme form	Location	Function	Result of inhibition	
COX-1 "good COX"	All tissues	1. Protect gastric mucosa 2. Support renal function 3. Promote platelet aggregation	1. Gastric erosion, ulceration 2. Renal impairment 3. Bleeding tendencies	BAD (usually)
COX-2 "bad COX"	Site of tissue injury, brain, kidneys, blood vessels, colon	1. Mediates inflammation 2. Mediates fever and reduces perception of pain 3. Promotes renal function 4. Promotes vasodilation 5. Contributes to colon cancer	1. Suppress inflammation 2. Alleviate pain, fever 3. Protect against colon cancer	GOOD

• **Fig. 9.1** Cyclooxygenase Inhibitors

NSAIDs – aspirin (ASA)

Non-Steroidal Anti-Inflammatory Drugs

Irreversible, nonselective COX inhibitor
Therapeutic uses:

COX-1	COX-2
Suppress platelet aggregation (protect against myocardial infarction, stroke)	• Analgesia • Antipyretic • Antiinflammatory • Dysmenorrhea • Cancer prevention • Alzheimer disease prevention

• **Fig. 9.2** NSAIDs—Aspirin (ASA)

Contraindications: Aspirin can cause Reye syndrome in children. Prescribers no longer recommend aspirin for routine pain, inflammation, or fever in children.

Adverse effects: Side effects of aspirin include GI distress, bleeding, renal impairment, and hypersensitivity reactions (Fig. 9.3). Aspirin can also cause salicylism, which results in tinnitus (ringing in the ears), sweating, headaches, and dizziness. In pregnant women, aspirin can cause anemia, postpartum hemorrhage, and prolonged labor.

NSAIDs – aspirin (ASA)

Adverse effects:

- Gastrointestinal (GI) effects
- Bleeding
- Renal impairment
- Salicylism: Tinnitus (ringing in the ears), sweating, headache, and dizziness
- Reye syndrome
- In pregnancy:
  - Anemia, postpartum hemorrhage; may prolong labor
- Hypersensitivity reaction

Most seen are from inhibiting COX enzymes

• **Fig. 9.3** NSAIDs—Aspirin (ASA) Adverse Effects

Later studies found that aspirin had cardiovascular benefits in low doses. Daily low-dose aspirin was then recommended for patients to prevent heart attacks and strokes. Recently, however, the recommendation to allow patients to take aspirin daily has been removed. Studies have found that the risk of bleeding outweighed the benefits aspirin provided in most cases. As such, it is now up to the provider to make the risk versus benefit calculation to determine if taking aspirin daily is a good choice.

Patient education and care: Patients should now consult a provider for instructions on taking aspirin. Aspirin interacts with many different drugs, including anticoagulants, glucocorticoids, alcohol, other NSAIDs, and angiotensin converting enzyme inhibitors (ACEIs) and angiotensin II receptor blockers (ARBs). Because of these interactions, a complete medication history is required before recommending aspirin.

Aspirin poisoning can occur if a patient takes the medication incorrectly. Signs and symptoms of acute aspirin poisoning include respiratory depression, hyperthermia, dehydration, and acidosis. Aspirin poisoning is serious and

NSAIDs – aspirin (ASA)

Drug interactions

- Anticoagulants
  - Warfarin and heparin
- Glucocorticoids
- Alcohol
- Ibuprofen
- Angiotensin-converting enzyme (ACE) inhibitors and angiotensin II receptor blockers (ARBs)

Acute poisoning signs

- Respiratory depression
- Hyperthermia
- Dehydration
- Acidosis

Serious! Life-threatening!

Notes:
Aspirin interacts with a lot of common things–be sure to get an accurate medication history!
Treatment for poisoning requires hospitalization but is supportive care

• **Fig. 9.4** NSAIDs—Aspirin (ASA) Drug Interactions and Poisoning Signs

life threatening; treatment for poisoning requires hospitalization. The poisoning cannot be reversed; therefore, treatment consists of supportive care only (Fig. 9.4).

SCENARIO 9.2. ASPIRIN

A patient asks a nurse practitionor if he should be taking a low dose of aspirin daily. He heard that his neighbor, who is a bit older than he is, was taking a low dose of aspirin to help prevent heart attacks. This patient has no history of heart problems, heart attacks, or strokes. Should this patient start a daily low-dose aspirin routine?

Answer: No, this patient has no indications for aspirin at this time. A low dose of aspirin daily is recommended for patients who have had a previous heart attack and/or stroke. There would be more harm than benefit if patients were to take a low dose of aspirin daily without a previous episode of heart attacks and/or strokes. After talking to the neighbor, it's likely that the neighbor's prescriber specifically recommended the aspirin based on the neighbor's health history.

First-Generation Nonaspirin NSAIDs

What defines first-generation NSAIDs is that, unlike aspirin, their inhibition of COX-1 and COX-2 is reversible. This reduces the risk of poisoning, and the GI, renal, and hemorrhagic side effects are lessened. However, unlike aspirin, they do not provide a protective effect to the heart. They have little or no antiplatelet activity.

For a mnemonic, sometimes we can look at the endings of drugs such as ibuprofen and naproxen, which both end with -en. However, the -en ending is common; thus, it is better to use -profen from ibuprofen; its recognized stem differs from -proxen in naproxen by only one letter. One of naproxen's brand names, Aleve, hints at alleviating pain.

Indications: We often see these NSAIDs for pain and inflammation in OA and RA conditions.

Patient education and care: When helping a patient, the choice often comes down to access and GI distress. Over-the-counter (OTC) first-generation NSAID choices include one that is shorter acting and one that is longer acting. A patient needs to take ibuprofen (Advil, Motrin) up to 4 times a day while naproxen (Aleve) can last 8 to 12 hours. Meloxicam (Mobic) requires a prescription and can last for

NSAIDs – ibuprofen naproxen, meloxicam

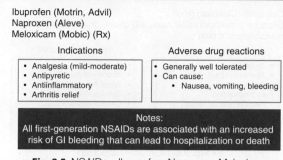

Ibuprofen (Motrin, Advil)
Naproxen (Aleve)
Meloxicam (Mobic) (Rx)

Indications

- Analgesia (mild-moderate)
- Antipyretic
- Antiinflammatory
- Arthritis relief

Adverse drug reactions

- Generally well tolerated
- Can cause:
  - Nausea, vomiting, bleeding

Notes:
All first-generation NSAIDs are associated with an increased risk of GI bleeding that can lead to hospitalization or death

• **Fig. 9.5** NSAIDs—Ibuprofen, Naproxen, Meloxicam

up to 24 hours. All of these choices have indications for mild or moderate pain, inflammation, fever, and arthritis. Some patients better tolerate NSAIDs than others, but all should eventually expect some degree of GI distress (Fig. 9.5).

SCENARIO 9.3. FIRST-GENERATION NONASPIRIN NSAIDS

A patient indicates she has arthritis pain that generally lasts throughout most of the day if she does not take her medicine. The medicine she takes now seems to help for a few hours, but then wears off. She asks if there is a medicine that will last longer so that she does not have to take so many pills.

Answer: Most likely, she is currently taking ibuprofen, which lasts for up to 6 hours. OTC naproxen should last longer and allow her to take fewer pills each day.

Second-Generation Nonaspirin NSAIDs

The main difference between first-generation and second-generation NSAIDs is that the second-generation NSAID will show a preference for COX-2 inhibition. The NSAID is just as effective as its first-generation cousins are; the advantage would include a lower risk for GI side effects. However, the renal effects remain, and a second-generation NSAID may lead to greater cardiovascular risk.

The –coxib suffix lets you know that celecoxib is a selective COX-2 inhibitor and it has several of the same letters as "celebrate." One can think that celecoxib is for *cele*brating relief from inflammatory conditions.

Indications: Its indications include many of those of the first-generation NSAIDs: OA, RA, acute pain, dysmenorrhea, and familial adenomatous polyposis.

Contraindications: Currently, celecoxib (Celebrex) is the only second-generation NSAID available for humans (Fig. 9.6). Veterinary medicine, however, has many COX-2 inhibitors. Celecoxib is not recommended for pregnant women or patients with a sulfonamide allergy.

Adverse effects: These include dyspepsia, abdominal pain, renal impairment, and its cardiovascular impact.

NSAIDs – celecoxib

Celecoxib (Celebrex) (Rx)
Because of cardiovascular risks, last-choice drug for long-term management of pain

Indications	Adverse drug reactions
• Osteoarthritis • Rheumatoid arthritis • Acute pain • Dysmenorrhea • Familial adenomatous polyposis	• Dyspepsia • Abdominal pain • Renal impairment • Sulfonamide allergy • Cardiovascular impact (stroke, myocardial infarction, and other serious events) • Use in pregnancy

• **Fig. 9.6** NSAIDs—Celecoxib

Patient education and care: Because of the cardiovascular risk, prescribers refrain from using celecoxib until they have carefully weighed the risks and benefits.

> #### SCENARIO 9.4. SECOND-GENERATION NONASPIRIN NSAIDS
>
> A patient with rheumatoid arthritis has a history of a past heart attack. Which NSAID would especially concern us for this patient?
>
> Answer: Celecoxib (Celebrex) is a second-generation NSAID that is known to have cardiovascular risk.

Acetaminophen

Acetaminophen (Tylenol), unlike NSAIDs, has no effect on inflammation (Fig. 9.7). Most patients take it for mild to moderate pain and/or fever. Because the liver processes acetaminophen using a similar pathway as that used for alcohol metabolism, we must reduce the dosage with patients who regularly use alcohol. Maximum daily dose is 3000 to 4000 mg for a healthy patient, but someone with liver disease or alcohol dependency would have an upper limit of 2000 mg daily. In the case of acetaminophen overdose, acetylcysteine (Mucomyst) can be given to reverse the effects.

The brand name Tylenol, generic name acetaminophen, and acronym APAP (pronounced A-PAP) all derive from the chemical name N-acetyl-para-amino-phenol.

N-ace*tyl*-para-amino-ph*enol* (Tylenol)
N-*acetyl*-para-*amino-phen*ol (acetaminophen)
N-*a*cetyl-*p*ara-*a*mino-*p*henol (APAP)

Acetaminophen, aspirin, and caffeine (Excedrin Extra Strength) are available in an OTC combination for headaches (Fig. 9.8). The acetaminophen and aspirin reduce pain, while the caffeine causes cerebral vasoconstriction, leading to headache relief.

> #### SCENARIO 9.5. ACETAMINOPHEN
>
> A patient has a fever and wants to know if acetaminophen will work. Previously, she tried ibuprofen, but it had hurt her stomach.
>
> Answer: Yes, acetaminophen would help reduce her fever, but it would not help for a patient who has inflammation.

Cyclooxygenase inhibitors – APAP

Acetaminophen (Tylenol)
Inhibits prostaglandin synthesis in central nervous system
<u>NO</u> antiinflammatory, antirheumatic properties, Reye syndrome

Indications	Adverse drug reactions

• Analgesic
• Antipyretic
• Arthritic pain (not inflammation)
	• Rare:
	  • Stevens-Johnson syndrome (SJS)
	  • Acute generalized exanthematous pustulosis (AGEP)
	  • Toxic epidermal necrolysis (TEN)

• **Fig. 9.7** Cyclooxygenase Inhibitors—APAP

Cyclooxygenase inhibitors – combos

Aspirin + acetaminophen + caffeine (Excedrin)

Caffeine causing cerebral vasoconstriction in the brain to relieve headaches

Indications	Warnings
• Headache	Persons under 18 should not use • ASA & Reye syndrome

• **Fig. 9.8** Cyclooxygenase Inhibitors—Combos

Opioid – receptors

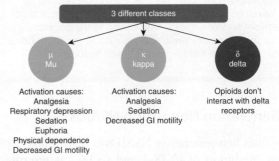

• **Fig. 9.9** Opioid—Receptors

Opioid Analgesics

Opioids act on opioid receptors and have morphine-like effects (Fig. 9.9). We usually use them for pain. There are three different opioid receptor classes that are especially important:

- μ (Greek letter mu [pronounced "myoo"]) opioid receptor—activation of this receptor can provide or cause analgesia, decreased GI motility, sedation, euphoria, physical dependence, and /or respiratory depression depending on the patient and dose.
- κ (Greek letter kappa) opioid receptor—activation can provide or cause analgesia, decreased GI motility, sedation.
- δ (Greek letter delta) opioid receptor—is one with which opioids do not interact.

Opioids vary in their addiction potential. To better classify them, the Drug Enforcement Administration (DEA)

DEA schedules

All medications that work on opioid receptors are controlled substances C-I have no medical use and are illegal

Name	Schedule
Heroin, marijuana, ecstasy	C-I
Fentanyl, oxycodone, Adderall, cocaine, hydrocodone	C-II
Acetaminophen/codeine, testosterone, anabolic steroids	C-III
Tramadol, Xanax, Ativan, Ambien	C-IV
Cheratussin, Lomotil, Lyrica	C-V

Abuse and dependence potential <u>decreases</u> as schedule number <u>increases</u>

• **Fig. 9.10** DEA Schedules

Opioids – morphine

Strong agonist for mu, kappa receptors

Opioid that all other opioids are measured against

Indications	Adverse drug reactions
• Relieves pain without affecting other senses: • sight, touch, smell, and hearing • No loss of consciousness	• Respiratory depression • Constipation • Urinary retention • Orthostatic hypotension • Emesis • Miosis • Cough suppression • Biliary colic • Tolerance and physical dependence

• **Fig. 9.11** Opioids—Morphine

Opioids – morphine ADRs

Miosis
- Pupillary constriction
- Toxic doses: Pupils may constrict to "pinpoint" size
  - Similar to pupils in bright lights
- Caused by morphine and other opioids

• **Fig. 9.12** Opioids—Morphine Adverse Drug Reactions

Opioids – fentanyl

Given via three routes:
- Parenteral:
  - Surgical anesthesia
- Transdermal (Duragesic*)
  - Patch: Heat acceleration
- Transmucosal
  - Lozenge on a stick (Actiq)
  - Buccal film (Onsolis*)
  - Buccal tablets (Fentora)
  - Sublingual tablets (Abstral)
  - Sublingual spray (Subsys)

100x more potent than morphine!

Lethal dose (2mcg) of Fentanyl

• **Fig. 9.13** Opioids—Fentanyl

uses roman numerals one through five (I, II, III, IV, V) to schedule controlled substances (Fig. 9.10). As the number increases, the abuse and dependence potential decreases. Thus, a medication that is Schedule II is more addicting than a drug that is Schedule III.

Morphine (Kadian, MS Contin) was the first opioid mass produced for medical use (Fig. 9.11). We use its potency as a standard by which we compare all others. Morphine is a strong agonist for μ and κ receptors. Patients will use it for moderate to severe pain relief. While side effects are similar for most opioids, we will review each in detail. The name morphine comes from the ancient Greek god of dreams, Morpheus. One brand name, Kadian, might derive from cir*cadian* (24-hour cycle), as Kadian is an extended-release formulation. MS Contin comes from *morphine sulfate contin*uous release.

Respiratory depression is a very dangerous opioid side effect. The respiratory system of a patient who has overdosed can eventually stop working, resulting in death. Younger patients as well as older patients are especially at risk. Other medications, such as central nervous system (CNS) depressant medications (e.g., benzodiazepines), can worsen this side effect. We also worry when the patient already has poor lung function, for example, an asthmatic.

Opioid-induced *constipation* is a common adverse reaction. It can lead to further complications, but we can readily treat the constipation with stimulant laxatives and/or stool softeners.

Opioids can also cause *euphoria* or *dysphoria*. Euphoria is when someone feels great; however, with opioids, this feeling is triggered artificially. Dysphoria is a sense of unease. We worry that when the pain goes away, patients will crave a feeling of euphoria and take an opioid without having any pain.

Sedation involves drowsiness. Because of this effect, patients should avoid driving while on opioids. *Miosis* is a contraction of the pupils of the eyes. Pinpoint pupils are a possible sign of opioid toxicity (Fig. 9.12).

Tolerance and physical dependence are related but distinct. *Tolerance* is when a provider has to increase the dose to get the same response from the patient. For example, a patient on morphine who feels pain after the receiving the same amount as the week before could be exhibiting tolerance to the dose. Tolerance to opioids develops for analgesia, respiratory depression, euphoria, and sedation. Tolerance does not affect miosis or constipation.

Physical dependence results in withdrawal symptoms if one removes the medication abruptly. Withdrawal from opioids can begin as early as 10 hours after the previous dose. The first symptoms include runny nose and sweating, but can progress to nausea and vomiting, abdominal cramps, muscle pain, and muscle spasms. Withdrawal lasts for a week to a week and a half if not treated. Withdrawal is very unpleasant.

Fentanyl (Duragesic*) is 100 times more potent than morphine and there are multiple routes that a provider can prescribe. One especially important form is the trans-dermal patch. Even after use, the patch can contain medication. Thus, these patches must be kept away from children and opioid-naïve people around them. We often reserve the patch for cancer patients, end-of-life care, and patients experiencing opioid tolerance. The brand name Duragesic* is a combination of two terms, long *dura*tion and anal*gesic* (Fig. 9.13).

Other DEA Schedule II Opioid Medications

- **Meperidine (Demerol)**—has a toxic metabolite; often used for short-term pain relief.

Nonopioid analgesic – tramadol

Tramadol (Ultram)

Has weak mu-receptor activity
• Most analgesia comes from norepinephrine/serotonin blockage

Indications	Adverse drug reactions
• Moderate-severe pain	• Sedation • Dizziness • Dry mouth • Constipation

Nursing considerations:
Lowers seizure threshold, making them more likely
Increases CNS depression when combined with opioids, benzodiazepines

• **Fig. 9.14** Nonopioid Analgesic—Tramadol

- **Methadone (Dolophine)**—used for moderate to severe pain; often used to treat opioid addiction.
- **Hydrocodone/acetaminophen (Vicodin*, Lortab)**—watch for other medications with acetaminophen and unintentionally going over daily recommended acetaminophen maximums.
- **Hydrocodone/ibuprofen (Vicoprofen)**—is an alternative to hydrocodone/acetaminophen that helps with inflammation and pain. The brand name Vicoprofen is a combination of the beginning letters of Vicodin with the ending letters of ibuprofen.
- **Oxycodone (OxyIR*, OxyContin)**—prescribed for severe pain, comes as an immediate-release or extended-release formulation. The brand name OxyIR indicates immediate release while OxyContin is continuous release.
- **Oxycodone/acetaminophen (Percocet)**—oxycodone with added acetaminophen. The -cet in Percocet indicates there is a*cet*aminophen in it.
- **Tram*adol* (Ultram)** is a weaker opioid (Schedule IV) medication with weaker μ-receptor affinity (Fig. 9.14). The analgesic effects actually come mostly from norepinephrine/serotonin reuptake inhibition. Tramadol is indicated for moderate to severe pain. Tramadol's adverse reactions include sedation, dizziness, dry mouth, and constipation. A concern is its ability to lower the seizure threshold and cause increased CNS depression when combined with benzodiazepines or opioids. The –adol stem indicates that tramadol is a mixed opioid analgesic.
- **Opioid antagonist—Naloxone (Narcan)** is an opioid antagonist. We can use it to reverse the action of opioid medications in overdose cases. It has a higher affinity or attraction for opioid receptors than opioid medications. This forces the medications off the receptor. This reversal will be very unpleasant. Naloxone should be used only for emergencies, and the patient will still need emergency medical treatment even after its use. Available dosage forms include IM injection, an intranasal spray, and an oral tablet. However, the tablet form is not effective for overdose, as it acts too slowly. The brand name Narcan is a combination of *narc*otic and *an*tagonist.

Migraine – pathology

Neurovascular disorder that involves dilation and inflammation of intracranial blood vessels

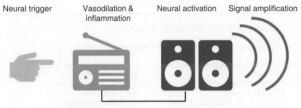

Neural trigger   Vasodilation & inflammation   Neural activation   Signal amplification

• **Fig. 9.15** Migraine—Pathology (Part 1

Migraine – pathology

Two compounds thought to be at play:

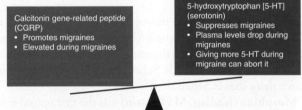

Calcitonin gene-related peptide (CGRP)
• Promotes migraines
• Elevated during migraines

5-hydroxytryptophan [5-HT] (serotonin)
• Suppresses migraines
• Plasma levels drop during migraines
• Giving more 5-HT during migraine can abort it

• **Fig. 9.16** Migraine—Pathology (Part 2)

Musculoskeletal Conditions and Treatment

Migraines

Migraines involve dilation and inflammation of intracranial blood vessels (blood vessels in the brain). Triggers, like bright lights or sounds, begin the process, which leads to an extreme headache and, in some cases, visual disturbances (Fig 9.15).

Two compounds are especially important in migraine treatment (Fig. 9.16; Table 9.2):

- Calcitonin gene-related peptide (CGRP) is thought to promote migraines; we find higher levels in patients during migraines.
- 5-hydroxytryptophan 1 (5-HT$_1$), a form of serotonin, suppresses migraines.

As such, we have two paths for treatment to either prevent a migraine from happening in the first place or to stop the migraine when it comes on (Fig. 9.17):

- **Prevention:** Scientists have discovered drugs that seem to have nothing to do with migraines that reduced migraine occurrences for patients with other conditions who were on these medicines; these patients experienced fewer attacks. For example, patients on the seizure medication

TABLE 9.2 Migraine Medications

Generic (Brand)	Drug Class	Common Dosage	Adverse Effects
Sumatriptan (Imitrex)	$5HT_{1B/1D}$ receptor agonists (triptan)	25–100 mg at migraine onset, no greater than 200 mg/day	Coronary vasospasm
Eletriptan (Relpax)	$5HT_{1B/1D}$ receptor agonists (triptan)	20–40 mg at migraine onset, no greater than 80 mg/day	Coronary vasospasm
Divalproex (Depakote ER)	Antiepileptic drug for migraine prophylaxis	500–1000 mg/day in divided doses	Lethargy, GI upset, depression, weight gain, alopecia
Amitriptyline (Elavil*)	Tricyclic antidepressant	10 mg at bedtime, up to 25–50 mg at night, max 150 mg/day	Headache, insomnia, dry mouth
Propranolol (Inderal)	Beta-blocker	60–120 mg/day	Dizziness, insomnia, fatigue, GI upset, respiratory distress

5HT, 5-hydroxytryptophan.

Migraine – treatment

Two options:

Abort ongoing attacks

Nonspecific analgesics
- Aspirin-like drugs
- Migraine-specific drugs
  - Serotonin 1B/1D receptor agonists

Prevent from occurring
- Antiepileptic drugs
  - **Divalproex (Depakote ER),** Gabapentin (Neurontin)
- Tricyclic antidepressants
  - **Amitriptyline (Elavil*)**
- Beta blockers:
  - **Propranolol (Inderal)**

• **Fig. 9.17** Migraine—Treatment

Migraine – triptans

Serotonin$_{1B/1D}$ receptor agonists (triptans)

Triptan family
- Suma*triptan* (Imitrex)*
- Nara*triptan* (Amerge)
- Riza*triptan* (Maxalt)
- Zolmi*triptan* (Zomig)
- Almo*triptan* (Axert)
- Frova*triptan* (Frova)
- Ele*triptan* (Relpax)*

*Most common

• **Fig. 9.18** Migraine—Triptans (Part 1)

divalproex reported fewer migraines. The same happened to patients on the tricyclic antidepressant amitriptyline and the blood pressure medicine propranolol. These happy "accidents" allowed many to avoid the pain of migraine.

- **Acute attacks:** When a migraine has already started its course, we look to the severity of the pain to guide treatment. For example, if the migraine is relatively mild, a patient might use an NSAID, or aspirin-like drugs, such as ibuprofen or naproxen. They might also consider migraine-specific drugs, including serotonin $5HT_{1B/1D}$ receptor agonists, also known as triptans.

Triptans—Triptans, named after the suffix in serotonin 5HT receptor agonists such as suma*triptan* (Imitrex) and ele*triptan* (Relpax), bind the serotonin receptors to vasoconstrict brain blood vessels, reducing pain and activating them, resulting in less pressure (Figs. 9.18 and 9.19). Triptans also suppress

Migraine – triptans

Serotonin$_{1B/1D}$ receptor agonists (triptans)

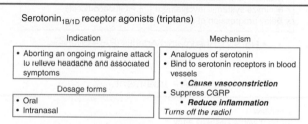

Indication
- Aborting an ongoing migraine attack to relieve headache and associated symptoms

Dosage forms
- Oral
- Intranasal

Mechanism
- Analogues of serotonin
- Bind to serotonin receptors in blood vessels
  - *Cause vasoconstriction*
- Suppress CGRP
  - *Reduce inflammation*
Turns off the radio!

• **Fig. 9.19** Migraine—Triptans (Part 2)

calcitonin gene-related peptide (CGRP), which reduces inflammation. These two actions combine to provide migraine relief.

The brand name **Relpax** combines "rel" for relief and "pax," the Latin word for peace. One can also think of a triptan as tripping up a headache.

Patient education and care: Make sure that patients are aware of potential adverse effects, including chest symptoms, such as heavy arms or chest pressure, and, of great concern, coronary vasospasm (Fig. 9.20). This can rarely result in chest pain or angina. There are many triptan dosage forms, including oral, intranasal, and subcutaneous. Thus, if one form is inconvenient, another may work better.

SCENARIO 9.7. TRIPTANS

A patient was self-treating her migraines with OTC NSAIDs, but this time, these medicines were not helping her current headache. Her prescriber ordered sumatriptan. How will this new medication work when the others did not?

Answer: Sumatriptan works as a serotonin 5-HT1 receptor agonist, which helps to relieve vasodilation and reduces inflammation by suppressing CGRP.

Rheumatoid Arthritis

RA is an autoimmune disease in which the immune system attacks the body. This results in joint inflammation and damage. There are two primary treatment goals: reduce symptoms and delay disease progression (Fig. 9.21).

Migraine – triptans

Serotonin$_{1B/1D}$ receptor agonists (triptans)

Adverse drug reactions

- Chest symptoms
  - Transient "heavy arms" or "chest pressure"
- Coronary vasospasm
  - Rare angina as a result of vasospasm
- Teratogenesis
- Others
  - Vertigo, malaise, fatigue, and tingling sensations
  - Very bad taste when taken in intranasal form

• **Fig. 9.20** Migraine—Triptans (Part 3)

Rheumatoid arthritis (RA) – overview

Autoimmune disorder that causes joint inflammation, damage, and pain

Treatment goals
- Relieve symptoms
- Maintain joint function
- Minimize systemic involvement
- Delay progression of disease

Drugs to treat
- NSAIDs
- DMARDs
- Glucocorticoids

• **Fig. 9.21** Rheumatoid Arthritis (RA)—Overview

RA – treatment

Overview
1. Start with a DMARD early
2. NSAIDs are given until DMARD is effective
3. Add other agents as necessary

• **Fig. 9.22** Rheumatoid Arthritis—Treatment

NSAIDs such as ibuprofen and meloxicam can reduce inflammation and pain; glucocorticoids, a type of steroid, can help with inflammation. It is the methotrexate, etanercept, and abatacept—disease-modifying antirheumatic drugs (DMARDs)—that can relieve symptoms *and* slow disease progression.

NSAIDs—Unlike OA, treatment for RA involves starting a DMARD as soon as possible. A DMARD takes some time to become effective; thus, providers prescribe NSAIDs in the interim. A doctor may add other medications for symptom management if needed (Fig. 9.22).

Glucocorticoids—A health professional can give glucocorticoids, or steroids, by a number of routes. Oral glucocorticoids can help with RA symptoms in the entire body. However, when the issue is localized to a specific joint, intra-articular injections are more beneficial. Long-term use includes toxic effects such as osteoporosis, gastric ulceration, and adrenal suppression (Fig. 9.23).

Traditional DMARDs can help with symptom control and slow disease progression. Methotrexate is the fastest-acting traditional DMARD; patients might improve within 3 to 6 weeks with 4 out of 5 seeing improvement overall (Fig. 9.24). Monitoring is required. Adverse reactions including hepatic fibrosis, bone marrow suppression, GI ulceration, and pneumonitis, which can be serious.

RA – glucocorticoids

Help with symptoms and slow disease progression

Generalized symptoms
(All over body)

Oral glucocorticoids

Localized symptoms
(one-two joints)

Intra-articular injections

Long-term use should be avoided due to toxicity:
- osteoporosis, gastric ulceration, adrenal suppression

• **Fig. 9.23** Rheumatoid Arthritis—Glucocorticoids

RA – methotrexate (MTX)

Fastest working DMARD

- Improvement between 3-6 weeks for patients
- At least 80% see improvement

Monitoring is required

Adverse drug reactions

Hepatic fibrosis
Bone marrow suppression
GI ulceration
Pneumonitis

• **Fig. 9.24** Rheumatoid Arthritis—Methotrexate (MTX)

Biologic DMARDs

Etanercept (Enbrel) is a type of biologic DMARD that works to inhibit tumor necrosis factor (TNF). **Abatacept (Orencia)** works a different way; its mechanism is as a T-cell activation inhibitor (Figs. 9.25 and 9.26). These types of medications can help with symptoms and slow disease progression by suppressing the immune system. However, there are risks of opportunistic infections. We try to reserve these medicines for patients with moderate to severe RA.

Side effects of etanercept include serious infections, severe allergic reactions, heart failure, hematologic disorders, liver injury, and CNS demyelinating disorders. Side effects of abatacept include headache, upper respiratory tract infection, nasopharyngitis, nausea, and serious infection.

While abatacept and etanercept have the same ending and it seems that they should work the same way, it is the infix, or middle letters, for these medications that provide their mechanism of action. The -ta- infix in abatacept means that it is going after T-cell receptors. The -ner- infix in etanercept points out that it reaches for tumor *ner*osis factor receptors.

SCENARIO 9.8. RHEUMATOID ARTHRITIS

A patient starts methotrexate and is clearly in pain. He asks how long it will take to start working. How long will it take for him to feel relief?

Answer: Methotrexate can improve symptoms in 3 to 6 weeks; as such, we would expect the prescriber to give NSAIDs or other medicines that act more quickly to help the patient in the interim.

Osteoporosis

Osteoporosis is a disease of low bone mass and bone fragility (Fig. 9.27). The bones are the greatest source of calcium

RA – biologics: enteracept (Enbrel)

Tumor Necrosis Factor inhibitor (TNFi)
Help with symptom control and slow progression

For use with moderate-severe RA

Adverse drug reactions

Serious infections
Severe allergic reactions
Heart failure
Hematologic disorders
Liver injury
Central nervous system (CNS) demyelinating disorders

• **Fig. 9.25** Rheumatoid Arthritis—Biologics: Enteracept (Enbrel)

RA – biologics: abatacept (Orencia)

T-cell activation inhibitor
Help with symptom control and slow progression

For use with moderate-severe RA

Adverse drug reactions

Headache
Upper respiratory infection
Nasopharyngitis
Nausea
Serious infections

• **Fig. 9.26** Rheumatoid Arthritis—Biologics: Abatacept (Orencia)

Osteoporosis – pathology

• Low bone mass and bone fragility
• Bone is the largest source of calcium in the body
• When body is low on calcium, osteoclasts (truck) break down bone structure to free calcium
• Osteoblasts (crane) build bone structure back up, using calcium in circulation

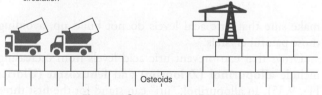
Osteoids

• **Fig. 9.27** Osteoporosis—Pathology

Osteoporosis – bisphosphonates

Analogues of pyrophosphate, incorporating into bone
Prevent osteoclasts from breaking down bone and releasing calcium

Indications	Drugs
Postmenopausal osteoporosis	Aldendronate (Fosamax)
Osteoporosis in men	Ibandronate (Boniva)
Paget disease	Tiludronate (Skelid*)
Glucocorticoid-induced osteoporosis	
Hypercalcemia of malignancy	

• **Fig. 9.28** Osteoporosis—Bisphosphonates

in the body. Osteoclasts break down bone and osteoblasts build them back up. Bisphosphonates such as **alendronate (Fosamax)** and **ibandronate (Boniva)** prevent the osteoclasts from breaking down the bone to release calcium, helping to strengthen the bones (Fig. 9.28).

Osteoporosis – alendronate

Alendronate (Fosamax)

Most common bisphosphonate used – dosed once weekly

Very poorly absorbed orally (less than 1%). Steps must be taken to maximize effectiveness:
• Must be taken on empty stomach
• Large glass of water (even coffee/juice can prevent absorption)

Nursing considerations:
Causes esophageal inflammation and ulceration (esophagitis)
Patient must be sitting/standing for at least 30 min after taking with large glass of water

• **Fig. 9.29** Osteoporosis—Alendronate

Osteoporosis – ibandronate

Ibandronate (Boniva)

Dosed once weekly or once monthly

Very poorly absorbed orally (less than 1%). Steps must be taken to maximize effectiveness:
• Must be taken on empty stomach
• Large glass of water (even coffee/juice can prevent absorption)

Nursing considerations:
Causes esophageal inflammation and ulceration (esophagitis)
Patient must be sitting/standing for at least 30 min after taking with large glass of water

• **Fig. 9.30** Osteoporosis—Ibandronate

Osteoporosis – OTC supplements

Primary prevention for development of osteoporosis

Calcium	Vitamin D
Citrate and carbonate both appropriate absorbed best in acidic environment	Cholecalciferol, ergocalciferol fat-soluble, toxicity is a concern

Nursing considerations:
Vitamin D toxicity is rare and involves large amounts to be taken
Regular weight-bearing exercise can be greatly beneficial as well

• **Fig. 9.31** Osteoporosis—OTC Supplements

While alendronate and ibandronate share the -dronate stem, it is simpler to remember that drone rhymes with bone. The brand name Fosamax looks like fossil, a mineralized bone (Figs. 9.29 and 9.30).

Patient education and care: Bisphosphonates are poorly absorbed orally. Thus, a patient must take them on an empty stomach. Even seemingly harmless orange juice or coffee can prevent their absorption; however, water is recommended. The patient also must avoid lying down for 30 minutes after taking the medicine because of the risk of esophagitis.

A step that patients can take is to use OTC supplements such as calcium and Vitamin D to maintain bone health (Fig. 9.31). This is a primary method for the prevention of the development of osteoporosis. While Vitamin D toxicity is rare, it can occur with very large doses. Many recommend weight-bearing exercise to improve patients' overall health.

SCENARIO 9.9. OSTEOPOROSIS

A patient started taking alendronate but lost the additional instructions the doctor provided to her. What two things must this patient know to make sure the medicine absorbs properly?

Answer: The patient can maximize absorption from alendronate by taking the medicine on an empty stomach and with a large glass of water.

Muscle spasm – cyclobenzaprine

Involuntary contraction of muscle or group of muscles

Cyclobenzaprine (Flexeril*)

Works at the brain stem to reduce tonic (muscle tone) motor activity

Nursing considerations:
Causes drowsiness – no driving after taking
Do not take with SSRI/SNRI due to risk of serotonin syndrome

• **Fig. 9.32** Muscle Spasm—Cyclobenzaprine

Muscle Spasms

Muscle relaxers help stop the involuntary contraction of muscles. A medicine such as **cyclobenzaprine (Flexeril*)** works at the brain center to reduce tonic or muscle-tone activity (Fig. 9.32). Use the brand name Flexeril to remember that it improves flexibility.

Patient education and care: Cyclobenzaprine can cause extreme drowsiness; thus, the patient should not drive and operate machinery after taking it. Certain antidepressants, such as selective serotonin reuptake inhibitors (SSRIs) and serotonin norepinephrine reuptake inhibitors (SNRIs), increase the risk of serotonin syndrome. With **diazepam (Valium)**, we are concerned with drowsiness again, but especially concerned if the patient mixes the medication with alcohol and other CNS depressants (Fig. 9.33).

SCENARIO 9.10. MUSCLE RELAXERS

A patient has back spasms and takes cyclobenzaprine for this condition. He also has a history of depression. What antidepressant classes are you especially concerned with him taking?

Answer: SSRIs such as fluoxetine (Prozac) and SNRIs venlafaxine (Effexor XR) could contribute to serotonin syndrome if taken with cyclobenzaprine.

Gout

Gout has the moniker "disease of kings" because the rich diet of kings might contribute to the uric acid buildup in many gout patients (Fig. 9.34). The most likely location for this buildup is in the big toe. Uric acid can crystallize, creating sharp, severe joint pain. The goal for treatment is to

Muscle spasm – diazepam

Involuntary contraction of muscle or group of muscles

Diazepam (Valium)

Reduces tonic motor activity, but always causes drowsiness to do so

Nursing considerations:
Causes drowsiness – no driving after taking
Do not mix with alcohol due to risk of CNS depression

• **Fig. 9.33** Muscle Spasm—Diazepam

Gout – pathology

"The disease of kings"
- Buildup of uric acid, usually in big toe
  - Uric acid crystallize
  - Sharp, severe joint pain occurs
- Chronic treatment involves decreasing uric acid levels
- NSAIDs used as first-line, acute, flare-up treatment

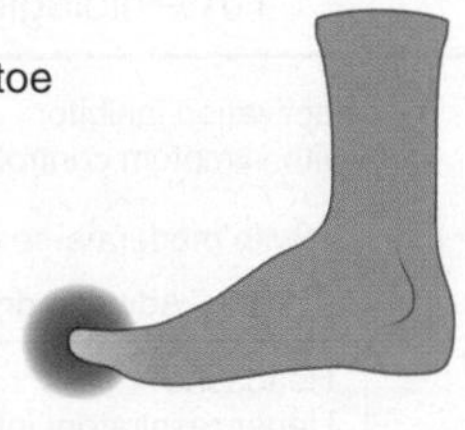

• **Fig. 9.34** Gout—Pathology

Gout – xanthine oxidase inhibitors

Prevent uric acid from being produced
Also break down any uric acid deposits/crystals that have been made

Allopurinol (Zyloprim)	Febuxostat (Uloric)
Cheap, generic can cause fatal hypersensitivity syndrome	Expensive, brand-only increase cardiovascular risk at higher doses

• **Fig. 9.35** Gout—Xanthine Oxidase Inhibitors

make sure that uric acid levels do not build up, avoiding those painful crystals.

Drugs that can prevent uric acid levels from increasing include **allopurinol (Zyloprim)** and **febuxostat (Uloric;** Fig. 9.35). In allopurinol, "uri" can stand for the first three letters of uric acid. Uloric might be a combination of *U* + *lo*wer + u*ric* acid.

Patient education and care: Like migraine treatment, we have preventative measures but also acute measures. If there is a gout flare-up, a patient might use an NSAID. Ensure that patients know which treatment regimen they are on and how they should take it. Preventative measures generally require daily treatment while acute therapy will need a dosage form only while the pain is there.

SCENARIO 9.11. GOUT

A patient experiences significant pain in his large toe. The prescriber diagnoses the pain as gout. What medication class would you expect for the acute pain? What medication class do you expect for prophylaxis for gout flare-ups and why?

Answer: The patient might use NSAIDs such as ibuprofen or naproxen for the acute pain and allopurinol or febuxostat as xanthine oxidase inhibitors for prophylaxis or gout prevention.

Summary

- Nonselective COX inhibitors such as ibuprofen, naproxen, and meloxicam inhibit both COX-1 and COX-2. Celecoxib affects COX-2 only; that selectivity should reduce the risk of GI distress.
- Daily low-dose aspirin had been recommended for patients to prevent heart attack or stroke. Recently, however, studies found the bleed risk to be significant. Now it is a prescriber who should decide whether a patient should take an aspirin daily.
- NSAID length of effect varies from ibuprofen, which a patient would take up to 4 times a day, naproxen, which can last 8 to 12 hours, and meloxicam, which can last 24 hours.
- A second-generation NSAID such as celecoxib will show a preference for COX-2 inhibition, possibly lowering GI side effects, but may lead to greater cardiovascular risk.
- Acetaminophen has no effect on inflammation but still helps with pain and fever. Patients with liver disease or alcohol dependency would have smaller daily limits.
- Two opioid side effects include respiratory depression and constipation. The provider can readily prevent the constipation but respiratory depression could require an opioid antagonist such as naloxone should the patient become toxic.
- Migraine-prevention medications include the antiepileptic divalproex, tricyclic antidepressant amitriptyline, and blood pressure medicine propranolol. Patients on these medicines reported migraine relief, helping researchers find novel solutions to prevent migraine. For acute migraine attacks, a patient might use an NSAID or combination medication such as aspirin/acetaminophen/caffeine (Excedrin Extra Strength). Severe migraines would warrant serotonin $5HT_{1B/1D}$ receptor agonists, also known as triptans.
- RA is an autoimmune disorder with two primary treatment goals: reduce symptoms and delay disease progression. NSAIDs can reduce inflammation and pain, steroids can help with inflammation, and DMARDs can relieve symptoms *and* slow disease progression.
- Osteoporosis is a disease of low bone mass and bone fragility. Bisphosphonates such as alendronate prevent the osteoclasts from breaking down the bone, allowing bones to strengthen.
- Muscle relaxers help stop the involuntary contraction of muscles. Muscle relaxers can cause extreme drowsiness; patients should not drive after taking them.
- In the case of acute gout attacks, we might use an anti-inflammatory, such as an NSAID. For prevention, we would look to xanthine oxidase inhibitors to reduce uric acid levels that can cause painful crystals, especially in the affected toe.

Review Questions

1. Which of the following medications is a selective COX-2 inhibitor?
   a. Acetaminophen (Tylenol)
   b. Ibuprofen (Advil, Motrin)
   c. Celecoxib (Celebrex)
   d. Meloxicam (Mobic)
2. To which DEA schedule do fentanyl, oxycodone, and morphine belong?
   a. C-II
   b. C-III
   c. C-IV
   d. C-V
3. To which opioid side effect would a patient likely not develop tolerance over time?
   a. Constipation
   b. Analgesia
   c. Dizziness
   d. Sedation
4. All of the following are opioid agonists *except*:
   a. Tramadol (Ultram)
   b. Naloxone (Narcan)
   c. Morphine (MS Contin)
   d. Fentanyl (Duragesic*)
5. Migraine medications either help with an acute attack or work for prophylaxis. Which medicine bests serves a patient having an acute attack?
   a. Sumatriptan (Imitrex)
   b. Propranolol (Inderal)
   c. Amitriptyline (Elavil*)
   d. Divalproex (Depakote)
6. NSAIDs help with inflammation and pain while DMARDs help to delay rheumatoid arthritis progression. Which medicine would one classify as a DMARD?
   a. Methotrexate (Rheumatrex*)
   b. Ibuprofen (Motrin, Advil)
   c. Naproxen (Aleve, Naprosyn)
   d. Meloxicam (Mobic)
7. How do osteoclasts and osteoblasts work with bone structure?
   a. Osteoclasts and osteoblasts both break down the bone structure.
   b. Osteoclasts and osteoblasts both build the bone structure.
   c. Osteoclasts build, while osteoblasts break down the bone structure.
   d. Osteoclasts break down, while osteoblasts build the bone structure.
8. Which OTC supplement combination would benefit an osteoporosis patient the most?
   a. Vitamin D and calcium
   b. Vitamin D and magnesium

c. Vitamin C and calcium

d. Vitamin A and Vitamin D

9. Identify the *correct* instructions for patients on cyclobenzaprine for muscle spasms?

    a. "Take on an empty stomach with a full glass of water."

    b. "Take once weekly to prevent muscle spasms."

c. "Do not drive or operate heavy machinery."

d. "Crush tablets before taking."

10. What is the drug class of allopurinol?

    a. 5-HT$_3$ agonist

    b. Xanthine oxidase inhibitor

    c. Nonsteroidal antiinflammatory drug

    d. Opioid

10

Respiratory

LEARNING OBJECTIVES

1. Discuss the stepwise management of respiratory conditions.
2. Describe the pathophysiology of common respiratory conditions.
3. Identify various medication classes in the therapeutic treatment of respiratory diseases.
4. Compare and contrast medicines within a given respiratory medication class.
5. Discuss the mechanisms of action, indications, drug interactions, and adverse effects of common respiratory medications.

Introduction to Respiratory Medications

In this chapter, we will review the medications that help improve the function of the respiratory system. Through antihistamines, decongestants, and nasal steroids, we can reduce the symptomatology of allergies. With antitussives and expectorants, we improve a patient's quality of life when that patient has a cough (Table 10.1). With asthma medications, we can restore much of a patient's activities of daily living, even in very severe cases. With anaphylaxis, a severe allergic reaction, we can reverse the effects of a hypersensitive response to an allergen. We will start by reviewing how antihistamines work.

Antihistamines

When the human body notices a foreign body, such as an allergen, the body releases histamine to remove it. In the body, we have two primary histamine receptors. Activating histamine-1 (H1) causes vasodilation, increased vascular permeability, and bronchoconstriction. These responses and fluid escaping the nasal capillaries cause runny nose and itchy eyes. When medicines, H1 antihistamines, block H1 receptors, they reverse or stop many of these physiologic effects.

By contrast, when the body activates histamine-2 (H2) receptors, gastric acid secretion increases (Fig. 10.1). H2 receptor antagonists include **ranitidine (Zantac)** and **famotidine (Pepcid)**. We cover them in detail in the gastrointestinal chapter.

We divide the H1 receptor antagonists into two generations. First-generation antihistamines, such as **diphenhydramine (Benadryl)**, often cause drowsiness while second-generation antihistamines, such as **cetirizine (Zyrtec)** and **loratadine (Claritin)**, minimize this side effect (Fig. 10.2).

Diphenhydramine (Benadryl) has no official suffix or stem but, often, electronic notecards on the Internet report that diphenhydramine's -ine is a stem because many antihistamines end in -ine. However, so does sertraline, an antidepressant, and about 20% of all generic names. Instead, use parts of Benadryl's brand as it *ben*efits a patient by *dry*ing up the patient's runny nose. Benadryl makes patients tired, and the letters b- e- d appear in *Ben*a*d*ryl as well to help you remember this drowsiness effect.

First-Generation Antihistamine

Diphenhydramine (Benadryl) is a first-generation H1 receptor antagonist (antihistamine) for treating nasal allergies and motion sickness, and can help with epinephrine treatment for anaphylaxis (Fig. 10.3). Diphenhydramine crosses the blood-brain barrier (BBB), which can lead to drowsiness.

Indications: Diphenhydramine can be used to relieve nasal allergies and dermatologic allergies, for motion sickness prevention and treatment, occasional insomnia, and management of Parkinsonian syndrome, including drug induced.

Contraindications: Hypersensitivity to antihistamines, breastfeeding, premature or newborn infants. Do not use over-the-counter (OTC) for children under 6 years old, to make a child sleep, or with other products that contain diphenhydramine.

Adverse effects: First-generation antihistamines, such as diphenhydramine, easily cross the BBB, resulting in drowsiness. These medicines can produce anticholinergic effects, opposing the neurotransmitter acetylcholine. Anticholinergic effects include anhidrosis (absence of sweat), blurry vision secondary to dry eyes, dry mouth, urinary retention, constipation, and tachycardia (rapid heart rate, above 100 beats per minute). Hyperactivity may occur in children.

TABLE 10.1   **Nonasthma Respiratory Medications**

Generic (Brand)	Drug Class	Common Dosage	Adverse Effects
Diphenhydramine (Benadryl)	First-generation antihistamine	25–50 mg up to 4 times daily	Drowsiness, dizziness
Loratadine (Claritin)	Second-generation antihistamine	10 mg daily	Headache, drowsiness, dry mouth
Cetirizine (Zyrtec)	Second-generation antihistamine	5–10 mg daily	Headache, drowsiness, dry mouth
Pseudoephedrine (Sudafed)	Oral decongestant	Immediate-release: 60 mg up to 4 times daily	Anxiety, headache, palpitations
Phenylephrine (Neo-Synephrine)	Nasal decongestant	Put drops in each nostril as needed	Possible rebound nasal congestion
Oxymetazoline (Afrin)	Nasal decongestant	2–3 sprays in each nostril twice daily	Mild dryness, stinging, headache, possible rebound nasal congestion
Triamcinolone (Nasacort 24HR)	Nasal steroid	2 sprays in each nostril once daily. Once symptoms are controlled, decrease to 1 spray in each nostril once daily. If relief is inadequate after 3 weeks (1 week OTC), discontinue use.	Headache, pharyngitis
Guaifenesin/ Dextromethorphan (Robitussin DM, Mucinex DM)	Expectorant/ antitussive	Guaifenesin: 200–400 mg/ Dextromethorphan 10–20 mg up to 6 times daily	Dizziness, drowsiness, nausea, vomiting

Histamine – A Tale of Two Receptors

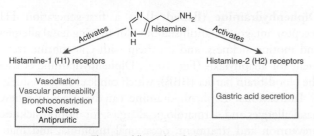

Biologically-active compound stored in mast cells and basophils released when allergen attaches to mast cells and basophils

• **Fig. 10.1** Histamine-2 receptors

Antihistamines – Types

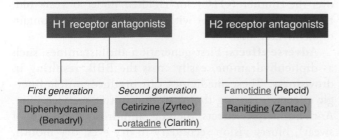

All antihistamines work best when started before symptoms appear

• **Fig. 10.2** Antihistamines—Types

Antihistamines – First-Generation H1

Diphenhydramine (Benadryl)
Crosses the blood-brain barrier easily, with high H1 receptor affinity in CNS

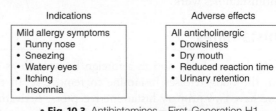

• **Fig. 10.3** Antihistamines—First-Generation H1

Patient education and care: Adults over 60 years old may experience more severe adverse effects from diphenhydramine and should exercise caution if taking it. Diphenhydramine may cause significant drowsiness. Thus, avoid driving or other tasks that require you to be alert until you know how it affects you.

Second-Generation Antihistamine

Second-generation antihistamines do not readily cross the BBB, reducing central nervous system (CNS) side effects, making these nondrowsy antihistamines (Fig. 10.4). Second-generation antihistamines cetirizine and loratadine have a longer half-life; thus, patients have to take some of these drugs only once daily.

Cetirizine (Zyrtec) has the letters -tir-, which we pronounce like "teardrop." Think of ce + tear + izine as protecting a patient from allergy eyes.

Lor*atadine* (Claritin) has the –atadine stem, which changed from –tadine. While we pronounce –tadine and –tidine similarly, the –atadine stem is an antihistamine stem, whereas the –tidine stem comes from the H2 receptor antagonists, such as **famotidine** and **ranitidine.** The Claritin brand name has all the letters from the word clear except the letter e, as in clearing allergies.

Cetirizine (Zyrtec) is a second-generation H1 receptor antagonist (antihistamine) for allergic rhinitis (nasal allergies) and conjunctivitis (itchy eyes). It is less likely to cross the BBB. This property means that it causes less drowsiness than first-generation antihistamines.

Indications: Allergic rhinitis and chronic spontaneous urticaria (hives).

Contraindications: Hypersensitivity to cetirizine or similar products.

Adverse effects: Drowsiness, headache, dry mouth.

Patient education and care: While cetirizine is less likely to cause drowsiness than diphenhydramine, patients should still avoid driving until they know how cetirizine affects them. Patients over 65 years may experience more severe adverse effects and should take cetirizine with caution.

SCENARIO 10.1. ANTIHISTAMINES

A patient thinks she has allergies and reports having a runny nose and itchy eyes. She drives a truck for a living and is concerned about becoming drowsy on the road. Which antihistamine medication might the patient use to solve both conditions?

Answer: Cetirizine or loratadine, second-generation antihistamines, can help the runny nose allergy symptom and are less likely to cause drowsiness than diphenhydramine.

Decongestants

Inflamed sinus vessels taking up excess fluids causes sinus congestion. These vessels expand, blocking airflow. Congestion can occurs without a runny nose. This mechanism is important because a patient will often mistake the treatment for congestion to be an antihistamine, which is the incorrect treatment. A better remedy is to reduce sinus inflammation by forcing fluid out with vasoconstriction. Decongestants produce this effect (Fig. 10.5).

Oral Decongestant

Pseudoephedrine (Sudafed) is an oral decongestant that acts as a sympathomimetic. The word sympathomimetic is a combination of the sympathetic nervous system, fight or flight, and mime, to mimic or copy. Pseudoephedrine's effect is to mimic the fight-or-flight system, activating alpha-1

Antihistamines – Second-Generation H1

Cetirizine (Zyrtec)
Lor*atadine* (Claritin)
Do not cross blood-brain barrier easily, reducing CNS side effects
Longer half-lives than first generation, dosed less frequently
(once daily)

Indications	Adverse Drug Reactions
Mild allergy symptoms • Runny nose • Sneezing • Watery eyes • Itching	Rarely: • Drowsiness

• **Fig. 10.4** Antihistamines—Second-Generation H2

Sinus Congestion – Pathology

Sinus blood vessels are inflamed
• Taken up excess fluid

Does not always cause runny nose

Treatment: reduce sinus inflammation by locally forcing fluid out of vessels
AKA: localized vasoconstriction

Decongestants cause vasoconstriction
• Shrinks vessels and membranes
• Fluid removed via drainage

• **Fig. 10.5** Sinus Congestion—Pathology

Decongestants – Pseudoephedrine

Pseudoephedrine (Sudafed)

Sympathomimetic action: activates alpha-1-adrenergic receptors

Indications	Adverse drug reactions
Allergic rhinitis congestion Nasal/sinus congestion	CNS excitement • Restlessness/insomnia • Anxiety Cardiovascular • Hypertension • Tachycardia

Decongestants should be avoided in those with cardiovascular diseases

• **Fig. 10.6** Decongestants—Pseudoephedrine

adrenergic receptors in blood vessels. We then see vasoconstriction that reduces sinus inflammation (Fig. 10.6).

Unfortunately, this fight-or-flight action also leads to side effects, including restlessness, insomnia, anxiety, and tachycardia (elevated heart rate). Another concern is that a possible increase in heart rate will lead to increased blood pressure. As such, providers do not recommend pseudoephedrine for cardiovascular patients.

One way to remember what pseudoephedrine (Sudafed) is for is to look at the end of **Suda*fed*** or the middle of **pseudo-e*phed*rine** and think a patient is "fed up" or "phed up" with congestion.

Decongestants – Pseudoephedrine

Drug of abuse, due to use in manufacturing of methamphetamine

Combat Methamphetamine Act of 2005 (national rules)	*Iowa Pseudoephedrine Control Law* (Iowa rules)
• Only available behind the counter	• Only available behind the counter
• Max of 9 grams per month AND	• Max of 7.5 grams per month AND
• Max of 3.6 grams on any one day	• Max of 3.6 grams on any one day
To any one person	To any one person

Manufacturers are formulating products with phenylephrine, another decongestant that doesn't have any restrictions on purchasing

• **Fig. 10.7** Decongestants—Pseudoephedrine Control

Decongestants – Phenylephrine

Phenylephrine (Sudafed PE)

Sympathomimetic action: activates alpha$_1$-adrenergic receptors

Indications	Adverse Drug Reactions
Allergic rhinitis congestion Nasal/sinus congestion	CNS excitement • Restlessness/insomnia • Anxiety Cardiovascular • Hypertension • Tachycardia

Decongestants should be avoided in those with cardiovascular diseases
Same mechanism, indication, and adverse drug reactions as pseudoephedrine
Doesn't work as well due to extensive liver metabolism (prevents it from getting into circulation)

• **Fig. 10.8** Decongestants—Phenylephrine

We worry about pseudoephedrine abuse because people can produce methamphetamine or "meth" from it. The *Combat Methamphetamine Act of 2005* restricts pseudoephedrine sales nationally (Fig. 10.7). As such, a person needs to ask at the pharmacy counter for the medicine. An individual can purchase only 3.6 g daily, or 9 g monthly. State laws may be more restrictive. For instance, Iowa puts the monthly per person sales cap at 7.5 g.

Phenylephrine (Sudafed PE) is another decongestant similar to pseudoephedrine that is useless in methamphetamine production. Why not use phenylephrine instead? The liver metabolizes phenylephrine extensively; thus, phenylephrine does not work as well. This disadvantage makes pseudoephedrine the better option for nasal congestion (Fig. 10.8).

Pseudoephedrine (Sudafed) decreases swelling in the nasal packages.

Indications: Pseudoephedrine resolves nasal congestion.

Contraindications: Avoid pseudoephedrine treatments within 2 weeks of using certain drugs for Parkinson disease and depression, called monoamine oxidase inhibitors (MAOIs).

Adverse effects: Common adverse effects are headache, nervousness, difficulty sleeping.

Patient education and care: Patients with high blood pressure should be careful when taking pseudoephedrine, as

Decongestants – Oxymetazoline

Oxymetazoline (Afrin)

Topical decongestant, delivered via nasal spray
• Also minimal side effects, as it doesn't go into circulation

Works very quickly (within minutes)

Notes:
Do not use nasal decongestants for longer then 5 days
Rebound congestion can occur

• **Fig. 10.9** Decongestants—Oxymetazoline

Antihistamine + Decongestants

Loratadine + D (Claritin-D)

Second-generation antihistamines are often combined with pseudoephedrine

Treats allergic rhinitis with congestion
• Reduces sneezing, runny nose, itchiness AND
• Reduces inflammation and congestion

• **Fig. 10.10** Antihistamine + Decongestants

the medication can increase already elevated blood pressure. Limit the use of caffeine, as this can cause shakiness and nervousness.

Oxymetazoline (Afrin) is a nasal spray decongestant. It has fewer side effects because it is topical. However, oxymetazoline can cause rebound congestion, that is, increased or more frequent congestion when the spray wears off. Thus, the instructions limit use to 72 hours or less (Fig. 10.9).

Nasal Decongestant

Oxymetazoline (Afrin) is an alpha-agonist nasal decongestant. It is available as a nasal spray.

Indications: Oxymetazoline clears nasal and sinus congestion and pressure due to colds and allergies.

Contraindications: OTC oxymetazoline use should not exceed more than 3 days to avoid rebound congestion.

Adverse effects: Oxymetazoline may cause rebound congestion if used for prolonged amounts of time, dry nose, and nasal irritation.

Patient education and care: Oxymetazoline (Afrin) is a nasal spray and may be harmful if swallowed. Advise patients to avoid using it for longer than 3 days, as it may cause rebound congestion.

Often, manufacturers combine decongestants and antihistamines for combination symptoms. Loratadine/pseudoephedrine (Claritin-D) is one such combination (Fig. 10.10). The second-generation antihistamine loratadine helps with allergy symptoms. Pseudoephedrine, the sympathomimetic, works to treat congestion. Together, they help a patient who has allergy symptoms and congestion.

A patient complains that he ran out of his loratadine/pseudoephedrine (Claritin-D) prescription over the weekend. He went to the 24-hour pharmacy and got the store brand from the shelf, but indicates it is not helping his stuffed-up nose. He shows you a box that reads "loratadine (Claritin)." What mistake did he make?

Answer: The patient had a prescription for Claritin-D, the combination of an antihistamine and decongestant. However, he likely did not realize that to get that same combination OTC, he would have to go to the pharmacy department. Instead, he mistakenly bought loratadine (Claritin) by itself. It worked only on his allergy symptoms, not congestion.

Nasal Steroids

Allergic rhinitis is an inflammation (-itis) of the nose (rhin-). One way to prevent, or at least lessen, the effects of seasonal allergies is to use a nasal steroid to avoid allergy symptoms. **Triamcinolone (Nasacort Allergy 24HR)** helps prevent these symptoms in a once-daily dose, but it can take 2 to 3 weeks to reach full effectiveness. It works by preventing inflammation in the allergic response.

There is no recognized steroid stem in **triamcinolone**. However, the -one, pronounced like I own something, matches the end of testoster*one*. This mnemonic may help one remember that they are both steroids. The brand name **Nasacort Allergy 24HR** outlines what it is for: Nasa- for nose, -cort for corticosteroid, Allergy for allergic rhinitis, and 24HR for how long it works.

Triamcinolone (Nasacort Allergy 24HR) is an alpha-agonist nasal decongestant. It is available as a nasal spray (Fig. 10.11).

Indications: Triamcinolone is for allergic rhinitis and upper respiratory allergies.

Contraindications: Do not use triamcinolone OTC for children under 2 years old or with hypersensitivity to the nasal spray's components.

Adverse effects: Adverse reactions can include dry nose and nosebleeds, as well as sore throat, headache, and a burning/itching sensation at the site of action.

Patient education and care: Caution patients to use triamcinolone (Nasacort Allergy 24HR) only as a nasal spray and avoid ingestion.

A patient had sinus congestion last year and had great results in just a few days by using a spray. However, he returned to his physician this season reporting that his steroid nasal spray is not working for his runny nose. The patient uses the spray every time he gets symptoms, yet he still has terrible allergies. Why is the medicine not working?

Answer: The patient needs to use triamcinolone (Nasacort Allergy 24HR) nasal spray daily for a few weeks before it will work to reduce his allergy symptoms. The decongestant spray from last year, possibly oxymetazoline (Afrin), worked immediately on congestion. The triamcinolone spray's medicine works differently to prevent seasonal allergies.

Nasal Glucocorticoids – Triamcinolone

Triamcinolone (Nasacort 24HR)

Dosed once daily
Can take up to 2–3 weeks to be fully effective
• Not great for PRN use

Adverse Drug Reactions

• Drying of nose
• Nosebleeds
• Burning/itching
• Sore throat
• Headache

Most effective medication for prevention and treatment of seasonal allergies

• **Fig. 10.11** Nasal Glucocorticoids—Triamcinolone

Antitussives – Dextromethorphan

Dextromethorphan

Activates opioid receptors in the cough center of the brain
• Suppresses the cough reflex
• Derived from codeine, but has minimal side effects at normal doses

Adverse drug reactions

(Similar to opioids)
• Dizziness
• Somnolence
• Fatigue

• **Fig. 10.12** Antitussives—Dextromethorphan

Expectorants – Guaifenesin

Guaifenesin

Increases the volume and decreases viscosity of respiratory mucus
• Makes it able to be coughed up more easily
• Often added with antitussives

Combination antitussive & expectorant	
Over-the-counter	Prescription-only
Guaifenesin/dextromethorphan (Robitussin DM)	Guaifenesin/codeine (Cheratussin AC)

• **Fig. 10.13** Expectorants—Guaifenesin

Antitussives/Expectorants

Dextromethorphan is an antitussive that can prevent cough (Fig. 10.12). It activates receptors in the brain to stop the cough reflex. There may be side effects, especially with higher doses, which can include dizziness, drowsiness, and fatigue.

Guaifenesin is an expectorant that can help remove mucus by increasing its volume and decreasing its viscosity or thickness (Fig. 10.13). We can see guaifenesin alone as brand **Mucinex** or in combination with dextromethorphan as Mucinex-DM or Robitussin-DM. We can find both OTC. If the cough is more severe, a prescriber might write a prescription for a combination with codeine, such as Cheratussin AC.

Guaifenesin/dextromethorphan aids in loosening phlegm and suppressing cough.

Indications: Guaifenesin/dextromethorphan can loosen phlegm and suppress the urge to cough.

Contraindications: Do not use while taking or within 2 weeks of receiving an MAOI, a particular drug class used for Parkinson disease and depression.

Adverse effects: Guaifenesin and dextromethorphan may cause drowsiness, dizziness, nausea, and stomach pain.

Patient education and care: Do not take more than the recommended dose or for longer than recommended. These products can contain sodium; therefore, keep this in mind for patients restricting sodium.

SCENARIO 10.4. ANTITUSSIVES/ EXPECTORANTS

A patient has a mild unproductive cough and chooses Mucinex for treatment. Does Mucinex have the medication she needs?

Answer: Guaifenesin (Mucinex) is an expectorant that increases respiratory mucus volume and decreases viscosity. However, to stop the cough, the patient needs guaifenesin with dextromethorphan and antitussive (Mucinex-DM).

Asthma

Asthma is a respiratory illness of chronic inflammation and often bronchoconstriction, a narrowing of the lung passages. Asthma attacks generally start with an allergen or trigger, such as cold air, exercise, or smoke inhalation. Inflammatory mediators such as histamine and leukotrienes respond to cause inflammation bronchial hyperactivity. The body is trying to protect itself by closing passages to the lungs, but this hyperreactive state can lead to difficulty breathing (Fig. 10.14). The treatment is to combat the inflammation and try to open the airways (Table 10.2).

Asthma – Pathology

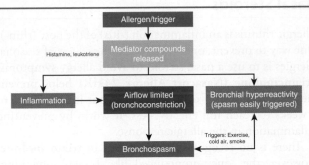

• **Fig. 10.14** Asthma—Pathology

TABLE 10.2 Asthma Respiratory Medications

Generic (Brand)	Drug Class	Common Dosage	Adverse Effects
Montelukast (Singulair)	Leukotriene receptor blocker	10 mg at bedtime	Drowsiness, dizziness
Omalizumab (Xolair)	Mast cell stabilizer	150–300 mg subcutaneously every 2–4 weeks	Headache, injection site reaction
Prednisone (Deltasone)	Oral steroid	Acute: 40–60 mg daily for 3–10 days Maintenance: 7.5–60 mg daily	Mood swings, hypertension
Methylprednisolone (Medrol)	Oral steroid	40–60 mg daily for 3–10 days	Mood swings, hypertension, hyperglycemia
Albuterol (ProAir)	Beta-2 agonist	2 inhalations every 4–6 hours as needed	Tachycardia, shakiness
Fluticasone/salmeterol (Advair)	Inhaled corticosteroid (ICS)/long-acting beta-agonist (LABA)	Fluticasone 100–500 mcg μg/ Salmeterol 50 μg	Thrush, upper respiratory tract infection (URTI), pneumonia
Budesonide/ formoterol (Symbicort)	ICS/LABA	Budesonide 80–160 μg/Formoterol 4.5 μg 2 inhalations twice daily	Headache, thrush, URTI
Ipratropium (Atrovent)	Short-acting muscarinic antagonist (SAMA)	MDI: 136 μg every 20 minutes for 3 hours Nebulizer: 500 μg every 20 minutes for 3 doses, then as needed	Bronchitis, headache, dizziness
Tiotropium (Spiriva)	Long-acting muscarinic antagonist (LAMA)	1.5–2.5 μg 2 inhalations twice daily	Dry mouth, upper respiratory infection, pharyngitis
Epinephrine (EpiPen)	Alpha-/beta-agonist for anaphylaxis	0.01 mg/kg IM every 5–15 minutes	Chest pain, arrhythmias

Leukotriene Receptor Blockers

Monte*lukast* (Singulair) is one preventative or prophylactic treatment for asthma that falls in the leukotriene receptor blocker class (Fig. 10.15). Montelukast is a maintenance medication for chronic treatment; it is not for treating an acute asthma attack. An allergen, or trigger, causes the body to release leukotrienes that form in leukocytes (white blood cells) and are responsible for bronchoconstriction, inflammation, and attracting other inflammatory mediators. By blocking their binding to receptors, montelukast (Singulair) prevents this inflammatory chain—reducing asthma episodes. This class can rarely produce an effect on mood, but its relative side-effect profile is safe. **Montelukast (Singulair)** has the -lukast stem, which has many of the leukotriene letters. The **Singulair** brand name comes from once-daily single dosing and opening of air passages.

Montelukast (Singulair) suppresses inflammation that causes asthma and other allergic conditions.

Indications: Singulair is for chronic treatment of asthma, allergic rhinitis, and prevention of exercise-induced bronchoconstriction.

Contraindications: Do not use montelukast if you are allergic to any components.

Adverse effects: Include drowsiness and dizziness.

Patient education and care: Montelukast is not for the treatment of intense asthma flare-ups. Reports of an infrequent adverse effect of suicidality are possible; providers will want to monitor the patient closely.

Monoclonal Antibodies

Omalizumab (Xolair) is an allergy-based monoclonal antibody for moderate to severe asthma (Fig. 10.16). Omalizumab complexes combine with immunoglobulin E (IgE) in the blood, reducing the amount available to mast cells. This mechanism, in turn, reduces the number of responding inflammatory mediators. The instructions restrict the medicine for patients age 12 and older. Side effects include injection site reactions, respiratory infections, and anaphylaxis. This drug is only for patients who have failed other therapies and is not first-line treatment.

Oma*lizumab* (Xolair) has a complicated stem that tells a lot about what the drug does. The -li- stands for immunomodulator, which affects the immune system. The -zu- stands for humanized or the source. The -mab stands for *monoclonal antibody*. This drug has a black box warning, which is a severe warning on the front page of the package insert about the possibility of anaphylaxis after the first dose. This reaction may occur even a year after the onset of treatment. As such, when a provider injects **omalizumab**, a medicine for treating anaphylaxis must be available. The brand name **Xolair** resembles "exhale" plus "air."

Omalizumab (Xolair) stabilizes mast cells so that they do not release histamine involved in allergies and asthma.

Indications: Patients with persistent asthma who are uncontrolled with an inhaled corticosteroid (ICS) and test

Asthma – Leukotriene Receptor Blockers

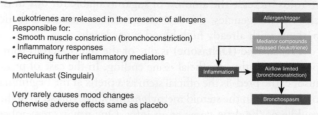

Leukotrienes are released in the presence of allergens
Responsible for:
- Smooth muscle constriction (bronchoconstriction)
- Inflammatory responses
- Recruiting further inflammatory mediators

Montelukast (Singulair)

Very rarely causes mood changes
Otherwise adverse effects same as placebo

• **Fig. 10.15** Asthma—Leukotriene Receptor Blockers

Asthma – Monoclonal Antibodies

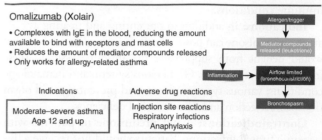

Omalizumab (Xolair)
- Complexes with IgE in the blood, reducing the amount available to bind with receptors and mast cells
- Reduces the amount of mediator compounds released
- Only works for allergy-related asthma

Indications	Adverse drug reactions
Moderate–severe asthma Age 12 and up	Injection site reactions Respiratory infections Anaphylaxis

• **Fig. 10.16** Asthma—Monoclonal Antibodies

Asthma – Oral Glucocorticoids

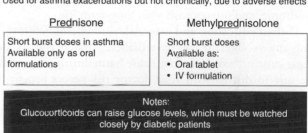

Oral steroids act through antiinflammatory actions
Used for asthma exacerbations but not chronically, due to adverse effects

Prednisone	Methyl*pred*nisolone
Short burst doses in asthma Available only as oral formulations	Short burst doses Available as: • Oral tablet • IV formulation

Notes:
Glucocorticoids can raise glucose levels, which must be watched closely by diabetic patients

• **Fig. 10.17** Asthma—Oral Glucocorticoids

positive for allergy to airborne allergens that are year-round. It is also for patients with chronic hives that do not respond to antihistamines.

Contraindications: Anyone with hypersensitivity to a drug component.

Adverse effects: Common adverse effects are injection site reactions and headaches.

Patient education and care: Do not use omalizumab for a severe asthma attack. Use a rescue inhaler instead. Pay attention to signs of a severe allergic reaction, such as fast and weak heart rate, anxiety, and chest and throat tightness.

Oral Glucocorticoids

Oral glucocorticoids also help prevent asthma attacks by reducing inflammation (Fig. 10.17). Prescribers can give *pred*nisone (Deltasone) or methyl*pred*nisolone (Medrol) in short bursts to lessen the damage after an acute asthma exacerbation. Unfortunately, chronic asthma treatment with oral steroids has many side effects. Glucocorticoids raise blood glucose levels. While it is good that our body's steroids increase the amount of sugar available for our muscles in emergencies, this is a danger for asthmatic diabetic patients with already high blood sugar levels.

***Prednisone* (Deltasone)** is one of the many steroid compounds with this unofficial -sone ending. In the case of prednisone, the pred- is the official stem as a prefix at the beginning of the word. In the steroid methyl*pred*nisolone, this stem in the middle of the drug name as an infix. One way to remember what the drug is for is to think of *pred*nisone and methyl*pred*nisolone as predators of inflammation; they eat it up.

Prednisone (Deltasone) is for many inflammatory and immune conditions.

Indications: In addition to preventing and treating asthma attacks, prednisone can positively affect many disease states that would benefit from suppressing the immune system. These include a variety of skin, GI, nervous system, and hematologic conditions; various types of cancer; and preventing solid organ transplant rejection and adrenocortical deficiency.

Contraindications: Avoid prednisone in patients with systemic fungal infections. Patients should not receive a live vaccine such as varicella or MMR (measles, mumps, and rubella) while taking immunosuppressive doses of prednisone. Do not use if allergic to any component of the drug.

Adverse effects: Prednisone may cause mood swings, hypertension, increased susceptibility to infection, Cushing syndrome, and osteoporosis with long-term use.

Patient education and care: Ask your doctor before getting any vaccines. If you have diabetes, watch your blood sugar closely. Prednisone may cause harm during pregnancy. Be sure to discuss with your doctor risk versus benefit of using prednisone while pregnant.

Inhaler Types

Asthma inhalers come in various types (Fig. 10.18). Individual patient considerations and cost are primary factors that separate them. There are four main inhaler types:
1. Metered-dose inhaler
   a. A propellant dispenses a single dose at a time
   b. Dexterity required: moderate to high
2. Dry powder inhaler
   a. Patient's breath helps to inhale the contents of a dry powder capsule
   b. Dexterity required: moderate
3. Respimat inhaler
   a. Creates a mist with the container's pressure
   b. Dexterity required: low
4. Nebulizer
   a. Machine creates the mist
   b. Dexterity required: minimal
   c. Note: Inconvenient, as nebulizers need a separate machine

Inhaled Corticosteroids

While oral steroids can cause significant systemic side effects, a solution is to deliver the steroid to the lungs directly.

Asthma – Inhaler Types

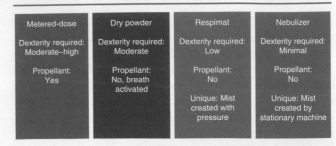

• **Fig. 10.18** Asthma—Inhaler Types

Asthma – Inhaled Corticosteroids (ICS)

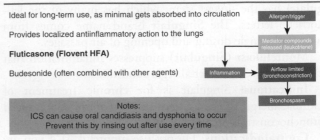

• **Fig. 10.19** Asthma—Inhaled Corticosteroids (ICS)

Asthma – Beta-2 Receptor Agonists

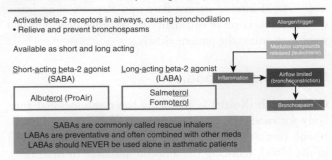

• **Fig. 10.20** Asthma—Beta-2 Receptor Agonists

Inhalers can contain ICS such as fluticasone (Flovent HFA) and budesonide (often in combined inhalers; Fig. 10.19). These provide localized anti-inflammatory action in the lungs. Even long-term, there is little to no systemic absorption. There are a few preventable side effects. ICS can cause thrush (oral candidiasis) or dysphonia (vocal cord spasm). A patient can prevent these by rinsing out the mouth after each use.

Beta-2 Agonists

Albuterol (ProAir HFA) is a drug that opens bronchi (air passages). We classify it as a beta-2 receptor agonist to identify the receptor it affects to cause this bronchodilation (Fig. 10.20). When the bronchi dilate, we see fewer bronchospasms. Beta-2 agonist inhalers come in short-acting forms, such as albuterol (ProAir), or long-acting formulations, such as **sal*meterol* (Serevent)** and **form*oterol*** (usually in combination with a steroid).

The -terol stem of **albuterol** indicates that it is a beta-2 adrenergic agonist for bronchodilation. However, the -terol stem does not help you know whether it is long-acting or short-acting, or how to distinguish it from sal*meterol*. One must memorize that distinction. The brand name **ProAir HFA** combines the word *pro*vide and *air*. The HFA stands for hydrofluoroalkane, the propellant that releases the medication.

Short-acting inhalers are rescue inhalers to rescue someone from an asthma attack immediately. Long-acting inhalers work prophylactically to prevent attacks. In asthma, we should not use long-acting beta-2 agonists (LABAs) alone because of possible side effects.

Albuterol (ProAir) relaxes the smooth muscle in the bronchii.

Indications: Bronchospasm treatment or prevention in patients with asthma or other reversible obstructive airway diseases. It prevents exercise-induced bronchospasm.

Contraindications: Do not use albuterol if allergic to milk protein, other sympathomimetics, or any component of the formulation.

Adverse effects: Nervousness, excitement, tremor, fast heart rate, pharyngitis

Patient education and care: Counsel patients on inhaler technique and pay attention to the dose counter to request refills before running out.

ICS/LABA Combinations

Fluticasone-Salmeterol (Advair) works by the anti-inflammatory, immunosuppressive, and antiproliferative properties of the ICS fluticasone and bronchial smooth muscle relaxation of salmeterol.

Indications: Advair is for treating asthma in patients 12 years old and older for all dosage forms and as young as 4 years old for Advair Diskus. It is also for chronic obstructive pulmonary disease (COPD).

Contraindications: It is not for use during an acute exacerbation of asthma or COPD attack or by anyone with an allergy to milk protein, corticosteroids, or sympathomimetics.

Adverse effects: Advair can cause headaches, upper respiratory tract infections, and pneumonia.

Patient education and care: Do not use Advair for an intense flare-up. Use a rescue inhaler instead. The patient should rinse the mouth with water after use to avoid thrush. Advair puts patients with COPD at increased risk for pneumonia.

Anticholinergic Agents

Other receptors that can relax bronchial smooth muscle are the cholinergic (muscarinic) receptors (Fig. 10.21). By blocking these receptors, anticholinergic agents prevent bronchoconstriction. Like the beta-agonists, we have short-acting muscarinic antagonists (SAMAs) and long-acting muscarinic antagonists (LAMAs). While we might see

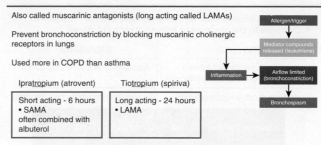

Asthma – Anticholinergics

Also called muscarinic antagonists (long acting called LAMAs)

Prevent bronchoconstriction by blocking muscarinic cholinergic receptors in lungs

Used more in COPD than asthma

Ipra*trop*ium (atrovent)
Short acting - 6 hours
• SAMA often combined with albuterol

Tio*trop*ium (spiriva)
Long acting - 24 hours
• LAMA

• **Fig. 10.21** Asthma—Anticholinergics

their uses in asthma, we often see anticholinergics more in COPD.

Short-Acting Muscarinic Antagonist

Ipra*trop*ium (Atrovent) is a short-acting muscarinic antagonist (SAMA) that can combine with albuterol. Instructors use **atropine** as the prototype drug for the anticholinergics, and you can see the -trop- stem in **a*trop*ine, ipra*trop*ium**, and **tio*trop*ium. Ipratropium (Atrovent)** causes bronchodilation by blocking acetylcholine receptors.

Indications: Ipratropium is for COPD. It is also used off label for acute exacerbation of asthma in combination with albuterol.

Contraindications: Allergy to any part of the formulation, including ipratropium and atropine.

Adverse effects: Ipratropium can cause bronchitis and sinusitis.

Patient education and care: Teach patients the correct inhaler technique.

Long-Acting Muscarinic Antagonist

Tio*trop*ium (Spiriva Respimat) is a LAMA that lasts for 24 hours. **Tiotropium** has the same -trop- stem as **ipratropium** and is the long-acting version. As with the -terols, the beta-2 receptor agonists, you have to memorize which anticholinergic is long acting versus short acting. **Spiriva** takes the "spir" from re*spir*ation.

Tio*trop*ium (Spiriva) causes bronchodilation by inhibiting muscarinic receptors.

Indications: Tiotropium is for both COPD and asthma maintenance. Only Spiriva Respimat is for treating asthma in adults and children over 6 years old.

Contraindications: Patients with an allergy to tiotropium, ipratropium, and atropine.

Adverse effects: Common adverse effects of tiotropium are dry mouth and upper respiratory tract infection.

Patient education and care: Do not use Spiriva for intense flare-ups. Use a rescue inhaler instead. Show the patient the correct inhaler technique.

Manufacturers often combine inhaled asthma agents to make administration easier (Fig. 10.22). To combat the inflammation and bronchospasm in asthma, we can expect a combination of ICS/LABA agents such as **fluticasone/sal*meterol* (Advair)** or **budesonide/formo*terol* (Symbicort)**. Just as with a solo ICS product, each patient must

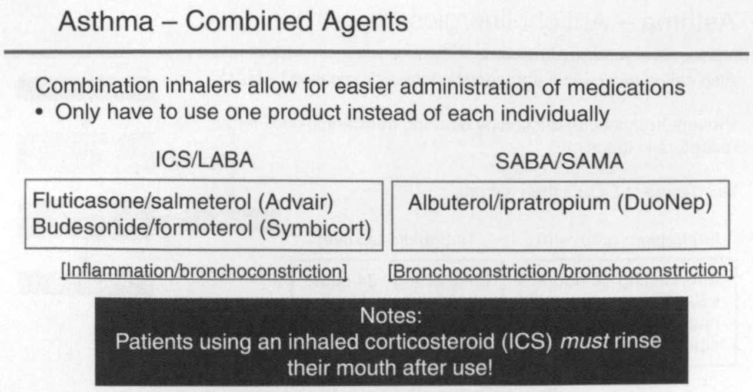

Asthma – Combined Agents

Combination inhalers allow for easier administration of medications
• Only have to use one product instead of each individually

ICS/LABA	SABA/SAMA
Fluticasone/salmeterol (Advair) Budesonide/formoterol (Symbicort)	Albuterol/ipratropium (DuoNep)
[Inflammation/bronchoconstriction]	[Bronchoconstriction/bronchoconstriction]

Notes:
Patients using an inhaled corticosteroid (ICS) *must* rinse their mouth after use!

• **Fig. 10.22** Asthma—Combined Agents

Anaphylaxis – Epinephrine

Allergens can cause severe allergic reactions, eventually anaphylaxis can occur within minutes
Alpha and beta receptors are effected, causing:
• Vasodilation
• Bronchoconstriction and bronchospasm

Epinephrine (EpiPen)
Acts rapidly on alpha and beta receptors throughout the body
Given as intramuscular injection

Patients should be taken to the emergency department after use of epinephrine to ensure safety if the medication is eliminated from the body before the allergen

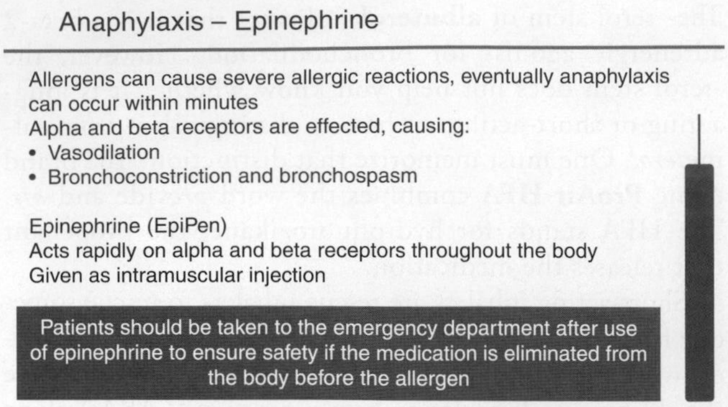

• **Fig. 10.23** Anaphylaxis—Epinephrine

rinse the mouth after each use. Combination SABA/SAMA products such as **albuterol/ipratropium (DuoNeb)** help with asthma. The brand name **DuoNeb** alludes to the *duo* of drugs in *neb*ulized form.

SCENARIO 10.5. ASTHMA

A patient is using budesonide/salmeterol (Symbicort) for keeping asthma controlled. What is the purpose of both components of Symbicort?

Answer: The budesonide is an ICS for inflammation. The formoterol is a beta-2 receptor agonist for bronchodilation. In combination, they help prevent or reduce the number of asthma attacks for the patient who has both inflammation and bronchoconstriction.

Anaphylaxis

Sometimes, allergens can trigger a very severe allergic reaction known as anaphylaxis. The eyes, lips, and throat might swell, making it hard for the patient to breathe. The lungs might also constrict, making it harder for air to get into the airway. An emergency medication, epinephrine (EpiPen), via an intramuscular injection, can reverse these physiologic actions (Fig. 10.23). It works quickly on alpha and beta receptors to save a patient's life. However, the patient should still go to the emergency department, as the body may eliminate epinephrine before eliminating the allergen. This concern is also why manufacturers always provide EpiPens in pairs. The patient may need a second dose on the way to the hospital to continue to facilitate breathing.

Epinephrine (EpiPen) has a Greek origin. "Epi" means "above," and "neph" means "kidney," referring to the adrenal gland that is above the kidney. One might hear the Latin version of **epinephrine**, which is adrenaline. Like the Greek, the "ad" means "above," and "renal" means "kidney."

The **EpiPen** brand name refers to the injector, which looks like a pen.

Epinephrine (EpiPen) causes bronchodilation, vasodilation, and heart rate increase by stimulating alpha, beta-1, and beta-2 adrenergic receptors.

Indications: Epinephrine can resolve type 1 hypersensitivity reactions such as anaphylaxis and hypotension from septic shock. Specific formulations can dilate eyes for surgery.

Contraindications: In an emergency, there are no absolute contraindications. In other situations, hypersensitivity to components of the drug and contraindications to vasopressors should be considered.

Adverse effects: Chest pain, hypertension, and arrhythmias are harmful effects of epinephrine.

Patient education and care: For anaphylaxis and allergies, inject the EpiPen into the muscle or fatty part of the skin, but not the buttocks. Educate anyone who may need to administer the drug for you on how to use it. Call emergency services after administration.

SCENARIO 10.6. ANAPHYLAXIS

A patient starts to have difficulty breathing, and you see that he just ate a peanut butter cookie. You recognize he is experiencing anaphylaxis. You find his health bracelet, which shows that he is allergic to peanuts. The patient has an EpiPen, but will the epinephrine (EpiPen) be given intravenously, intramuscularly, or subcutaneously?

Answer: Inject epinephrine (EpiPen) intramuscularly. The proper technique includes pushing the auto-injector firmly into the patient's thigh (even through pants) at a 90-degree angle until it "clicks." One holds the pen securely in place for 3 seconds, then removes it. A call to 911 should send the patient to the emergency department.

Summary

• We divide antihistamines, also known as H1 receptor antagonists, into two generations. The first-generation antihistamines, such as **diphenhydramine**, often cause drowsiness. Second-generation antihistamines, such as **cetirizine** and **loratadine**, cause little drowsiness.

- Frequently, patients will mistake the treatment for a runny nose (antihistamine) for that of a congested nose (decongestant). However, a combination product such as loratadine/pseudoephedrine can help with both. The second-generation antihistamine loratadine helps with allergy symptoms; pseudoephedrine, the sympathomimetic, treats congestion.
- Allergic rhinitis is chronic nasal inflammation. A nasal steroid can prevent allergy symptoms in a once-daily dose, but it can take 2 to 3 weeks to reach full effectiveness. Adverse reactions can include dry nose and nosebleeds.
- Guaifenesin is an expectorant that can help remove mucus by increasing its volume and decreasing its viscosity or thickness. We can see guaifenesin alone or in combination with the antitussive cough-suppressant dextromethorphan, such as Mucinex-DM or Robitussin-DM. We can find both OTC. If the cough is severe, a prescriber might prescribe a codeine-based medicine, such as Cheratussin AC.
- Albuterol is a beta-2 receptor agonist that provides bronchodilation to relieve an asthmatic's bronchoconstriction. Beta-2 agonist inhalers come in short-acting forms, such as albuterol, or long-acting formulations, such as salmeterol, and formoterol, usually combined with an ICS. These provide localized anti-inflammatory action in the lungs. An ICS can cause thrush or dysphonia, but a patient can prevent these by rinsing the mouth after each use.
- In some patients, allergens can trigger anaphylaxis, a severe allergic reaction. The eyes, lips, and throat might swell, making it hard for the patient to breathe. An emergency medication, epinephrine (EpiPen), via an intramuscular injection, can reverse these physiologic responses.

Review Questions

1. All of these medicines block a histamine receptor. Which one is a minimally sedating, second-generation H1 antihistamine?
   a. Famotidine (Pepcid)
   b. Loratadine (Claritin)
   c. Ranitidine (Zantac)
   d. Diphenhydramine (Benadryl)
2. A patient can find each of these medicines OTC or behind the counter. Which is a nasal spray that will relieve congestion quickly?
   a. Oxymetazoline (Afrin)
   b. Pseudoephedrine (Sudafed)
   c. Triamcinolone (Nasacort 24HR)
   d. Phenylephrine (Sudafed PE)
3. Which of the following medications is an OTC antitussive?
   a. Dextromethorphan
   b. Triamcinolone (Nasacort 24HR)
   c. Guaifenesin (Mucinex)
   d. Codeine
4. Which medication is a monoclonal antibody for allergic asthma prophylaxis?
   a. Infliximab (Remicade)
   b. Montelukast (Singulair)
   c. Albuterol (ProAir)
   d. Omalizumab (Xolair)
5. Which inhaler type requires patients to use their breath to inhale the active medication?
   a. Metered-dose inhaler
   b. Respimat inhaler
   c. Nebulizer
   d. Dry powder inhaler
6. Which asthma medicine contains a long-acting beta-2 agonist?
   a. Albuterol (ProAir)
   b. Fluticasone/salmeterol (Advair)
   c. Fluticasone (Flovent HFA)
   d. Tiotropium (Spiriva)
7. Which respiratory drug or drug combination contains a short-acting muscarinic antagonist?
   a. Albuterol/ipratropium (DuoNeb)
   b. Tiotropium (Spiriva)
   c. Albuterol (ProAir)
   d. Triamcinolone (Nasacort 24HR)
8. Which of the following is a possible inhaled corticosteroid side effect if a patient fails to rinse out the mouth after each use?
   a. Oral candidiasis
   b. Bradycardia
   c. Chest pain
   d. Diarrhea
9. Which medication or medication pair contains a long-acting beta-2 agonist?
   a. Albuterol (ProAir)
   b. Tiotropium (Spiriva)
   c. Albuterol/ipratropium (DuoNeb)
   d. Fluticasone/salmeterol (Advair)
10. An anaphylactic patient just took a dose of epinephrine. She is sitting upright and breathing well on her own. The patient asks if she still needs to go to the emergency department. You respond:
    a. No, this patient is stable and can go home
    b. No, the patient can drive herself to the emergency department since she is stable
    c. Yes, call 9-1-1 as this patient may experience another anaphylactic episode when the epinephrine wears off
    d. Yes, but we should wait for the epinephrine to take full effect before calling for an ambulance

11

Immune

1. Discuss the management of immune conditions.
2. Describe the pathophysiology of common immune conditions.
3. Identify various medication classes in the therapeutic treatment of immune diseases.
4. Compare and contrast medicines within a given immune medication class.
5. Discuss the mechanisms of action, indications, drug interactions, and adverse effects of common immune medications.

Antimicrobial Introduction

Antimicrobial means "against microbes." We can often divide these medications into three broad categories: antibiotics (drugs for bacteria), antifungals (drugs for mycoses or fungi), and antivirals (drugs for viruses). In this chapter, we will first review general properties of microorganisms and then dive into bacteria, fungi, and viruses.

Gram Positive Versus Gram Negative

As we look at microbes, those organisms we see under a microscope, we find that our understanding of them helps us choose the correct antibiotic. Prescribers choose antibiotic treatment often knowing whether the organism is **Gram positive (Gram +)** or **Gram negative (Gram –;** Fig. 11.1). A Gram stain test will either color (Gram +) or fail to color (Gram –) the organism. Gram + bacteria have fewer layers taking up the stain, while an extra layer in the Gram – bacteria prevents the stain from staying on.

While our intuition tells us that Gram – bacteria have better protection, this does not necessarily mean that our treatments will be more potent. Rather, different antibiotics simply better affect a Gram + or Gram – bacterium.

Bacteriostatic Versus Bactericidal

We can also classify the medications into different groups as **bacteriostatic** or **bactericidal**. Bacteriostatic antibiotics keep the bacteria from replicating. Bactericidal antibiotics kill the bacteria outright. While it makes sense that killing the bacteria outright would be better, bactericidal antibiotics are not always the better option. Often an antibiotic kills the target bacteria as well as some of the host's good bacteria.

Antibiotic Class Examples

Different antibiotic classes (Figs. 11.2 and 11.3) disrupt different bacterial cellular processes:
- Inhibition of cell wall synthesis
  - Penicillins
  - Cephalosporins
  - Vancomycin
- Inhibition of DNA/RNA synthesis
  - Fluoroquinolones
- Inhibition of protein synthesis (bacteriostatic)
  - Tetracyclines
  - Macrolides
  - Lincosamides
  - Linezolid
- Inhibition of protein synthesis (bactericidal)
  - Aminoglycosides

Broad Versus Narrow Spectrum

We can divide antibiotics subjectively into **broad-spectrum** and **narrow-spectrum** categories (Fig. 11.4). A broad-spectrum antibiotic covers a wide range of organisms. This is a good choice when a provider is working against an unknown organism. However, there is collateral damage in that more good bacteria would suffer. We might also see antibiotic resistance develop. Narrow-spectrum antibiotics cover specific microbes. Nevertheless, to use them effectively, we need to know which organism is causing the infection. These will generally cause less resistance. We can often employ a technique known as empiric therapy, or making an educated guess, based on where the infection is and using the clinician's past experience. Then, when the lab later identifies the microbe, the prescriber can switch the patient to a narrow-spectrum antibiotic.

---

*Brand discontinued, now available only as generic
†Naming conventions can vary between prescription and OTC formulations

Bacterial Resistance

Bacteria can form resistance in four ways (Fig. 11.5): (1) reduce the site of action-drug concentration by either pumping the drug out or preventing it from entering at the site of action, (2) create an antagonist that works to block a site of action, (3) alter the drug target to a shape that no longer allows the antibiotic to fit, or (4) inactivate the drug entirely.

Superinfections

A supervisor, the leader, is above a subordinate, the employee. In the same way, a superinfection is above the original infection (Fig. 11.6). We see these infections more commonly with broad-spectrum antibiotics. For example, if a physician treats an ear infection with a broad-spectrum antibiotic, it can lead to a vaginal yeast infection, oral thrush, or a dangerous infection such as *Clostridium difficile* (*C. diff*). *C. diff* is already in the gut but, generally, the good bacteria keep it from proliferating. However, a broad-spectrum antibiotic might wipe out some of the gut's normal flora. When this happens, it opens the door for *C. diff* to take hold.

Methicillin-Resistant *Staphylococcus aureus*

Methicillin-resistant *Staphylococcus aureus* (MRSA) is a resistant strain of bacteria that many common antibiotics cannot kill (Fig. 11.7). This resistant bacterium changes penicillin-binding proteins, or PBPs, where penicillins normally bind. This reduces the affinity or attraction of the penicillins and cephalosporins to target sites, making them

Gram Positive vs Gram Negative

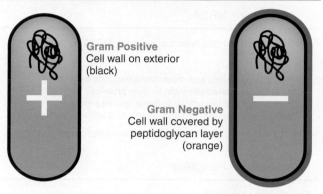

Gram Positive
Cell wall on exterior
(black)

Gram Negative
Cell wall covered by
peptidoglycan layer
(orange)

• **Fig. 11.1** Gram Positive Versus Gram Negative

Antimicrobials – Targets

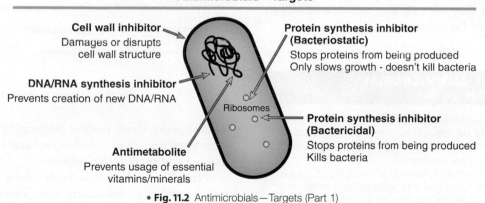

Cell wall inhibitor
Damages or disrupts
cell wall structure

DNA/RNA synthesis inhibitor
Prevents creation of new DNA/RNA

Ribosomes

Antimetabolite
Prevents usage of essential
vitamins/minerals

**Protein synthesis inhibitor
(Bacteriostatic)**
Stops proteins from being produced
Only slows growth - doesn't kill bacteria

**Protein synthesis inhibitor
(Bactericidal)**
Stops proteins from being produced
Kills bacteria

• **Fig. 11.2** Antimicrobials—Targets (Part 1)

Antimicrobials – Targets

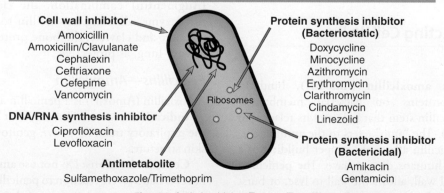

Cell wall inhibitor
Amoxicillin
Amoxicillin/Clavulanate
Cephalexin
Ceftriaxone
Cefepime
Vancomycin

DNA/RNA synthesis inhibitor
Ciprofloxacin
Levofloxacin

Ribosomes

Antimetabolite
Sulfamethoxazole/Trimethoprim

**Protein synthesis inhibitor
(Bacteriostatic)**
Doxycycline
Minocycline
Azithromycin
Erythromycin
Clarithromycin
Clindamycin
Linezolid

**Protein synthesis inhibitor
(Bactericidal)**
Amikacin
Gentamicin

• **Fig. 11.3** Antimicrobials—Targets (Part 2)

Antimicrobial – Spectrums

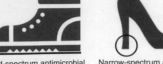

Broad-spectrum antimicrobial Cover against a lot of different microbes "Jack of all trades, master of none"	Narrow-spectrum antimicrobial Cover very specific type of microbes Hard-hitters Preferred once microbe type is known

• **Fig. 11.4** Antimicrobial—Spectrums

Antimicrobials – Resistance Mechanisms

Microbes develop resistance by spontaneous mutation and conjugation (sharing). Resistance has 4 mechanisms:

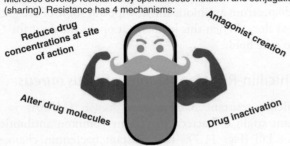

Reduce drug concentrations at site of action

Antagonist creation

Alter drug molecules

Drug inactivation

• **Fig. 11.5** Antimicrobials—Resistance Mechanisms

less effective or ineffective. MRSA then requires treatment by other antibiotics that do not depend on this binding protein. Usually, there will be a protocol to guide prescribers to make sure that they use only anti-MRSA antibiotics to reduce the potential for resistance.

SCENARIO 11.1. ANTIMICROBIAL INTRODUCTION

A provider treats a patient who has a sinus infection but the provider has not yet determined the actual bacteria causing the infection. What is a way this provider could make sure that the patient gets the best treatment?

Answer: By using empiric therapy and making an educated guess, the provider could give a broad-spectrum antibiotic. When the lab results return, the provider could change the antibiotic to a narrow-spectrum antibiotic that would decrease the likelihood of resistance.

Antibiotics Affecting Cell Walls

Penicillins

Penicillins, such as **amoxicillin (Amoxil*)**, bind to penicillin-binding proteins on bacterial membranes. Amoxicillin has the -cillin stem that indicates its relation to penicillins (Fig. 11.8). The "amo" refers to the amino penicillin subtype. Amoxicillin affects the proper building of a cell wall, something humans do not have. The penicillin, by weakening the cell wall, allows the wall to lyse, or burst like a balloon, killing the bacterium. Penicillins work well

Antimicrobials – Superinfections

A new infection that starts when treating a current one

Most commonly occur after using broad-spectrum antibiotics

Examples: Treating ear infection with broad-spectrum antibiotic and one of the following develops:

Vaginal yeast infection	Oral thrush	*Clostridium difficile*

• **Fig. 11.6** Antimicrobials—Superinfections

Antibiotics – MRSA

<u>M</u>ethicillin-<u>r</u>esistant *Staphylococcus* <u>a</u>ureus (MRSA)

Resistant to penicillins and most cephalosporins through its ability to create altered penicillin-binding proteins
- Antibiotics have low affinity to these altered proteins
- Serious infection that requires strong antibiotics to eliminate

• **Fig. 11.7** Antibiotics— Methicillin-Resistant *Staphylococcus aureus*

Antibiotics – Penicillins

Amoxicillin (Amoxil*)

Bind to penicillin-binding proteins on bacterial cytoplasmic membranes

Prevent creation of new cell wall structure
- Cell walls weaken and eventually cause lysing (burst, like balloons)

Effective against mostly Gram-positive bacteria

Bacteria have mutated to become resistant

MRSA coverage: None

• **Fig. 11.8** Antibiotics—Penicillins

against many Gram-positive bacteria (Table 11.1). However, since penicillins have been around a long time, bacterial resistance is often a possibility.

Penicillins and cephalosporins have a chemical structure known as a beta-lactam ring. This ring is a target of the bacterial enzyme beta-lactamase. The enzyme fundamentally alters the ring structure, making the drug useless (Fig. 11.9). However, with the **amoxicillin/clavulanate (Augmentin)** combination, the clavulanate "distracts" the enzyme, allowing amoxicillin to work. Think of clavulanate and clavicle, the bone protecting the upper part of your lung, as protective.

Penicillins—Amoxicillin

Amoxicillin (Amoxil*) is a penicillin antibiotic.

Indications: Amoxicillin can treat bacterial infections of the respiratory tract, *H. pylori*, genitourinary, and skin and skin structures.

Contraindications: Do not use amoxicillin if the patient has ever had a severe reaction to penicillins, other beta-lactam antibiotics, or any component of the drug.

TABLE 11.1 Cell Wall Inhibitors, Classes, Dosages, and Adverse Reactions

Generic (Brand)	Drug Class	Common Dosage	Adverse Effects
Amoxicillin (Amoxil*)	Penicillin	500–1000 mg	Diarrhea, vaginal infection
Amoxicillin-clavulanate (Augmentin)	Penicillin	500–875 mg	Diarrhea, candidiasis
Cephalexin (Keflex)	Cephalosporin (first-generation)	250–1000 mg every 6 hours	Abdominal pain, diarrhea
Cefuroxime (Ceftin*)	Cephalosporin (second-generation)	250–500 mg twice daily	Diarrhea
Ceftriaxone (Rocephin*)	Cephalosporin (third-generation)	1–2 g IV/IM daily	Irritation at injection site, diarrhea
Cefepime (Maxipime)	Cephalosporin (fourth-generation)	1–2 g IV every 8–12 hours	Diarrhea
Ceftaroline (Teflaro)	Cephalosporin (fifth-generation)	600 mg IV every 12 hours	Diarrhea, vomiting, nausea
Vancomycin (Vancocin)	Glycopeptide	Oral: 125–500 mg 4 times daily IV: 15–20 mg/kg/dose every 8–12 hours; max dose 2 g	IV: red man syndrome Oral: nausea, hypokalemia

Antibiotics – Beta-Lactamase inhibitors

Amoxicillin/clavulanate (Augmentin)

Scientists developed compounds to distract the beta-lactamases
• Called beta-lactamase inhibitors

Added to beta-lactams, and the antibiotic still is effective
• Beta-lactamase inhibitors "distract" the enzyme, allowing the active drug to sneak by

• **Fig. 11.9** Antibiotics—Beta-Lactamase Inhibitors

Antibiotics – Cephalosporins

All have a β-lactam ring like penicillins
Work the same as penicillins—still inhibit cell wall synthesis

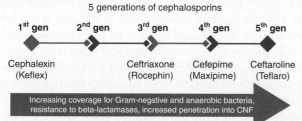

• **Fig. 11.10** Antibiotics—Cephalosporins (Part 1)

Adverse effects: Diarrhea, vaginal infection, and headache are adverse effects of amoxicillin.

Patient education and care: Hormonal contraceptives may not work as well while you are taking amoxicillin. Use a nonhormonal backup method, such as condoms, during therapy. Amoxicillin may cause secondary infections if not taken as prescribed.

Antibiotics – Cephalosporins

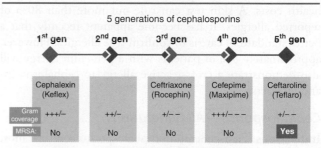

• **Fig. 11.11** Antibiotics—Cephalosporins (Part 2)

Cephalosporins

Cephalosporins resemble penicillins in their mechanisms of action and both have beta-lactam rings. We divide cephalosporins into five generations (Fig. 11.10). Three important attributes change as the generations increase.

Drugs gain more Gram-negative and anaerobic coverage, more resistance to beta-lactamases, and increased central nervous system (CNS) penetration. This means they have a different spectrum of action, have more endurance to resistance, and can reach areas of the body that lower generations cannot. For example, a first-generation cephalosporin such as **cephalexin (Keflex)** has excellent Gram-positive coverage but little Gram-negative coverage. Third-generation **ceftriaxone (Rocephin*)** and fourth-generation **cefepime (Maxipime)** have Gram-positive and Gram-negative coverage. Fifth-generation cephalosporins such as **ceftaroline (Teflaro)** lose some Gram coverage, but they do cover MRSA, making them very valuable (Fig. 11.11).

Patient allergies to cephalosporins and penicillins, known as beta-lactam allergies, are similar (Fig. 11.12). Unfortunately, the allergies are often overreported and poorly documented. While 10% of patients report a penicillin

Antibiotics – β-Lactam Allergies

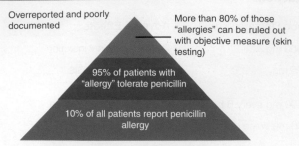

• **Fig. 11.12** Antibiotics—Beta-Lactam Allergies

allergy, 95% would tolerate the drug. This is important because sometimes a penicillin, with fewer side effects and more effectiveness, is often the very best medication for an infection.

However, because of an incorrectly reported allergy, patients do not get the penicillin. Instead, they receive a medication that might cause more side effects or not work as well to treat the infection. These beta-lactam allergies ultimately lead to poorer health outcomes and higher health costs. A skin test can rule out more than 80% of reported allergies. It has become apparent recently that a better standard of care is to confirm true allergies. However, approximately 5% of patients with a penicillin allergy will also demonstrate a cross-reactive allergy to cephalosporins and vice versa.

Cephalosporins—All Generations

Indications: First-generation cephalosporins can treat most Gram-positive cocci infections and some Gram-negative infections. Second-generation cephalosporins cover additional Gram-negative species. Third-generation cephalosporins have less Gram-positive coverage but cover more Gram-negative species than previous generations. Fourth-generation cephalosporins can treat additional species of resistant Gram-negative bacteria. Fifth-generation cephalosporins can treat resistant Gram-positive bacteria, such as MRSA.

Contraindications: Patients with a cephalosporin allergy should not take any cephalosporin. A patient with an allergy to any component of a given drug should not take it. Do not use cefuroxime or cefepime in patients with penicillin or other beta-lactam allergies. Do not give ceftriaxone to newborns with high bilirubin. Do not administer ceftriaxone formulations containing lidocaine into a vein.

Adverse effects: Diarrhea is a common adverse effect and ceftaroline may cause nausea and vomiting. Ceftriaxone may cause irritation at the injection site.

Patient education and care: Take cephalosporins as prescribed to avoid secondary infections and tell your doctor about all medications that you are taking. For example, probenecid may interact with cephalexin. Cefuroxime may decrease birth control pill efficacy; thus, use a backup method such as condoms to prevent pregnancy.

Antibiotics – Glycopeptide

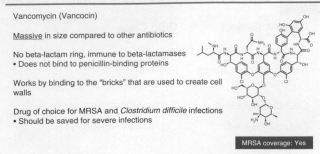

• **Fig. 11.13** Antibiotics—Glycopeptide (Part 1)

Antibiotics – Glycopeptide

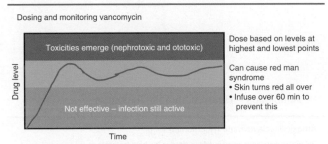

• **Fig. 11.14** Antibiotics—Glycopeptide (Part 2)

Glycopeptides

Vancomycin (Vancocin), a glycopeptide antibiotic, works like beta-lactam antibiotics and prevents cell wall synthesis (Fig. 11.13). Glycopeptides are large molecules that lack a beta-lactam ring, making them immune to beta-lactamases. This is one reason vancomycin is a drug of choice for resistant infections such as MRSA and *C. diff*. Hospital protocols often limit drug use to reduce the possibility of resistance.

Vancomycin has a narrow therapeutic window, which means that the window between the toxic level and effective level is very narrow (Fig. 11.14). If the vancomycin dose is too low, the bacteria remains alive. If the dose is too high, vancomycin can damage the kidney (nephrotoxicity) and/or ears (ototoxicity). As such, providers closely monitor the blood levels at the highest and lowest points. Rarely, vancomycin infusion triggers a hypersensitivity reaction known as red man syndrome. Red man syndrome causes severe swelling and rash. To avoid this dangerous reaction, we use a slow infusion, around 60 minutes or more.

Glycopeptide—Vancomycin

Vancomycin (Vancocin) is a glycopeptide antibiotic.

Indications: Vancomycin taken orally treats bacterial infections of the gastrointestinal (GI) tract, such as *C. diff* and enterocolitis. Vancomycin injection treats and prevents endocarditis and various *Staphylococcus* infections.

Contraindications: Patients with allergies to vancomycin or its components should not take it.

TABLE 11.2	Bacterial Protein Inhibitors, Classes, Dosages, and Adverse Reactions		
Generic (Brand)	**Drug Class**	**Common Dosage**	**Adverse Effects**
Doxycycline (Doryx)	Tetracyclines	100–200 mg daily in 1 or 2 divided doses	Tooth discoloration, diarrhea, stomach pain
Azithromycin (Zithromax, Z-Pak)	Macrolides	250–500 mg daily	Diarrhea, nausea
Clindamycin (Cleocin)	Lincosamides	600–1800 mg daily divided into 2–4 doses	*Clostridium difficile*, metallic taste
Linezolid (Zyvox)	Oxazolidinones	600 mg every 12 hours	Diarrhea, decreased white blood cell count
Gentamicin (Garamycin*)	Aminoglycosides	Usual dosing: 3–5 mg/kg/day every 8 hours	Dizziness, vertigo
Ciprofloxacin (Cipro)	Fluoroquinolones	400–750 mg every 12 hours	Diarrhea, nausea, musculoskeletal effects in children

Bacteriostatic vs Bactericidal

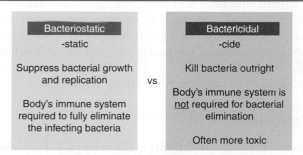

• **Fig. 11.15** Bacteriostatic Versus Bactericidal

Bacteriostatic – Bacterial Ribosomes

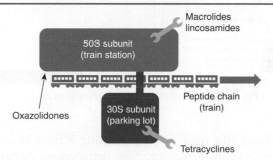

• **Fig. 11.16** Bacteriostatic—Bacterial Ribosomes

Adverse effects: Headache, stomach pain, diarrhea, and nausea are common adverse effects. If red man syndrome occurs, reduce the infusion rate.

Patient education and care: Take exactly as prescribed to prevent a secondary infection and tell the prescriber if you are pregnant. Some products may be harmful in pregnancy.

SCENARIO 11.2. ANTIBIOTICS AFFECTING CELL WALLS

Why might a patient need vancomycin (Vancocin) rather than amoxicillin (Amoxil) for skin infections like MRSA?

Answer: MRSA can inactivate penicillins by attacking the beta-lactam ring. Vancomycin lacks a beta-lactam ring, which makes it optimal for MRSA.

Bacteriostatic Protein Synthesis Inhibitors

Bacteriostatic antibiotics suppress bacterial growth and reproduction (Table 11.2). The suffix -static means to stop. This allows the immune system to catch up and kill the bacteria. **Bactericidal** antibiotics kill bacteria outright (Fig.

11.15). The stem -cidal means to kill. These agents do not require the body's immune system to kill the bacteria. Using a bacteriostatic antibiotic might allow the infection to go longer but also better preserves the body's good (beneficial) bacteria. Bactericidal medicines can damage the bad as well as good bacteria.

Ribosomes connect amino acids to build or synthesize proteins. As such, antibiotics that are protein synthesis inhibitors will act on one of two subunits of the ribosomes, which manufacture proteins (Fig. 11.16). Macrolides, lincosamides, and oxazolidinones act on the 50S subunit, which is like a train station where other passengers (amino acids) get on the protein train. However, tetracycline acts on the 30S subunit of the ribosome. We can think of this as the parking lot where amino acids arrive as passengers and add to the train.

Tetracyclines

Tetracyclines such as **minocycline (Minocin)** and **doxycycline (Doryx)** bind to the 30S subunit of the ribosome (Fig. 11.17). They prevent the binding of transfer RNA (tRNA) to messenger RNA (mRNA). That is, the amino acids on the tRNA cannot get out of the parking lot. In turn, the

Bacteriostatic – Tetracyclines

Minocycline (Minocin)
Doxycycline (Doryx)

- Bind to 30S ribosomal subunit
- Prevent binding of transfer RNA to messenger RNA
  - People can't get out of the parking lot
- Peptide chain production is halted
  - Train can't leave the station without passengers

MRSA coverage: Yes

• **Fig. 11.17** Bacteriostatic—Tetracyclines (Part 1)

Bacteriostatic – Macrolides

Azithromycin (Zithromax, Z-Pak)
Clarithromycin (Biaxin*)
Erythromycin (E-mycin*)

Bind to the 50S ribosomal subunit (train station)
Prevent amino acids from being added to the peptide
- Passengers can't get on the train

Erythromycin is a CYP450 inhibitor, leading to lots of drug interactions

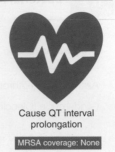

Cause QT interval prolongation

MRSA coverage: None

• **Fig. 11.19** Bacteriostatic—Macrolides

Bacteriostatic – Tetracyclines

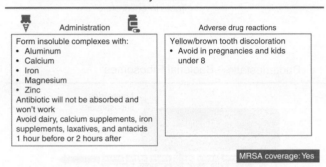

Administration	Adverse drug reactions
Form insoluble complexes with: • Aluminum • Calcium • Iron • Magnesium • Zinc Antibiotic will not be absorbed and won't work Avoid dairy, calcium supplements, iron supplements, laxatives, and antacids 1 hour before or 2 hours after	Yellow/brown tooth discoloration • Avoid in pregnancies and kids under 8

MRSA coverage: Yes

• **Fig. 11.18** Bacteriostatic—Tetracyclines (Part 2)

peptide chain (the train) stops, preventing it from leaving the station without passengers. Note, tetracyclines do have MRSA coverage.

Unfortunately, tetracyclines can chelate (pronounced KEY-late) to form insoluble complexes with certain cationic elements. A cationic element is one with a plus charge, such as calcium (Ca^{+2}) on the Periodic Table of Elements. Other cationic elements also cause this issue, such as aluminum, magnesium, iron, and zinc.

This interaction matters because we find these types of elements in dairy, calcium supplements, iron supplements, and certain antacids. Patients should avoid taking an antacid, for example, 1 hour before or 2 hours after taking the tetracycline. Avoid tetracyclines in pregnant women and children under 8 years of age to avoid a possible permanent tooth discoloration in those children (Fig. 11.18).

Use the "d" in doxycycline to remember that dentists use it to treat periodontal disease under the Doryx brand name. Also, the -cycline stem helps classify this group as a tetracycline.

Tetracyclines—Doxycycline

Doxycycline (Doryx) is a tetracycline antibiotic.

Indications: Doxycycline treats a variety of Gram-negative bacterial infections, such as *Escherichia coli*. It also treats certain Gram-positive infections, such as susceptible *Streptococcus*, and can be used along with other medications to treat amebiasis. It is used to prevent malaria, among other indications.

Contraindications: Do not take doxycycline if allergic to any component of the drug. Certain formulations (Periostat and Apprilon) should not be used in pregnancy, breast-feeding, or children under 8 years old.

Adverse effects: Doxycycline can cause tooth discoloration, diarrhea, and stomach pain.

Patient education and care: Doxycycline may cause sun sensitivity. Avoid sun exposure or use sunscreen and adequate clothing while taking this medication. Doxycycline may cause hormonal contraceptives such as birth control pills to become less effective. Use a backup nonhormonal method such as condoms while taking doxycycline.

Macrolides

Macrolides include **azithromycin (Zithromax, Z-Pak), clarithromycin (Biaxin*)**, and **erythromycin (E-Mycin**; Fig. 11.19). They bind to the 50S ribosomal subunit in bacteria, preventing the train from adding passengers (amino acids).

Frequently, how often a patient takes a medicine affects how well that patient takes the medicine. We usually dose erythromycin 4 times daily, clarithromycin twice daily, and azithromycin once daily. Therefore, azithromycin should have the best patient compliance.

Macrolides can cause a prolongation of the QT interval, which is a danger to the heart. Use caution in patients with heart issues or those taking other QT-prolonging medications. Erythromycin can inhibit a liver-enzyme family, CYP450, which is instrumental in drug metabolism, causing many drug interactions.

Macrolides—Azithromycin

Azithromycin (Zithromax) is a macrolide antibiotic.

Indications: Azithromycin treats a variety of bacterial infections. These include susceptible respiratory, skin and skin structure, and sexually transmitted infections. It is effective against *Haemophilus influenzae*, *Moraxella catarrhalis*, *Streptococcus pneumoniae*, *Streptococcus* species, *Staphylococcus* species, chlamydia, gonorrhea, and other infections.

Contraindications: Do not take azithromycin if allergic to any component of the drug or any other macrolide. If taking azithromycin has caused liver dysfunction in the past, do not take it.

Bacteriostatic – Lincosamides

Clindamycin (Cleocin)

Bind to the 50S subunit and prevent protein synthesis
• Passengers can't get onto the train

MRSA coverage: None

• **Fig. 11.20** Bacteriostatic—Lincosamides

Bacteriostatic – Oxazolidinones

Linezolid (Zyvox)

Binds to the 50S subunit and prevents formation of initiation complex
• Prevents the train from coming into the station

Unique mechanism (preventing initiation complex), leading to very little resistance

Interacts with SSRIs/SNRIs, potentially causing serotonin syndrome

MRSA coverage: Yes

• **Fig. 11.21** Bacteriostatic—Oxazolidinones

Adverse effects: The most common adverse effects are diarrhea and nausea.

Patient education and care: Do not take azithromycin with antacids that contain magnesium or aluminum. Finish the full course of azithromycin as prescribed, even if you feel better.

Lincosamides

Lincosamides such as **clindamycin (Cleocin)** act like macrolides and bind to the 50S subunit of bacterial ribosomes (Fig. 11.20). Systemic clindamycin can be toxic, including causing a superinfection such as *C. diff.* Therefore, clindamycin as a topical medication, often for acne, is more prevalent. Macrolides and lincosamides lack MRSA coverage.

Oxazolidones

Similar to macrolides and lincosamides, the oxazolidones, such as **linezolid (Zyvox)**, bind to the 50S subunit of bacterial ribosomes (Fig. 11.21). However, they act in a unique way. They prevent the initiation complex from forming or, continuing with the analogy, they do not allow the train to come to the station. This unique mechanism, along with careful use, has resulted in little bacterial resistance. Linezolid works against MRSA and vancomycin-resistant enterococcus (VRE). A concern is that linezolid interacts with selective serotonin reuptake inhibitors (SSRI) and serotonin norepinephrine reuptake inhibitors (SNRI) antidepressants, potentially causing serotonin syndrome. Careful patient monitoring is necessary.

Oxazolidinones—Linezolid

Linezolid (Zyvox) is an oxazolidinone antibiotic.

Bactericidal – Bacterial Ribosomes

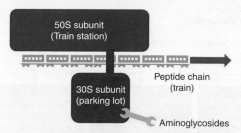

• **Fig. 11.22** Bactericidal—Bacterial Ribosomes

Indications: Linezolid treats bacterial infections such as VRE infections, susceptible community-acquired and hospital-acquired pneumonia, and susceptible complicated and uncomplicated skin and skin structure infections.

Contraindications: Do not take linezolid if allergic to any component of it. Do not take it within 2 weeks of taking a monoamine oxidase inhibitor.

Adverse effects: Common adverse effects of linezolid are headache, diarrhea, and upset stomach.

Patient education and care: Continue to take linezolid as prescribed, even if you feel better. Avoid certain foods, such as red wine and cheeses, to prevent high blood pressure.

SCENARIO 11.3. BACTERIOSTATIC PROTEIN SYNTHESIS INHIBITORS

A patient has a bacterial infection resistant to vancomycin called vancomycin-resistant enterococcus (VRE). What medication class might the provider call on to treat this infection?

Answer: Linezolid (Zyvox) is a bacteriostatic antibiotic that binds to the 50S subunit of bacterial ribosomes, preventing initiation complex formation. Linezolid has activity against VRE.

Bactericidal Protein Synthesis Inhibitors

Aminoglycosides such as **amikacin (Amikin*)** and **gentamicin (Garamycin)** are two bactericidal protein synthesis inhibitors. They bind to 30S subunits, causing three disruptions in the bacteria. Aminoglycosides inhibit protein synthesis (i.e., the train cannot leave the station). They cause premature termination of protein synthesis (i.e., canceling the train departure). Finally, they produce abnormal proteins (i.e., the wrong train leaves the station; Fig. 11.22).

Aminoglycosides are bactericidal against Gram-negative aerobes (bacteria that use oxygen) but require close monitoring against toxicity (Figs. 11.23 and 11.24). These antibiotics can cause nephrotoxicity that can lead to permanent kidney damage. Aminoglycosides can also cause ototoxicity (ear damage). We attribute toxicity to high trough levels.

Bactericidal – Aminoglycosides

Amikacin (Amikin*)
Gentamicin (Garamycin)

Bactericidal against Gram-negative aerobes

Bind to 30S subunit and cause 3 different events:

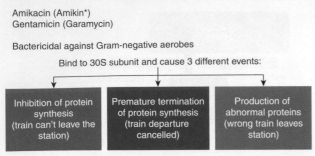

| Inhibition of protein synthesis (train can't leave the station) | Premature termination of protein synthesis (train departure cancelled) | Production of abnormal proteins (wrong train leaves station) |

• **Fig. 11.23** Bactericidal—Aminoglycosides (Part 1)

Aminoglycosides—Gentamicin

Gentamicin (Garamycin) is an aminoglycoside antibiotic.

Indications: Gentamicin treats serious bacterial infections. Specifically, it treats susceptible meningitis, sepsis, bone, endocardial, skin and skin structure, urinary tract, peritoneal, and respiratory tract infections.

Contraindications: Do not take gentamicin if allergic to any component of the drug or other aminoglycosides.

Adverse effects: Even at typical doses, gentamicin may cause neurologic, hearing, and kidney damage. Staying well hydrated will decrease these effects.

Patient education and care: Stay hydrated by drinking plenty of liquids unless told otherwise. This medication is available only as injection into the muscle or vein.

SCENARIO 11.4. BACTERICIDAL PROTEIN SYNTHESIS INHIBITORS

A patient arrives to the inpatient floor on amikacin (Amikin*). What are the two side effects and toxicities that concern a provider?

Answer: Amikacin is an aminoglycoside that is notorious for nephrotoxicity (kidney damage) and ototoxicity (ear damage).

DNA/RNA Synthesis Inhibitors

An antibiotic can affect the production of nucleic acids such as DNA and RNA. DNA gyrase and topoisomerase IV, both enzymes, coil and uncoil DNA for replication (Fig. 11.25). Coiled DNA is ready for storage. Uncoiled DNA is ready for replication. Fluoroquinolones, broad-spectrum antibiotics, such as **levofloxacin (Levaquin*)** and **ciprofloxacin (Cipro)**, inhibit this coiling and uncoiling process (Fig. 11.26). Adverse reactions include phototoxicity, confusion, and superinfections that are often fungal. A rare but serious side effect is Achilles tendon rupture, especially in the elderly.

We sometimes call fluoroquinolones floxacins after their infix -fl- + suffix -oxacin. Like tetracyclines, fluoroquinolones cause photosensitivity, which is an increased sensitivity

Bactericidal – Aminoglycosides

Amikacin (Amikin)
Gentamicin (Garamycin)

Require intense monitoring due to main toxicities

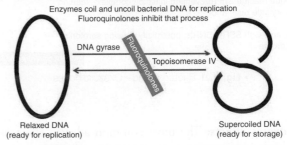

| Nephrotoxicity Leads to increased ototoxicity and permanent kidney damage | Otoxicity Hearing damage and potential balance issues | *Both produced by high trough levels over time* |

MRSA coverage: None

• **Fig. 11.24** Bactericidal—Aminoglycosides (Part 2)

DNA/RNA Synthesis Inhibitors

Enzymes coil and uncoil bacterial DNA for replication
Fluoroquinolones inhibit that process

DNA gyrase   Fluoroquinolones   Topoisomerase IV

Relaxed DNA (ready for replication)   Supercoiled DNA (ready for storage)

• **Fig. 11.25** DNA/RNA Synthesis Inhibitors (Part 1)

DNA/RNA Synthesis Inhibitors

Ciprofloxacin (Cipro)
Levofloxacin (Levaquin*)

Broad-spectrum antibiotics

Adverse drug reactions	Administration
Phototoxicity Superinfections (usually fungal) Confusion **Rare but serious: tendon rupture**	Avoid dairy, vitamins at same time • Cause chelation-like tetracyclines

MRSA coverage: None

• **Fig. 11.26** DNA/RNA Synthesis Inhibitors (Part 2)

to burning from sunlight and chelation, the binding to cations such as Ca++ in milk and dairy.

Fluoroquinolones

Ciprofloxacin (Cipro) is a fluoroquinolone antibiotic.

Indications: Ciprofloxacin treats or prevents bacterial infections. It specifically treats urinary tract infections, infectious diarrhea, typhoid, hospital-acquired pneumonia, bone and joint infections, and prostate infections. It can be used to prevent anthrax progression and plague.

Contraindications: Do not take ciprofloxacin if allergic to any component of the drug or other quinolones. Do not take while taking tizanidine.

TABLE 11.3 Miscellaneous Antibiotics, Classes, Dosages, and Adverse Reactions

Generic (Brand)	Drug Class	Common Dosage	Adverse Effects
Sulfamethoxazole (SMX)/ trimethoprim (TMP) (Bactrim)	Antimetabolite	Single strength tablet: 400 mg SMX/80 mg TMP Double strength tablet: 800 mg SMX/160 mg TMP Dose is dependent on indication	Nausea, diarrhea, headache, high potassium
Metronidazole (Flagyl)	Nitroimidazole	500–750 mg every 8 hours	Headache, nausea, vaginitis

Adverse effects: Common adverse effects include diarrhea, nausea, and vomiting. It may also cause nerve problems and tendon irritation and rupture.

Patient education and care: Ciprofloxacin increases your sensitivity to the sun. Wear sunscreen or protective clothing to prevent sunburn. Do not take ciprofloxacin with dairy products unless it is with a full meal. Take ciprofloxacin at least 2 hours before or 6 hours after taking antacids or other divalent and trivalent cations.

SCENARIO 11.5. DNA/RNA SYNTHESIS INHIBITORS

After treatment for a severe urinary tract infection, a patient reports warmth in his Achilles tendon when he got back to running. What antibiotic and antibiotic class might the patient be on?

Answer: Levofloxacin and ciprofloxacin are both fluoroquinolones, which have a black box warning for tendon rupture. Black box warnings are special warnings at the start of the package insert alerting the provider to a must-see interaction or concern.

Miscellaneous Antibiotics

Human and bacterial cells require folate for DNA, RNA, and protein production (Table 11.3). However, mammals can eat folate as part of their diet. Bacteria must produce their own. This allows antibiotics to selectively hurt bacteria and not mammals. A folate building block is para-aminobenzoic acid (PABA). Sulfamethoxazole antibiotics are chemically similar to PABA and the bacteria uses them instead. This stops folate manufacture, stopping proper bacterial DNA, RNA, and protein synthesis (Fig. 11.27).

Sulfamethoxazole/trimethoprim (Bactrim) combines two chemicals to prevent bacterial folate synthesis at separate steps of the process (Fig. 11.28). We often see this medicine in treating urinary tract infections. The most common side effect is sun sensitivity. However, more serious side effects are possible, such as Stevens-Johnson syndrome, hemolytic anemia, kernicterus, crystalluria, and renal damage. The brand name Bactrim has is derived from "bacterium."

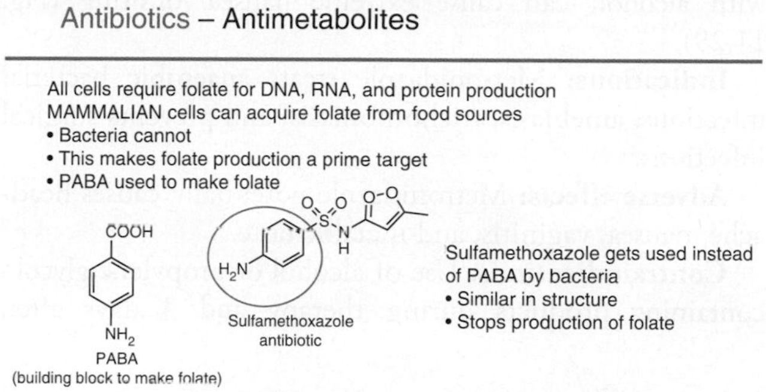

Antibiotics – Antimetabolites

All cells require folate for DNA, RNA, and protein production MAMMALIAN cells can acquire folate from food sources
• Bacteria cannot
• This makes folate production a prime target
• PABA used to make folate

Sulfamethoxazole gets used instead of PABA by bacteria
• Similar in structure
• Stops production of folate

COOH

NH₂
PABA
(building block to make folate)

Sulfamethoxazole antibiotic

• **Fig. 11.27** Antibiotics—Antimetabolites

Antimetabolites – Sulfamethoxazole

Sulfamethoxazole/trimethoprim (Bactrim)
Both work to prevent folate from being used to create more DNA/RNA, proteins

In a drug class called dihydrofolate reductase inhibitors

Serious adverse drug reactions
• Stevens-Johnson syndrome
• Hemolytic anemia
• kernicterus
• renal damage from crystalluria

Causes sun sensitivity

MRSA coverage: Yes

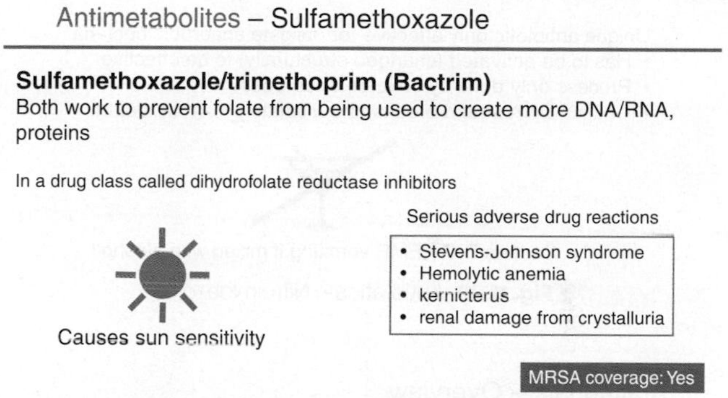

• **Fig. 11.28** Antimetabolites—Sulfamethoxazole

Antimetabolites

Sulfamethoxazole/trimethoprim (Bactrim) is a sulfonamide antibiotic.

Indications: Oral formulations treat susceptible bacterial infections, including urinary tract infections, ear infections, chronic obstructive pulmonary disease (COPD) exacerbations, and traveler's diarrhea. Intravenous formulations treat more severe bacterial infections, such as Pneumocystis pneumonia (PCP) shigellosis, and severe or complicated urinary tract infections.

Contraindications: Do not use this drug for a patient with a sulfa allergy or hypersensitivity to any drug component. Do not use if any component of this drug has caused low thrombocytes or megaloblastic anemia in the past. Do not use in infants under 2 months old. Do not use if currently taking dofetilide.

Adverse effects: Common adverse effects are nausea, loss of appetite, diarrhea, and vomiting.

Patient education and care: This drug increases sun sensitivity. Wear sunscreen and protective clothing outdoors. Watch for rare reactions. If you notice a rash or blisters, get in contact with your physician immediately or go the emergency department.

Nitroimidazoles

Metronidazole (Flagyl) is specific for obligate anaerobic bacteria and needs to be activated to be effective. It causes DNA strand breaks and microbe death. Metronidazole has what is called a disulfiram-like reaction that, when mixed with alcohol, can cause extreme nausea/vomiting (Fig. 11.29).

Indications: Metronidazole treats anaerobic bacterial infections, amebiasis, trichomoniasis, and prevents surgical infections.

Adverse effects: Metronidazole potentially causes headache, nausea, vaginitis, and metallic taste.

Contraindications: Use of alcohol or propylene glycol–containing products during therapy and 3 days after, disulfiram use within 2 weeks, first trimester of pregnancy with trichomoniasis, allergy to any component of the formulation.

Patient education and care: Metronidazole reacts with alcohol to cause extreme vomiting. Patients should be advised to avoid alcohol and propylene glycol, even small hidden amounts, during therapy with metronidazole and for 3 days after discontinuation.

SCENARIO 11.6. MISCELLANEOUS ANTIBIOTICS

A patient who is on metronidazole mentions he is going to a wedding this weekend and wanted to know if it is okay to have "just one" alcoholic drink. What concerns you about this request?

Answer: Disulfiram (Antabuse*) is a medicine used to help alcoholics quit drinking. When an alcoholic drinks, that individual experiences terrible nausea and possibly vomiting. In the same regard, a patient who takes metronidazole with alcohol will experience the same disulfiram-like effect, causing nausea and vomiting.

Antibiotics – Nitroimidazoles

Metronidazole (Flagyl)

Unique antibiotic only effective for obligate anaerobic bacteria
- Has to be activated (changed structurally) to be effective
- Process only done by obligate anaerobes
- Causes DNA strand breaks and ultimately microbe death

Causes EXTREME vomiting if mixed with alcohol!

• **Fig. 11.29** Antibiotics—Nitroimidazoles

Antifungals – Overview

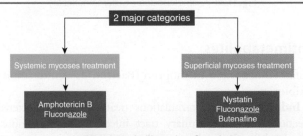

• **Fig. 11.30** Antifungals—Overview

Antifungal Medications

Antifungals are effective for fungal infections rather than bacterial or viral. We can divide antifungals into two major categories (Fig. 11.30). First, there are antifungals for systemic mycoses treatment, such as amphotericin and fluconazole. Second, we can use antifungals for superficial mycoses—often, skin infections or thrush—with nystatin, fluconazole, and butenafine (Table 11.4).

Polyene antifungals such as **amphotericin B (Fungizone)** and **nystatin (Mycostatin*)** bind to sterols in cell membranes, increasing their permeability (porousness; Fig. 11.31). This allows monovalent cations such as potassium (K+) and sodium (Na+) to leak out. Some antifungals are fungistatic, slowing growth. Other antifungals are fungicidal, killing the fungi. The difference between fungistatic and fungicidal action often comes from the drug concentration.

Many antifungal drugs are toxic when used systemically because the sterols they bind look a lot like human sterols, like cholesterol.

Amphotericin B is a systemic medication. Providers usually use it for serious fungal infections. Nystatin is a topical

TABLE 11.4	Antifungals, Classes, Dosages, and Adverse Reactions			
Generic (Brand)	Drug Class	Common Dosage		Adverse Effects
Fluconazole (Diflucan)	Azole antifungal	100–800 mg daily		Headache, nausea
Amphotericin B (Lipid complex; Abelcet)	Polyene antifungal	5 mg/kg daily		Chills, fever
Nystatin	Polyene antifungal	400,000–1,000,000 units 3–4 times daily		Diarrhea, nausea

Antifungals – Polyenes

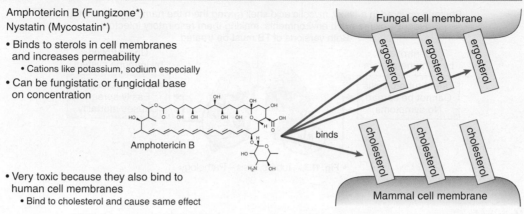

Amphotericin B (Fungizone*)
Nystatin (Mycostatin*)

- Binds to sterols in cell membranes and increases permeability
  - Cations like potassium, sodium especially
- Can be fungistatic or fungicidal base on concentration

Amphotericin B

- Very toxic because they also bind to human cell membranes
  - Bind to cholesterol and cause same effect

• **Fig. 11.31** Antifungals—Polyenes

Antifungals – Azoles

Fluconazole (Diflucan)

Inhibits ergosterol synthesis, preventing cell membrane formation and causes increased membrane permeation

Used for both systemic and superficial fungal infections

Polyenes	Azoles
• Work on outside of membrane to bind to sterols and increase permeation • Very toxic due to mammal sterol binding	• Work on inside of cell to prevent sterol formation and increase permeation • Minimal toxicity due to only fungal uptake

• **Fig. 11.32** Antifungals—Azoles

Antifungals – OTC Options

Butenafine (Lotrimin Ultra)
Topical antifungal used to treat superficial mycoses

Causes the fungus to create excessive squalene, which is normally converted to ergosterol
- Large amount of squalene is toxic to fungi

• **Fig. 11.33** Antifungals—Over-the-Counter Options

antifungal that is relatively safe, so much so that prescribers use it for thrush in young children.

Azole antifungals such as **fluconazole (Diflucan)** inhibit ergosterol synthesis in fungi, preventing membranes from forming and increasing membrane permeability (Fig. 11.32). The main difference between polyenes and azole antifungals is where they work. Polyenes work outside of membranes. Their toxicity comes from their interaction with cholesterol in the mammals' membranes. Azole antifungals work inside membranes. Selective fungal uptake limits their toxicity. Fluconazole is unusual in that a doctor can prescribe it for systemic and superficial fungal infections.

Butenafine (Lotrimin) is an over-the-counter (OTC) antifungal medication for superficial mycoses (Fig. 11.33). It causes increased fungal squalene synthesis. Generally, the

fungi use squalene to create ergosterol for the cell membrane. However, too much squalene is toxic. Butenafine is for topical fungal infections such as tinea corporis (ringworm), tinea cruris (jock itch), and tinea pedis (athlete's foot).

Azoles

Fluconazole (Diflucan) is an azole antifungal.

Indications: Fluconazole treats fungal infections, particularly those caused by candida (yeast). It treats both systemic and localized infections. Fluconazole also treats cryptococcal meningitis and prevents fungal infection in patients receiving a stem cell transplant.

Contraindications: Do not use fluconazole in anyone who is allergic to any component of the drug. Use caution with other azole antifungal allergies. If taking 400 mg or more, do not give terfenadine or any CYP3A4 substrates that cause QT interval prolongation.

Adverse effects: Headache, dizziness, and nausea are fluconazole's most common adverse effects.

Patient education and care: Take fluconazole exactly as prescribed to avoid secondary infection.

Polyenes

Amphotericin B Lipid Complex (Abelcet) is a polyene antifungal.

Indications: Abelcet treats invasive fungal infection in anyone for whom amphotericin B deoxycholate did not work or it could not be tolerated.

Contraindications: Do not use Abelcet in anyone allergic to amphotericin or any other component of the drug.

Adverse effects: Fever and chills are the most common adverse effects. To alleviate nonanaphylactic infusion reactions, premedicate 30 to 60 minutes before the infusion with NSAIDs with or without diphenhydramine or acetaminophen with diphenhydramine.

Patient education and care: Abelcet is administered as an infusion into the vein.

Tuberculosis – Pathology

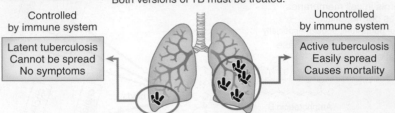

Bacteria covered in a waxy, mycolic acid shell (giving them the name *myco*bacteria)
Require oxygen-rich environments, making them respiratory infectors
Both versions of TB must be treated:

Controlled
by immune system

Latent tuberculosis
Cannot be spread
No symptoms

Uncontrolled
by immune system

Active tuberculosis
Easily spread
Causes mortality

• **Fig. 11.34** Tuberculosis—Pathology

Topical Antifungals

Butenafine (Lotrimin Ultra) is a topical antifungal.

Indications: Butenafine treats tinea versicolor, athlete's foot (tinea pedis), jock itch (tinea cruris), and ringworm (tinea corporis).

Contraindications: Do not use butenafine if allergic to any component of the drug. Do not use on nails, scalp, for vaginal yeast infection, or near the eyes or mouth.

Adverse effects: Burning and stinging are common adverse effects.

Patient education and care: Apply butenafine topically. Seek medical help if swallowed.

SCENARIO 11.7. ANTIFUNGAL MEDICATIONS

A child has thrush (oral candidiasis). Which antifungal medication is the prescriber likely to give—mycostatin (Nystatin) or amphotericin B (Fungizone*)?

Answer: Mycostatin* (Nystatin) is a medication that a parent could administer to the child safely for thrush. Amphotericin B is for systemic infections and too toxic for this situation. Nystatin (Mycostatin*) is a polyene antifungal that binds to sterols in cell membranes, increasing the membrane's permeability. This leads to leakage of monovalent cations such as potassium (K+) and sodium (Na+).

Antimycobacterial Agents

A waxy, mycolic acid shell covers mycobacteria such as tuberculosis (TB; Fig. 11.34). These bacteria need oxygen-rich environments; thus, we find them in the respiratory tract. The two common forms of TB are latent TB and active TB. The immune system controls the mycobacteria in latent TB and the patient exhibits no symptoms. In contrast, the immune system does not control active TB and it is highly contagious. The patient can suffer severe symptoms and die. Multiple antimycobacterial agents will form the treatment regimen.

TB reproduces slowly, but many antibiotics target fast-replicating cells. This slow replication means that TB readily resists a single medication. As such, we treat TB with multidrug regimens. Remember the drugs with the RIPE

Antimycobacterial – Options

Multiple medications are used at the same time (usually 3–4) to prevent inadequate drug therapy

- TB can become resistant to a single med very easily
  - Leads to multi-drug resistance
- TB grows very slowly, and most antibiotics target fast-replicating cells

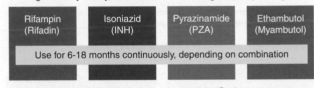

| Rifampin (Rifadin) | Isoniazid (INH) | Pyrazinamide (PZA) | Ethambutol (Myambutol) |

Use for 6-18 months continuously, depending on combination

• **Fig. 11.35** Antimycobacterial—Options

Antimycobacterial Agents

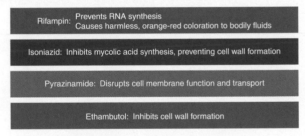

Rifampin: Prevents RNA synthesis
Causes harmless, orange-red coloration to bodily fluids

Isoniazid: Inhibits mycolic acid synthesis, preventing cell wall formation

Pyrazinamide: Disrupts cell membrane function and transport

Ethambutol: Inhibits cell wall formation

• **Fig. 11.36** Antimycobacterial Agents

mnemonic, as in the TB test induration (raised skin) is ripe. (Figs. 11.35 and 11.36; Table 11.5).

R. **Rifampin (Rifadin)** prevents RNA synthesis and can cause a harmless, red-orange coloration to bodily fluids. Use the letter 'r' in rifampin and 'r' in red to remember.

I. **Isoniazid (INH)** Inhibits mycolic acid synthesis, which prevents the formation of a cell wall.

P. **Pyrazinamide (PZA)** disrupts cell membrane transport and function.

E. **Ethambutol (Myambutol)** inhibits the formation of a cell wall.

Antitubercular Agents

Rifampin (Rifadin), **isoniazid**, **pyrazinamide**, and **ethambutol** are antitubercular agents.

TABLE 11.5 — Antimycobacterial Agents, Classes, Dosages, and Adverse Reactions

Generic (Brand)	Drug Class	Common Dosage	Adverse Effects
Rifampin (Rifadin)	Rifamycin; antitubercular agent	Dosing varies depending on indication. 300 mg twice daily is common.	Diarrhea, discoloration of bodily fluids
Isoniazid	Antitubercular agent	Dosing varies depending on indication. Common dosing is 5 mg/kg/dose once daily	Nausea, vomiting, injection site reaction for intramuscular
Pyrazinamide	Antitubercular agent	Dosing depends on weight and frequency may be daily, 3 times weekly, or twice weekly.	Muscle pain, nausea, tiredness
Ethambutol (Myambutol)	Antitubercular agent	Dosing depends on weight and frequency may be daily, 3 times weekly, or twice weekly.	Nausea, headache, loss of strength and energy

Indications: Antitubercular agents treat infection with *Mycobacterium tuberculosis*. In an active TB infection, all four of these medications may be used in the beginning to prevent bacterial resistance. Rifampin and isoniazid may be continued after initial treatment and may also be used to treat latent TB. Rifampin also treats *Neisseria meningitidis* in patients who carry it without symptoms.

Contraindications: Do not take antitubercular agents if allergic to any component of the drugs or similar drugs within the same class. Do not use rifampin in combination with certain protease inhibitors (human immunodeficiency virus [HIV] treatment). Do not use ethambutol in a patient who cannot report eyesight changes and avoid pyrazinamide during a gout attack.

Adverse effects: Rifampin may cause diarrhea and discoloration of fluids. Isoniazid may cause nausea, vomiting, and injection site reaction. Pyrazinamide and ethambutol may cause nausea and loss of energy. Although rare, watch out for signs of liver problems with isoniazid and vision loss with ethambutol.

Patient education and care: Rifampin causes bodily fluids to change color, which may stain contact lenses. Hormonal birth control methods such as birth control pills may be less effective while taking rifampin. Use a backup method such as condoms during therapy. Avoid alcohol while taking antitubercular agents. Get regular eye exams while taking ethambutol and report any vision changes. Some patients may need to take vitamin B6 while on isoniazid.

SCENARIO 11.8. ANTIMYCOBACTERIAL AGENTS

A patient with active tuberculosis says that once she started taking her four medications, rifampin, isoniazid, pyrazinamide, and ethambutol, she thought she saw blood in her urine. One of these medicines turns urine red/orange. Which is it?

Answer: Rifampin (remember with the letter "r") turns urine red-orange. It is not blood; rather, it is a harmless effect of the drug.

Antivirals – Targets

Viruses are obligate parasites, making them challenging to treat
• Rely entirely upon host cells and synthetic commands for replication

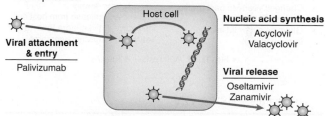

• **Fig. 11.37** Antivirals—Targets

Non-HIV Antiviral Agents

We call viruses obligate parasites because they cannot reproduce without another organism. They use the host cell; because of this, they are difficult to treat. The medicine often targets a normal part of the cell, causing unwanted toxicity (Fig. 11.37). Three ways that non-HIV antivirals can work are by preventing viral attachment/entry, nucleic acid synthesis, or viral release (Table 11.6).

Docosanol

This is a topical antiviral for cold sores caught and treated early. While a patient could take oral medications and go to the physician, the convenience of an OTC solution such as docosanol makes it more likely that the patient will use the medicine. The brand name Abreva takes part of the word abbreviate, as the medicine will abbreviate or shorten the infection time.

Influenza

The best treatment for any infection is prevention when possible. We hope to prevent influenza with an injectable such as **Fluzone Quadrivalent**. Just as a college quadrangle has

TABLE 11.6   Non-HIV Antivirals, Classes, Dosages, and Adverse Reactions

Generic (Brand)	Drug Class	Common Dosage	Adverse Effects
Docosanol (Abreva)	Topical antiviral agent	Apply 5 times daily to affected area on face or lips. Continue until healed.	Skin irritation, allergic reaction
Influenza virus vaccine (Fluzone Quadrivalent)	Inactivated vaccine	0.5 mL per dose 1 dose per flu season	Injection site irritation, muscle pain
Oseltamivir (Tamiflu)	Neuraminidase inhibitor, antiviral	Treatment: 75 mg twice daily Prophylaxis: 75 mg once daily	Headache, vomiting, nausea
Acyclovir (Zovirax)	Antiviral	400 mg 3 times daily, although dosing may change based on indications and immune function	Tiredness, nausea, vomiting
Palivizumab (Synagis)	Monoclonal antibody	15 mg/kg once monthly during respiratory syncytial virus season	Fever, skin rash

Antivirals – Influenza

Prevention
Yearly influenza vaccine (Fluzone, Flumist)
- Changes yearly to best predict prevalent strains
- Given as either IM injection or intranasal mist

Treatment (neuraminidase inhibitors)
- Oseltamivir (Tamiflu)
- Zanamivir (Relenza)
  - *Inhalation delivery*
- Prevent viral release from host cell
- Ineffective if given more than 48 hours after showing symptoms

• **Fig. 11.38** Antivirals—Influenza

Antivirals – HSV & VZV

Herpes Simplex Virus (HSV)
Varicella-Zoster Virus (VZV)

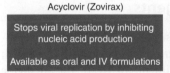

Acyclovir (Zovirax)
- Stops viral replication by inhibiting nucleic acid production
- Available as oral and IV formulations

Valacyclovir (Valtrex)
- Same mechanism as acyclovir
- Only available as oral tablets

• **Fig. 11.39** Antivirals—Herpes Simplex Virus and Varicella-Zoster Virus

Antivirals – RSV

Respiratory Syncytial Virus (RSV)
Virus which causes respiratory infections, usually seasonally

Palivizumab (Synagis)

Monoclonal antibody

Prevents RSV in premature infants and young children with chronic lung diseases

Monthly injection given through winter months

• **Fig. 11.40** Antivirals—Respiratory Syncytial Virus

four sides, a quadrivalent vaccine stimulates the immune system against four viruses. The most current recommendation allows children 6 to 35 months to get 0.25 mL or 0.5 mL for each dose. Children 3 years old and older and adults should get a 0.5-mL dose. When giving a shot is difficult, **Flumist**, a live attenuated influenza vaccine nasal spray for those 2 to 49 years old, is an option (Fig. 11.38).

These flu vaccines prepare the body to better fight the flu infection using either a weak or killed form of the virus. Because influenza can change its form quickly, manufacturers change the flu shot each year to best combat the predicted strains.

If a patient already has the flu, then a prescriber can give neuraminidase inhibitors, such as **oseltamivir (Tamiflu)** and **zanamivir (Relenza)**. These prevent the cell from releasing the virus. However, the patient must act fast, as these drugs are ineffective more than 48 hours after symptoms start. The medicine reduces symptoms and/or the infection's duration.

Acyclovir (Zovirax) and **valacyclovir (Valtrex)** stop viral production by inhibiting nucleic acid production in herpes simplex virus (HSV) and varicella-zoster virus (VZV). Acyclovir has oral and IV forms, while valacyclovir is available only in oral tablets (Fig. 11.39).

We unfortunately see respiratory syncytial virus (RSV) each season, which can cause significant issues for premature infants and young children (Fig. 11.40). A monoclonal antibody, **palivizumab (Synagis)**, can help prevent children from acquiring the virus, especially those who have compromised lung function. Providers generally give the monthly injection during the winter.

Topical Antiviral Agents

Docosanol (Abreva) is a topical antiviral agent.

Indications: Docosanol (Abreva) treats cold sores on the face and lips.

Contraindications: Do not use docosanol if allergic to any component of it.

Adverse effects: Skin irritation and allergic reaction are the most common adverse effects.

Patient education and care: Docosanol (Abreva) should be applied topically to the affected area, not swallowed. If ingested, contact a poison control center. Docosanol (Abreva) should not be given to children under 12 years old unless discussed with a doctor.

Inactivated Vaccine

Influenza virus vaccine (Fluzone Quadrivalent) is an inactivated vaccine.

Indications: The influenza vaccine prevents illness from influenza virus subtypes A and B. Fluzone Quadrivalent, among other vaccine products, may be given to patients 6 months of age and older.

Contraindications: Do not receive the influenza vaccine if severely allergic to any component of it. Individual manufacturers list severe egg allergy as a contraindication. However, the Advisory Committee on Immunization Practices (ACIP) and National Advisory Committee on Immunization (NACI) do not consider egg allergy a contraindication to receiving the influenza vaccine.

Adverse effects: Common adverse effects are injection site pain, headache, and muscle and joint pain.

Patient education and care: The influenza vaccine protects for one flu season and should be administered every year. It does not treat the flu and may not protect everyone who receives it. The inactive influenza vaccine does not cause the flu.

Neuraminidase Inhibitor

Oseltamivir (Tamiflu) is a neuraminidase inhibitor antiviral.

Indications: Tamiflu treats influenza A and B in adults and children over 2 weeks old who have had symptoms for less than 48 hours. Tamiflu also prevents influenza A and B in adults and children over 1 year old.

Contraindications: Do not take oseltamivir if allergic to any component of the drug.

Adverse effects: Diarrhea, nausea, vomiting, and headache are the most common adverse effects of oseltamivir.

Patient education and care: Although it prevents the flu, Tamiflu should not replace your annual flu shot. Tamiflu does not stop you from spreading the flu to others. Continue to stay away from others while sick.

Antiviral Agent

Acyclovir (Zovirax) is an antiviral agent.

Indications: Oral acyclovir treats initial and recurrent episodes of genital herpes simplex virus, shingles, and chickenpox. Injectable acyclovir treats infections of higher severity.

Contraindications: Do not use acyclovir if allergic to acyclovir, valacyclovir, or any component of the drug.

Adverse effects: Acyclovir's most common adverse effects are nausea, vomiting, and energy loss.

Antivirals – HIV replication cycle

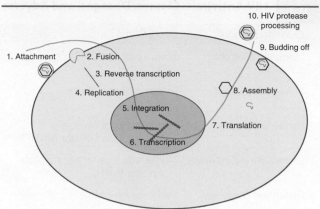

• **Fig. 11.41** Antivirals—Human Immunodeficiency Virus Replication Cycle

Patient education and care: Acyclovir does not cure genital herpes and does not stop it from spreading to others. Always use a latex or polyurethane condom.

Monoclonal Antibody

Palivizumab (Synagis) is a monoclonal antibody.

Indications: Palivizumab prevents RSV in infants and children who were born prematurely (less than 35 weeks' gestational age) and are less than 6 months old at the start of RSV season. They can still receive palivizumab if 24 months old at the start of RSV season if they received treatment for bronchopulmonary dysplasia in the past 6 months or have congenital heart disease.

Contraindications: Do not use palivizumab if allergic to any component of the medication.

Adverse effects: Fever and rash are the most common adverse effects of palivizumab.

Patient education and care: During RSV season, your child's medical staff will administer palivizumab into the muscle every month. Your child does not need any more doses for the current RSV season if your child contracts RSV.

SCENARIO 11.9. NON-HIV ANTIVIRAL AGENTS

A patient presents to a walk-in clinic complaining of flu-like symptoms. He says he has been sick for almost a week. He shows a positive test for influenza; would oseltamivir (Tamiflu) be a good choice for treatment? Why or why not?
Answer: It has been more than 48 hours since the symptoms started; oseltamivir (Tamiflu) would not help someone who has had the flu for this long.

HIV Antivirals

HIV is a virus that has 10 primary steps involved in the infection and release of the virus to other cells: (1) attachment, (2) fusion, (3) reverse transcription, (4) replication, (5) integration, (6) transcription, (7) translation, (8)

TABLE 11.7   HIV Antivirals, Classes, Dosages, and Adverse Reactions

Generic (Brand)	Drug Class	Common Dosage	Adverse Effects
Maraviroc (Selzentry)	Entry inhibitor; CCR5 antagonist	300 mg twice daily. Adjust dose based on other medications.	Infection, fever, rash
Enfuvirtide (Fuzeon)	Fusion protein inhibitor	90 mg subcutaneously twice daily	Injection site reaction, diarrhea, nausea
Efavirenz (Sustiva)	Non-nucleoside reverse transcriptase inhibitor (NNRTI)	600 mg daily. Adjust dose based on other medications	CNS toxicity, rash, increased cholesterol
Emtricitabine (Emtriva)	Nucleoside reverse transcriptase inhibitor (NRTI)	200 mg daily	Hyperpigmentation, diarrhea, nausea
Raltegravir (Isentress)	Integrase inhibitor	400 mg twice daily or 1200 mg once daily	Increased ALT, headache
Darunavir (Prezista)	Protease inhibitor	800 mg daily or 600 mg twice daily depending on patient-specific factors. Co-administer with cobicistat or ritonavir.	Skin rash, diarrhea, cholesterol increase

HIV antivirals – Preventing Entrance to Cell

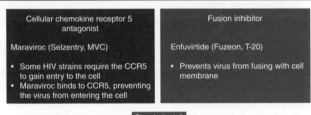

• **Fig. 11.42** HIV Antivirals—Preventing Entrance to Cell

assembly, (9) budding off, and (10) HIV protease processing (Fig. 11.41). HIV drugs aim to stop many of these steps (Table 11.7).

CCR5 Antagonists and Fusion Inhibitors

Cellular chemokine receptor 5 (CCR5) antagonists act by preventing step 2: fusion. HIV requires the CCR5 to access a cell. With a CCR5 antagonist such as **maraviroc (Selzentry)**, it binds to CCR5, preventing the virus from entering the cell (Fig. 11.42). Fusion inhibitors such as **enfuvirtide (Fuzeon)** also prevent entry to the cell by stopping the fusion of the virus with the cell membrane.

CCR5 Antagonist

Maraviroc (Selzentry) is a CCR5 antagonist.

Indication: Maraviroc treats infection of CCR5-tropic HIV-1 in adults and children over 2 years old and weighing at least 10 kg. Use in combination with other antiretrovirals.

Contraindications: Patients should not take maraviroc if they have low kidney function and are taking CYP3A inhibitors or inducers.

Adverse effects: Common adverse effects of maraviroc are fever, rash, abdominal pain, constipation, diarrhea, and common cold symptoms.

Patient education and care: Maraviroc does not cure HIV. Continue to see your doctor. You can still spread HIV to others. Use latex or polyurethane condoms and do not share needles, toothbrushes, razors, or similar products. Rise slowly to avoid passing out. Do not run out of this medication.

Fusion Protein Inhibitor

Enfuviritide (Fuzeon) is a fusion protein inhibitor.

Indications: Enfuviritide treats infection with HIV-1 if it continues to replicate despite other treatments. Use enfuviritide in combination with other antiretrovirals.

Contraindications: Do not take enfuviritide if allergic to any component of it.

Adverse effects: The most common adverse effects of enfuviritide are injection site reaction, nausea, and diarrhea.

Patient education and care: Enfuviritide does not cure HIV. Continue to see your doctor. You can still transmit HIV to others. Use latex or polyurethane condoms and do not share needles, toothbrushes, razors, or similar products. Do not run out of this medication.

HIV Medicines Working on Enzymes

To improve compliance with multidrug regimens, drug manufacturers often combine multiple drugs. **Atripla** is a combination of three drugs (efavirenz, emtricitabine and tenofovir) working in two different ways. This stops step 3 of the process: reverse transcription. Non-nucleotide reverse transcriptase inhibitor (NNRTI) **efavirenz** binds to the enzyme responsible for reverse transcriptase. This deforms the structure of newly formed DNA. Nucleotide reverse

HIV antivirals – NNRTI/NRTIs

Non-nucleotide reverse transcriptase inhibitor (NNRTI) with nucleotide reverse transcriptase inhibitor (NRTI)

efavirenz/emtricitabine/tenofovir (Atripla)

Efanvirenz (EFV)	Emtricitabine (FTC)	Tenofovir (TDF)
NNRTI	NRTI	NRTI
Binds to enzyme responsible for reverse transcriptase, changing structure of new DNA formed to be faulty	Incorporated into DNA at the reverse transcription step and causing faulty DNA to be produced	

Step halted: 3

• **Fig. 11.43** HIV Antivirals—Non-nucleotide Reverse Transcriptase Inhibitors/Nucleotide reverse transcriptase inhibitors

HIV antivirals – Integrase Strand Transfer Inhibitor

Raltegravir (Isentress, RAL)

Integrase is an enzyme used by HIV virus to insert its viral DNA into host DNA and take over host production machinery

Integrase strand transfer inhibitors halt this process

Step halted: 5

• **Fig. 11.44** HIV Antivirals—Integrase Strand Transfer Inhibitor

HIV antivirals – Protease Inhibitors

Darunavir (Prezista, DRV)

The last step in HIV replication is processing by HIV protease
• Without protease, the virus is inert and unable to infect other host cells

Protease inhibitors prevent viral maturation and very effective

Step halted: 10

• **Fig. 11.45** HIV Antivirals—Protease Inhibitors

transcriptase inhibitors (NRTIs) such as **emtricitabine** and **tenofovir** work at the reverse transcription step, causing production of poor DNA (Fig. 11.43).

The integrase strand transfer inhibitor **raltegravir (Isentress)** acts on integrase, an enzyme that HIV uses to insert its viral DNA into host DNA to take over the host apparatus (Fig. 11.44). Raltegravir stops step 5: integration.

Darunavir (Prezista) is a protease inhibitor that works in one of the last steps of HIV replication (Fig. 11.45). Without this final step, the virus is unable to infect other host cells after viral maturation.

Non-nucleotide Reverse Transcriptase Inhibitors

Efavirenz (Sustiva) is a non-nucleotide reverse transcriptase inhibitor.

Indications: Efavirenz treats infection with HIV-1 in adults and children over 3 months old and weighing at least 3.5 kg. Use efavirenz in combination with other antiretrovirals.

Contraindications: Do not take efavirenz if allergic to any component of it. Do not take it with elbasvir or grazoprevir.

Adverse effects: Common adverse effects of efavirenz are CNS toxicity, skin rash, and high cholesterol.

Patient education and care: Use effective birth control while taking efavirenz and for a long time after stopping efavirenz. Some types of hormonal birth control might not work as well while taking efavirenz. Efavirenz does not cure HIV, and you may be able to spread it to others. Use latex or polyurethane condoms and do not share needles, razor blades, or similar products. Do not run out of this medication.

Nucleoside Reverse Transcriptase Inhibitor

Emtricitabine (Emtriva) is a nucleoside reverse transcriptase inhibitor.

Indications: Emtricitabine treats infection with HIV-1. Use it in combination with other antiretrovirals.

Contraindications: Do not use emtricitabine if allergic to any of its components.

Adverse effects: Common adverse effects of emtricitabine are hyperpigmentation, diarrhea, and nausea.

Patient education and care: Emtricitabine does not cure HIV. You may be able to spread HIV to others. Use latex or polyurethane condoms and do not share needles, razor blades, or similar products. Do not run out of this medication.

Integrase Inhibitor

Raltegravir (Isentress) is an integrase inhibitor.

Indications: Raltegravir treats infection with HIV-1. Use it in combination with other antiretrovirals.

Contraindications: Do not use raltegravir if allergic to any of its components.

Adverse effects: Common adverse effects of raltegravir are increased alanine transaminase (ALT; a liver function test) and headache.

Patient education and care: Raltegravir does not cure HIV. You may be able to spread HIV to others. Use latex or polyurethane condoms and do not share needles, razor blades, or similar products. Do not run out of this medication.

Protease Inhibitor

Darunavir (Prezista) is a protease inhibitor.

Indications: Darunavir treats infection with HIV-1 in adults and children over 3 years old. Use darunavir with ritonavir. Use in combination with other antiretrovirals.

Contraindications: Do not use darunavir if taking medications that are cleared by CYP3A4. Do not use darunavir if taking other drugs with narrow therapeutic index. Do not use darunavir without ritonavir as it will not be effective.

Adverse effects: Common adverse effects of darunavir are skin rash, diarrhea, and rise in cholesterol.

Patient education and care: Some hormonal birth controls might not work as well while taking darunavir. Darunavir does not cure HIV, and you may be able to spread it to others. Use latex or polyurethane condoms and do not share needles, razor blades, or similar products. Darunavir must be taken with ritonavir or cobicistat in order to work properly. These medications interact with numerous other medications. Tell your provider about all medications that you are currently taking and before starting any new ones. Do not run out of this medication.

SCENARIO 11.10. HIV ANTIVIRALS

While some HIV medications work on the enzymes involved in the replication process, two work by preventing entry into the cell. What are two examples of these types of medications?
   Answer: Maraviroc is a CCR5 antagonist that prevents binding to a receptor. Enfuvirtide is a fusion inhibitor preventing fusion of the virus to the cell membrane.

Summary

- We can separate organisms using the Gram stain. Gram-positive (Gram +) bacteria take up the stain because they have fewer layers; Gram-negative (Gram –) organisms do not because of an extra protective layer.
- We can classify antibiotics as broad spectrum or narrow spectrum. A broad-spectrum antibiotic covers many organisms. A narrow-spectrum antibiotic is much more specific.
- Penicillins, such as amoxicillin (Amoxil*), bind to penicillin-binding proteins and affect the cell walls of bacteria. If the bacteria develop a beta-lactamase enzyme against the amoxicillin, adding clavulanate as amoxicillin/clavulanate (Augmentin) may help.

- As we go up the cephalosporin generations from first to fourth, these drugs generally gain more Gram-negative and anaerobic coverage, more resistance to beta-lactamases, and increased CNS penetration. They have a different spectrum of action, have more endurance to resistance, and can reach body areas that lower generations cannot.
- Bacteriostatic antibiotics suppress bacterial growth and reproduction while bactericidal antibiotics kill bacteria outright. A reason to use a bacteriostatic antibiotic includes preserving more good bacteria in the body.
- An antibiotic can affect the production of DNA and RNA. DNA gyrase and topoisomerase IV, both enzymes, coil and uncoil DNA for replication. Fluoroquinolones, broad-spectrum antibiotics, such as levofloxacin (Levaquin*) and ciprofloxacin (Cipro) inhibit this coiling and uncoiling process.
- Antifungals are effective for fungal infections over bacterial or viral. We can divide antifungals into two major categories: (1) for **systemic mycoses** treatment, such as amphotericin; and (2) for **superficial mycoses**, such as thrush treatment with nystatin.
- The slow replication of TB means that TB readily resists a single medication. As such, we treat TB with multidrug regimens. Remember the drugs with the RIPE mnemonic, as in the TB test induration (raised skin) is ripe: R, Rifampin; I, isoniazid; P, pyrazinamide; and E, ethambutol.
- We might prevent influenza with an injectable such as Fluzone Quadrivalent or Flumist, an influenza vaccine nasal spray. Because influenza can change annually, manufacturers change the flu shot each year.
- HIV is a virus that has 10 primary steps; medications work on some of those steps. Either an HIV medication prevents the passage of the virus into the cell, as with CCR5 antagonists or fusion inhibitors, or it affects important viral enzymes—reverse transcriptase, integrase, and protease.

Review Questions

1. Which antibiotic drug class inhibits DNA/RNA synthesis?
   a. Penicillins
   b. Fluoroquinolones
   c. Aminoglycosides
   d. Macrolides
2. Fill in the two blanks. As you _____ in cephalosporin generations, Gram-negative coverage _____.
   a. Increase, decreases
   b. Decrease, decreases
   c. Decrease, increases
   d. Increase, increases
3. Which of the following antibiotics would not cover for methicillin-resistant *Staphylococcus aureus* (MRSA)?
   a. Linezolid (Zyvox)
   b. Clindamycin (Cleocin)

   c. Sulfamethoxazole/trimethoprim (Bactrim)
   d. Ceftaroline (Teflaro)
4. The following medication is not bacteriostatic:
   a. Azithromycin (Z-Pak)
   b. Amikacin (Amikin*)
   c. Minocycline (Minocin)
   d. Linezolid (Zyvox)
5. All of the following antibiotics work on the 30S ribosomal subunit *except*?
   a. Linezolid (Zyvox)
   b. Doxycycline (Doryx)
   c. Amikacin (Amikin*)
   d. Gentamycin (Garamycin)
6. Which atypical antibiotic can a prescriber use only for obligate anaerobic bacteria?
   a. Metronidazole (Flagyl)

b. Sulfamethoxazole/trimethoprim (Bactrim)
c. Fluconazole (Diflucan)
d. Amphotericin B (Fungizone*)

7. This polyene antifungal is available as a topical agent for thrush:
a. Metronidazole (Flagyl)
b. Fluconazole (Diflucan)
c. Nystatin (Mycostatin*)
d. Amphotericin B (Fungizone*)

8. Respiratory syncytial virus (RSV) prophylaxis involves which of the following medications?
a. Palivizumab (Synagis)
b. Acyclovir (Zovirax)
c. Valacyclovir (Valtrex)

d. Infliximab (Remicade)

9. What are the four drugs in the multidrug regimen of tuberculosis treatment?
a. Rifampin, Isentress, Pyrazinamide, and Efavirenz
b. Rifampin, Isoniazid, Pyrazinamide, and Emtricitabine
c. Rifampin, Isoniazid, Pyrazinamide, and Ethambutol
d. Rifampin, Isentress, Pyrazinamide, and Ethambutol

10. In which class would darunavir (Prezista) fall?
a. Cellular chemokine receptor 5 antagonists
b. Non-nucleotide reverse transcriptase inhibitor
c. Integrase strand transfer inhibitor
d. Protease inhibitor

12

Neuropsychology

1. Discuss the neurotransmitters and their importance in the management of neurologic and psychological conditions.
2. Describe the pathophysiology of common neurologic and psychotherapeutic conditions.
3. Identify various medication classes in the therapeutic treatment of neurologic and psychological conditions
4. Compare and contrast medicines within a given medication class as they relate to receptors and generations.
5. Discuss the mechanisms of action, indications, drug interactions, and adverse effects of common neurologic and psychological conditions.

Introduction

Neuropharmacology is a combination word that translates to the study of drugs that affect the nervous system. The drugs either work on the peripheral nervous system (PNS) or the central nervous system (CNS). Neurons, or nerve cells, transmit information through electrical impulses to message another neuron, a muscle cell, or a secretary gland cell. The electrical signal takes two steps: axonal conduction and synaptic transmission.

Axonal Conduction

The signal travels from the soma on the left moving the action potential to the end of the axon (Fig. 12.1).

Axonal conduction drugs, such as lidocaine (Solarcaine), are used as local anesthetics that can dull pain. Note the following:
- These drugs are not selective.

- There are more adverse effects.
- There are few medication classes.

Synaptic Transmission

- First, the action potential reaches the nerve terminal.
- Neurotransmitter releases.
- The transmitter binds to the receptor at the postsynaptic cell ("post" means "after" and "synaptic" means "the gap").

This helps us understand the two broad categories of medications and their targets.

Synaptic transmission drugs, such as fluoxetine (Prozac), are used as antidepressants, which we will see later in the chapter, that work specifically on serotonin (Fig. 12.2). Note the following:
- The drugs are selective.
- You can "choose" adverse effects.
- There are many medication classes.

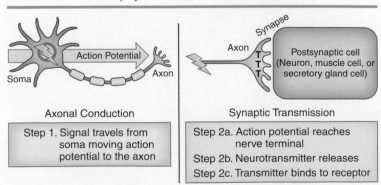

Neuropsych – Neuronal Transmission

Action Potential

Soma · Axon

Synapse

Axon · Postsynaptic cell (Neuron, muscle cell, or secretory gland cell)

Axonal Conduction

Step 1. Signal travels from soma moving action potential to the axon

Synaptic Transmission

Step 2a. Action potential reaches nerve terminal
Step 2b. Neurotransmitter releases
Step 2c. Transmitter binds to receptor

• **Fig. 12.1** Neuronal Transmission

---

* Brand discontinued, now available only as generic
† Naming conventions can vary between prescription and OTC formulations

Over-the-Counter Local Anesthetics (Axonal Conduction)

There are two major classes of local anesthetics named after the molecules in the middle of their structures: esters and amides. Esters, such as **benzocaine (Anbesol)**, are generally found in topical agents because, when given by injection, they are more allergenic (cause allergic reactions). Amides are less allergenic; therefore, **lidocaine**, an amide, is usually well tolerated when injected. Most students know of **cocaine** and remember that these amides are local anesthetics through the -caine ending association among the three names: **benzocaine**, **lidocaine**, and cocaine. The axon looks a little like the hook of a candy cane to help you remember the association between -caine and axonal conduction (Table 12.1).

Benzocaine and Lidocaine

Benzo*caine* (Anbesol) has the -caine stem, indicating that **benzocaine** is a local anesthetic that is in the ester type, a bit less safe and generally used topically (Fig. 12.3). **Lido*caine*** is often used topically and is available over-the-counter (OTC) to treat sunburns, hence the brand name **Solarcaine** Cool Aloe Burn Relief Formula Pain. Injectable and patch forms of **lidocaine** are also available by prescription. It would be the safer of the two because it is an amide type. In French, *ami* means friend; thus, think of the amide type local anesthetic as more friendly.

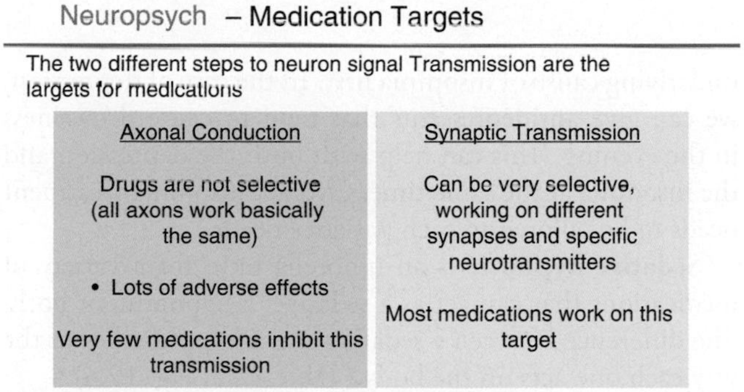

Local Anesthetics
Benzocaine

Benzocaine (Anbesol) is a topical analgesic or local anesthetic.

Indications: Generally, we use benzocaine for minor relief of skin irritation, such as cuts, scrapes, minor burns, and poison ivy and sumac. We can use the oral formulations for toothaches and cold sores. The oral sprays can help with sore throats and decrease the gag reflex.

Contraindications: Be careful not to use benzocaine on deep wounds and cuts, infections, or serious burns. Watch out for allergies to any component of the drug, other -caine anesthetics, or para-amino-benzoic acid (PABA).

Adverse effects: Include a tingling, burning, or stinging sensation.

Patient education and care: Be careful not to breathe in this drug. It can cause serious harm if inhaled. If using for the mouth, do not eat while your mouth is numb. It may cause you to bite your tongue. Keep it away from clothing, as it can cause staining. Do not swallow formulations meant for the rectum or skin, as this can cause serious harm.

Lidocaine

Lidocaine is a local anesthetic or topical analgesic.

Indications: We can use lidocaine for topical pain and irritation relief. Some examples of this are mouth sores, skin irritation such as eczema, intubation procedures, hemorrhoids, nerve diseases, and pain from shingles.

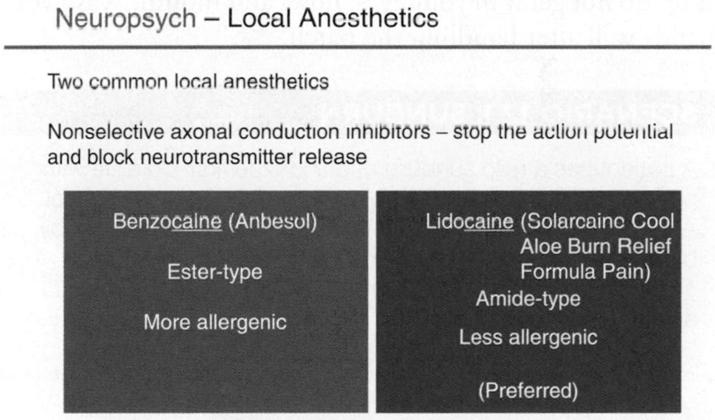

Neuropsych – Medication Targets

The two different steps to neuron signal Transmission are the targets for medications

Axonal Conduction	Synaptic Transmission
Drugs are not selective (all axons work basically the same)	Can be very selective, working on different synapses and specific neurotransmitters
• Lots of adverse effects	Most medications work on this target
Very few medications inhibit this transmission	

• **Fig. 12.2** Medication Targets

Neuropsych – Local Anesthetics

Two common local anesthetics

Nonselective axonal conduction inhibitors – stop the action potential and block neurotransmitter release

Benzocaine (Anbesol) Ester-type More allergenic	Lidocaine (Solarcaine Cool Aloe Burn Relief Formula Pain) Amide-type Less allergenic (Preferred)

• **Fig. 12.3** Local Anesthetics

TABLE 12.1 Local Anesthetics—Classes, Dosages, and Adverse Effects

Generic (Brand)	Drug Class	Dosage	Adverse Effects
Benzocaine (Anbesol)	Topical analgesic, local anesthetic	Use specific product labeling. Common dosage: Spray: Use 1 spray up to 4 times daily Ointment: Apply a thin layer to affected area up to 4 times daily	Tingling, burning, or stinging sensation
Lidocaine (Solarcaine Cool Aloe Burn Relief Formula Pain)	Topical analgesic, local anesthetic	Use specific product labeling. Common dosage: Cream: Apply a thin layer topically 2–3 times daily as needed	Swelling, redness

TABLE 12.2   Sedative-Hypnotics—Classes, Dosages, and Adverse Effects

Generic (Brand)	Drug Class	Dosage	Adverse Effects
Acetaminophen/ diphenhydramine (Tylenol PM)	Analgesic/first-generation antihistamine	1–2 tablets every 6 hours	Fatigue, anxiety
Eszopiclone (Lunesta)	Hypnotic	1 mg at bedtime, max 3 mg daily	Headache, altered taste
Zolpidem (Ambien)	Hypnotic	ER: 6.25 mg females, 6.25–12.5 males IR: 5 mg females, 5–10 mg males	Headache, dizziness, drowsiness
Ramelteon (Rozerem)	Melatonin receptor agonist	8 mg daily 30 minutes before bedtime	Drowsiness, dizziness, fatigue

ER, Extended release; *IR,* immediate release.

Contraindications: Be careful not to use lidocaine on broken skin or mucous membranes. Do not use it on an infection. Do not use in patients who have an allergy to any component of lidocaine or other amide type local anesthetics.

Adverse effects: Skin irritation, redness, and swelling are common adverse effects.

Patient education and care: Lidocaine should not be used for teething. Do not use for children under 3 years old unless told to by a doctor. If using a formulation for the skin, do not get it in your eyes, nose, and mouth. Wash your hands well after handling the patch.

SCENARIO 12.1. SUNBURN

A patient has a mild sunburn and finds the first-aid aisle with pain relief products. She chooses lidocaine (Solarcaine Cool Aloe Burn Relief Formula Pain). Would this medicine work by blocking axonal conduction or by synaptic transmission?

Answer: Axonal conduction—lidocaine is a local anesthetic.

Sedative-Hypnotics (Sleeping Pills)

The diagnosis of **insomnia** can vary from patient to patient, but the important part of the diagnosis is the impact on daytime activities. Some people can sleep for 4 hours and feel fine; others need 8 hours of sleep or they will be miserable in the morning. The benchmark for diagnosis is: "Is it affecting your activities of daily living?"

If lack of sleep is keeping the patient from completing tasks during the day, the patient would be diagnosed with insomnia. In addition, the patient's symptoms and causes of insomnia are going to be considered when creating a treatment plan. Insomnia can have a variety of causes, including depression and anxiety. The insomnia can also be called idiopathic, which is a fancy way of saying that we don't know what is causing it. Often, it is better to treat the

Sedative-Hypnotics – Overview

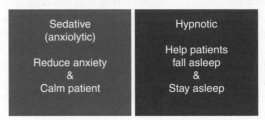

Some medications are sedative of hypnotic, others are both

• **Fig. 12.4** Sedative-Hypnotics Overview

underlying cause of insomnia first. In the case of depression, we can give antidepressants that tend to cause drowsiness in the evening. This can help with both the depression and the insomnia at the same time. Overall, insomnia treatment needs to be tailored to each patient's needs.

Sedative-hypnotic is an umbrella term for a variety of medications that can act as a sedative, a hypnotic, or both. The difference between a sedative and a hypnotic lies in the way each one acts on the body (Table 12.2, Fig. 12.4).

Sedatives act as an anxiolytic. The anxio- root of the word relates to anxiety, and the -lytic root means "to break apart." This just means that sedatives are used to reduce anxiety and calm the patient down. Hypnotics, on the other hand, are designed to help the patient fall asleep, stay asleep, or both.

You can think of **hypnotics** as being related to hypnosis in their relationship with sleep. While hypnotics are very useful for sleep disorders, the timing is critical. If a hypnotic doesn't last through the night, the patient may wake up in the middle of the night. If it lasts too long, it can cause drowsiness in the morning. The goal is to have the medication last just the right amount of time. Some patients may only have trouble falling asleep; some may only have trouble staying asleep. It is important that the hypnotic is tailored to the patient. We will talk about a specific class of sedative-hypnotics here: benzodiazepines.

Sedative-Hypnotics – Antihistamines

The first-generation antihistamine diphenhydramine produces drowsiness

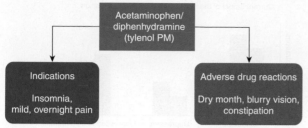

Tolerance to drowsiness builds within 1–2 weeks, but ADRs continue

• **Fig. 12.5** Sedative-Hypnotics Antihistamines

Sedating Antihistamines

Something as common as a first-generation antihistamine such as **diphenhydramine**, which has the side effect of drowsiness, and **acetaminophen**, a nonnarcotic analgesic that helps relieve pain, can improve a patient's sleep. Together, they form **acetaminophen/diphenhydramine (Tylenol PM Extra Strength)**, with the PM standing for the nighttime dosing with the added diphenhydramine ingredient (Fig. 12.5). Tolerance to drowsiness tends to build up for diphenhydramine; thus, this isn't a long-term solution. Also, dry mouth, blurry vision, and constipation are possible side effects. This choice is especially poor for the elderly because of the risk of falls.

Analgesic and First-Generation Antihistamine

Acetaminophen/diphenhydramine (Tylenol PM Extra Strength) is an analgesic and first-generation antihistamine combination.

Indications: We can use acetaminophen/diphenhydramine to treat aches and pains accompanied by insomnia. It can be used for headache, arthritis, fever, muscle pain, and other pains when someone is having trouble sleeping.

Contraindications: Avoid this product in children under 12 years old. Do not take it with other products that contain acetaminophen or diphenhydramine, including topical treatments, as this can lead to overdose. Do not use in someone with an allergy to any component of the drug.

Adverse effects: Fatigue and anxiety are common adverse effects.

Patient education and care: Do not take more of this drug than what is recommended. Be careful that you are not taking other products that contain acetaminophen or diphenhydramine. Overdose can be very dangerous. Be careful while driving and avoid driving until you know how this drug affects you. It may cause you to be very drowsy.

Benzodiazepine-Like Drugs

A class of drugs related to benzodiazepines, called the benzodiazepine-like drugs (Fig. 12.6), we generally refer

Sedative-Hypnotics – Benzo-Like

Structurally different than benzodiazepines BUT same mechanism of action; produce only *hypnotic* effects

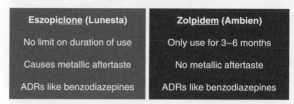

• **Fig. 12.6** Sedative-Hypnotics—Benzodiazepine-Like

to as just "hypnotic." **Eszopiclone (Lunesta)** has a generic stem -clone and will put you in the sleeping zone. Some students point to the "z" in **eszopiclone** for getting your z's. For **zolpidem (Ambien, Ambien CR)** use the -pidem stem to remember **zolpidem** as a sedative-hypnotic. *Controlled Release* **zolpidem (Ambien CR)** works for people who have difficulty maintaining sleep *and* those who have difficulty falling asleep. The regular version works only for those having trouble falling asleep. There are some sharp differences between eszopiclone and zolpidem. A patient should use zolpidem from 3 to 6 months only rather than eszopiclone, which has no limit. Eszopiclone has a metallic aftertaste that some patients find unpleasant. Both have adverse drug reactions (ADRs) similar to those of a benzodiazepine.

Hypnotics

Eszopiclone (Lunesta) is a hypnotic.

Indications: We can use eszopiclone to treat insomnia.

Contraindications: Anyone who has experienced complex sleep behavior, such as sleep walking or driving, should not take eszopiclone. Do not take eszopiclone if allergic to any component of it.

Adverse effects: Common adverse effects include headache and bad taste in your mouth.

Patient education and care: Take eszopiclone as you are going to bed. It may cause sleep walking, sleep driving, and other actions while not fully awake. Stop taking eszopiclone if this happens to you.

Zolpidem (Ambien) is a hypnotic.

Indications: We can use zolpidem to treat insomnia. Depending on the formulation, it can help with going to sleep and/or staying asleep.

Contraindications: Do not use zolpidem in someone who has experienced complex sleep behaviors such as sleep walking while taking it.

Adverse effects: Headache, drowsiness, and dizziness are the most common adverse effects.

Patient education and care: Take zolpidem as you are about to go to bed. Do not drive until you feel awake. Zolpidem may cause sleep walking, sleep driving, and other actions while not fully awake. Stop taking zolpidem if this happens to you.

Melatonin: Brain produces hormone to induce sleep

Ramelteon (Rozerem)

Binds to melatonin receptors to cause drowsiness

No abuse potential like benzodiazepines and benzo-likes

No limit on length of use

ADRs equal to placebo

• **Fig. 12.7** Sedative-Hypnotics—Melatonin Agonists

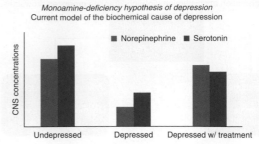

Monoamine-deficiency hypothesis of depression
Current model of the biochemical cause of depression

• **Fig. 12.8** Depression—Pathology

Melatonin Receptor Agonist

The body naturally produces a brain hormone called melatonin to help a person sleep. Ra*melteon* (Rozerem) binds to melatonin receptors to cause drowsiness (Fig. 12.7). It does not have abuse potential, like benzodiazepines and benzodiazepine-like drugs, and there is no limit on its length of use. The adverse drug reactions are about the same as a placebo. The -melteon stem in **ramelteon** lets you know it's a melatonin agonist. There are many letters from melatonin in that suffix ending.

Melatonin Receptor Agonist

Ramelteon (Rozerem) is a melatonin agonist.

Indications: We can use ramelteon for patients who have trouble falling asleep.

Contraindications: Do not use ramelteon with fluvoxamine or with serious allergy to ramelteon.

Adverse effects: Adverse effects are feeling tired, dizzy, and weak.

Patient education and care: Take ramelteon 30 minutes before bedtime. Do not take ramelteon if you can't get at least 7 to 8 hours of sleep.

SCENARIO 12.2. INSOMNIA

A patient has insomnia for the first time and is looking for something OTC to help him sleep. Which would better match what he wants, acetaminophen/diphenhydramine (Tylenol PM Extra Strength) or eszopiclone (Rozerem)?

Answer: Acetaminophen/diphenhydramine (Tylenol PM Extra Strength) is an OTC product and a combination of a nonnarcotic analgesic for pain and a first-generation antihistamine for drowsiness. Eszopiclone (Rozerem) is prescription only.

Antidepressants

One of the main theories of the pathology of depression is the monoamine-deficiency hypothesis of depression (Fig. 12.8). This is a fancy academic way of saying that we think the cause of depression is that the levels of two neurotransmitters, serotonin and norepinephrine (both are monoamines), are too low. This is the currently accepted model of depression. Healthy individuals have higher levels of serotonin and norepinephrine, while depressed individuals have lower levels of these transmitters. When we treat depression, we expect these levels to go up. Therefore, antidepressant agents aim to increase the level of one or both of these neurotransmitters (Table 12.3)

All antidepressants work to increase the levels of these monoamines in one way or another. Selective serotonin reuptake inhibitors (SSRIs) act to keep serotonin in the synapse, while serotonin norepinephrine reuptake inhibitors (SNRIs) do the same and also act on norepinephrine. Tricyclic antidepressants (TCAs) are named after the shape of their molecule, but they also act on serotonin and norepinephrine. Finally, monoamine oxidase inhibitors (MAOIs) act by inhibiting monoamine oxidase, an enzyme that breaks down serotonin and norepinephrine (Fig. 12.9).

SSRIs and SNRIs carry the names of the neurotransmitters they affect. The TCA class name comes from the chemical structure's three rings. **Amitriptyline (Elavil*)** is an example (Fig. 12.10). The last group of antidepressants includes the MAOIs. A word that ends in -ase is usually an enzyme; thus, if an antidepressant blocks the enzyme that breaks a neurotransmitter down, then there are more neurotransmitters (the monoamines, in this case) available to elevate the patient's mood. An example of an MAOI is **isocarboxazid (Marplan)**.

Dosing at the right time can minimize adverse effects seen with serotonergic agents. For example, fluoxetine might give the patient energy and paroxetine might cause drowsiness, even though they are in the same SSRI drug class. Seeing a patient's chart with the evening dose as fluoxetine or morning dose as paroxetine should be a red flag (Fig. 12.11).

Selective Serotonin Reuptake Inhibitors

The SSRI class includes drugs such as **citalopram (Celexa), escitalopram (Lexapro), sertraline (Zoloft), paroxetine (Paxil)**, and **fluoxetine (Prozac)**. These medications selectively inhibit reuptake (breakdown) of serotonin within neurons. Increased serotonin levels can improve a patient's mood.

TABLE 12.3 Antidepressants—Classes, Dosages, and Adverse Effects

Generic (Brand)	Drug Class	Dosage	Adverse Effects
Fluoxetine (Prozac)	Selective serotonin reuptake inhibitor (SSRI)	10–60 mg daily, depending on indication	Insomnia, headache, anxiety
Duloxetine (Cymbalta)	Serotonin/norepinephrine reuptake inhibitor (SNRI)	Initial: 30–40 mg daily for 1 week Maintenance: 60 mg daily	Nausea, headache, dry mouth
Amitriptyline (Elavil*)	Tricyclic antidepressant (TCA)	MDD: 100–300 mg daily, starting at 25 mg daily Dose varies by indication.	Fatigue, dry mouth, nausea
Isocarboxazid (Marplan)	Monoamine oxidase inhibitor (MAOI)	Initial: 10 mg twice daily Maintenance: 40–60 mg daily	Dizziness, dry mouth, constipation, trouble sleeping, fatigue

MDD, Major depressive disorder.

Neuropsych – Antidepressants

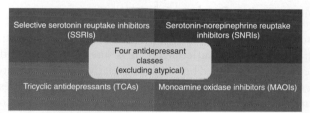

• **Fig. 12.9** Antidepressants—Five Classes

Neuropsych – Antidepressants

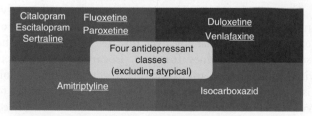

• **Fig. 12.10** Antidepressants—Examples in Five Classes

Serotonergic Agents Timing

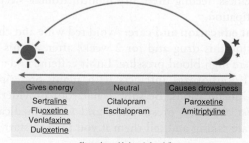

*Isocarboxazid given twice daily

• **Fig. 12.11** Serotonergic Agents Timing

Fluoxetine was the first SSRI to make it to market. The -oxetine ending is supposed to be for **fluoxetine**-like entities, but you will see -oxetine on the SNRI **dul*oxetine*** (**Cymbalta**) and attention deficit hyperactivity disorder (ADHD) medication **atom*oxetine*** (**Strattera**), so be careful. When **fluoxetine** gained a new indication, for premenstrual dysphoric disorder (PMDD), it also gained a new brand name: **Sarafem*** —"Sara" like the girl's name and "fem" for feminine. The highest ranked angels are Sera-p-h-i-m; thus, combatting PMDD is the work of angels.

Par*oxetine* is similar to the SSRI **flu*oxetine***, with the same -oxetine stem. **Paxil** derives from **par*oxetine***. The controlled-release (CR) version of **Paxil** is supposed to have fewer initial side effects and be a little easier to dose. Sertraline is known for having severe gastrointestinal effects and may affect a patient's willingness to take it.

Escitalopram has the same es- prefix (added onto **citalopram**) discussed with the proton pump inhibitors **esomeprazole** and **omeprazole,** in which the sinister "S" form is superior.

Selective Serotonin Reuptake Inhibitor

Fluoxetine (Prozac) is an SSRI.

Indications: We can use fluoxetine in major depressive disorder (MDD), bipolar depression, obsessive-compulsive disorder, panic disorder, premenstrual dysphoric disorder (Sarafem only), bulimia nervosa, and treatment-resistant depression.

Contraindications: Do not start fluoxetine within 2 weeks of taking an MAOI. Do not start an MAOI or thioridazine within 5 weeks of taking fluoxetine. Do not start fluoxetine if taking linezolid, pimozide, or IV methylene blue. Avoid in anyone with an allergy to any component.

Adverse reactions: Headache, anxiety, and insomnia are common adverse reactions.

Patient education and care: Do not stop taking fluoxetine suddenly. Talk to your doctor about how to slowly stop taking it to avoid side effects. Fluoxetine may increase thoughts of suicide. Be sure to watch for signs of this in anyone beginning fluoxetine. Call your doctor if this happens to you.

Serotonin-Norepinephrine Reuptake Inhibitors

Similar to the SSRIs are the SNRIs **duloxetine (Cymbalta)** and **venlafaxine (Effexor XR)**. Be careful—**duloxetine** is an SNRI, yet has the -oxetine stem of some SSRIs (**flu***oxetine*, par*oxetine*).

Dul*oxetine* (**Cymbalta**) affects serotonin and norepinephrine. One can think of the "du" as duo (two). It's especially useful for patients with chronic pain. Next is venla*faxine* (**Effexor XR**). Remember this drug by its stem -faxine. Take with food daily and do not skip doses.

Selective Serotonin and Norepinephrine Reuptake Inhibitor

Duloxetine (Cymbalta) is a selective serotonin and norepinephrine reuptake inhibitor.

Indications: We can use duloxetine for MDD, generalized anxiety disorder, diabetic peripheral neuropathy, and chronic musculoskeletal pain. The delayed-release particle capsules can be used for fibromyalgia.

Contraindications: Do not start duloxetine within 14 days of taking an MAOI. Do not start an MAOI within 5 days of taking duloxetine. Do not start duloxetine if taking linezolid or IV methylene blue. Avoid in anyone with an allergy to any component.

Adverse reactions: Nausea, headache, dry mouth, and drowsiness are the more prevalent adverse reactions.

Patient education and care: Get up slowly from a reclining or sitting position to avoid dizziness and falls. Tell your doctor if you are experiencing suicidal thoughts.

Tricyclic Antidepressants

Ami*triptyline* (**Elavil***)—the "tri" in **ami***triptyline* helps students remember this is a TCA, or tricyclic antidepressant. It "trips" up depression. At the same time that its mechanism of action blocks serotonin and norepinephrine reuptake to help the patient, it also blocks histamine and alpha-adrenergic receptors and shows anticholinergic effects creating significant adverse effects. This is why we rarely see TCAs in practice for depression (Fig. 12.12).

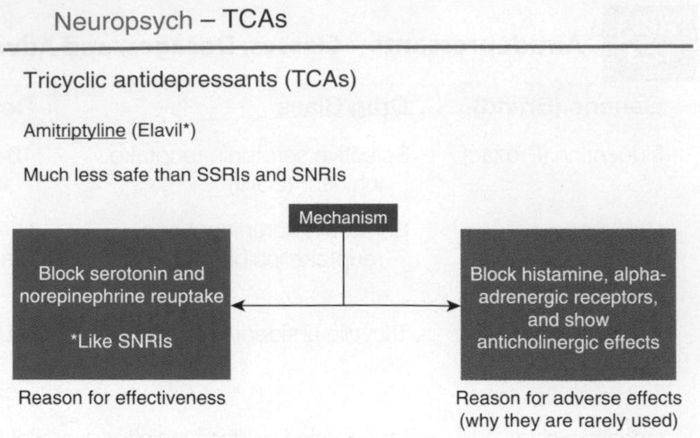

Amitriptyline

Amitriptyline (Elavil*) is a TCA.

Indications: We can use amitriptyline for MDD.

Contraindications: Be careful of taking amitriptyline within 14 days of taking an MAOI or with cisapride. Avoid it during recovery from a heart attack. Do not take amitriptyline if allergic to any component of it.

Tricyclic antidepressants (TCAs)

Amitriptyline (Elavil*)

Much less safe than SSRIs and SNRIs

• **Fig. 12.12** Tricyclic Antidepressants (TCAs)

Adverse reactions: Constipation, dry mouth, dizziness, and anxiety are common adverse effects.

Patient education and care: Be careful of drowsiness while taking amitriptyline and do not drive until you know how it affects you. Drink plenty of water while taking amitriptyline.

Monoamine Oxidase Inhibitors

Isocarboxazid (Marplan) is more known for its adverse effects than therapeutic effects. It is one of the first antidepressants developed but is not safe relative to newer agents. A serious interaction with tyramine can elevate blood pressure. Tyramine appears in foods such as aged cheese, chocolate, red wine, and craft beers; combining these foods with an MAOI can result in hypertensive crisis.

Isocarboxazid

Isocarboxazid (Marplan) is a monoamine oxidase inhibitor.

Indications: We can use isocarboxazid to treat depression.

Contraindications: Do not use isocarboxazid in anyone with high blood pressure, headaches, or history of heart, cerebrovascular, or liver disease. It should not be used with poor kidney function. Isocarboxazid interacts with multiple medications. Be sure to get a full medication history from the patient, including OTC medications, to avoid interactions. Some medications, such as SSRIs, need to be discontinued for at least 2 weeks before starting isocarboxazid. Do not use it in anyone with allergies to any drug component.

Adverse reactions: Common adverse reactions are headache, dizziness, feeling tired, dry mouth, trouble sleeping, and constipation.

Patient education and care: Avoid red wine and cheese while taking this drug and for 2 weeks after, as this may cause severe high blood pressure. Limit caffeine and avoid alcohol. Isocarboxazid interacts with many prescription and OTC medications. Be sure to tell your provider and pharmacist about all prescription and OTC medication that you are taking and tell them if you plan to start anything new.

TABLE 12.4	Smoking Cessation Aids—Classes, Dosages, and Adverse Effects		
Generic (Brand)	**Drug Class**	**Dosage**	**Adverse Effects**
Bupropion (Zyban*)	Smoking cessation aid	Initial: 150 mg daily for 3 days. Maintenance: 150 mg twice daily	Insomnia, headache, dry mouth, agitation, nausea and vomiting
Varenicline (Chantix)	Partial nicotine agonist, smoking cessation aid	0.5 mg once daily days 1–3, 0.5 mg twice daily days 4–7, then 1 mg twice daily	Nausea, nightmares, headache, insomnia

SCENARIO 12.3. ANTIDEPRESSANT TIMING

The chart shows that a patient is on sertraline (Zoloft) at bedtime. However, the patient has complained about insomnia and not being able to sleep. What SSRI would you expect to see instead of sertraline for a bedtime dose?

Answer: Paroxetine (Paxil) is an SSRI that would likely cause drowsiness. Along with the fact that sertraline is energizing, giving an SSRI such as sertraline, which causes gastrointestinal distress, at bedtime, is also a concern.

Nicotine cessation – Rx options

Two FDA-approved medications for smoking cessation

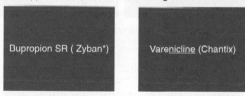

Bupropion SR (Zyban*)   Varenicline (Chantix)

• **Fig. 12.13** Prescription Options for Nicotine Cessation

Smoking Cessation

There are many OTC nicotine replacement products on the market, which we'll cover in another chapter. Here, we'll focus on two tablets used by prescription that help patients quit smoking: **bupropion** (**Wellbutrin, Zyban***), an atypical antidepressant, and **varenicline** (**Chantix**), a partial nicotinic receptor agonist (Table 12.4, Fig. 12.13).

Bupropion (Wellbutrin, Zyban*) was first marketed as **Wellbutrin**, an atypical antidepressant, one that didn't fit into the SSRIs, SNRIs, TCAs, or MAOIs. We're not necessarily sure how it works. However, reports must have come in that patients stopped smoking while taking it; thus, the company repackaged the drug with the new brand name **Zyban***, to put a "ban" on smoking. The sustained release (SR) form is the only one approved for smoking because it lasts much longer. There is some risk with this medication, especially in patients with a history of seizures, because it can lower the seizure threshold, making an epileptic event more likely. Bupropion works to reduce the discomfort of withdrawal symptoms, such as anxiety, irritability, and so forth (Fig. 12.14).

Nicotine Cessation – Bupropion

Bupropion sustained-release (Zyban*)
• Only SR formulation approved for smoking cessation

Atypical antidepressant – exact mechanism is unknown

Decreases the urge to smoke

Reduces withdrawal symptoms
• Anxiety, irritability, etc.

Adverse drug reactions

> Insomnia
> Agitation
> Dry mouth
> Headache

• **Fig. 12.14** Nicotine Cessation—Bupropion

Nicotine Cessation – Varenicline

Varenicline (Chantix)

Partial nicotinic receptor agonist
• Prevents withdrawal symptoms
• Blocks nicotine reward pathway

Most effective medication for smoking cessation

Adverse drug reactions

> Nausea
> Insomnia
> Abnormal dreams
> Headache
> Skin rash

Nausea ADR is dose-dependent (30–40% of patients)

• **Fig. 12.15** Nicotine Cessation—Varenicline

Varenicline (Chantix), another smoking cessation medication, has caused distressing dreams, suicidal thoughts, and other adverse effects, such as insomnia, nausea, headache, and skin rash (Fig. 12.15). One way to think of what varenicline does is to say, "With **varenicline**, 'I'm vary incline ta quit.'" It blocks the pathway that rewards someone for smoking; quitting in a few days is not unheard of.

Dopamine and Norepinephrine Reuptake Inhibitor Smoking Cessation Aid

Bupropion (Zyban*) is a dopamine and norepinephrine reuptake inhibitor smoking cessation aid.

Indications: We can use Zyban* for smoking cessation. Other forms of bupropion (Wellbutrin, Aplenzin) can prevent seasonal affective disorder and treat MDD.

Contraindications: Do not use bupropion in anyone with a history of seizures, anorexia, or bulimia. If someone

TABLE 12.5   Benzodiazepines—Classes, Dosages, and Adverse Effects

Generic (Brand)	Drug Class	Dosage	Adverse Effects
Alprazolam (Xanax)	Benzodiazepine	IR: 2–6 mg daily in 3–4 divided doses. Start at 0.25 mg 3–4 times daily.	Drowsiness, fatigue, sedation
Diazepam (Valium)	Benzodiazepine, anticonvulsant	2–10 mg every 3–6 hours as needed, max 40 mg daily	Drowsiness
Lorazepam (Ativan)	Benzodiazepine, anticonvulsant	0.5–2 mg every 4–6 hours as needed, max 10 mg/day	Drowsiness, sedation, agitation (paradoxical)
Midazolam (Versed*)	Benzodiazepine, anticonvulsant	Intranasal: 0.1 mg/kg IM: 0.07–0.08 mg/kg IV: Start at 0.5–2 mg every 2–3 minutes until effective (usually 2.5–5 mg total)	Slow breathing, shallow breathing

IM, Intramuscular; *IR*, immediate release; *IV*, intravenous.

has abruptly stopped a sedative drug such as benzodiazepines or alcohol, do not use bupropion. Do not use with linezolid, IV methylene blue, or within 2 weeks of taking an MAOI. If allergic to any component of bupropion, do not use it.

Adverse reactions: Insomnia, headache, weight loss, and agitation are common adverse reactions.

Patient education and care: Start taking bupropion 1 week before your quit date. Bupropion may cause mood changes such as anger, fury, and agitation. It may also cause thoughts of suicide or murder. If any of these changes happen, tell your doctor. Do not stop taking this drug suddenly. Follow instructions from your doctor on how to slowly stop the drug. Avoid alcohol.

SCENARIO 12.4. THE DEPRESSED SMOKER

A depressed patient wants to quit smoking. However, he is worried about being anxious and irritable all the time. Of varenicline and bupropion, which would be the best choice?

Answer: As bupropion is both an antidepressant and smoking cessation aid, this might be the better choice, allowing the patient to take one medicine instead of two. The bupropion will help with the anxiety and irritability as well.

Smoking Cessation Aid, Partial Nicotine Agonist

Varenicline (Chantix) is a partial nicotine agonist used for smoking cessation.

Indications: We can use varenicline as a smoking cessation aid.

Contraindications: Do not use varenicline if allergic to any component of the drug.

Adverse reactions: Nightmares, trouble sleeping, and headache are common adverse effects of varenicline.

Patient education and care: You may choose a fixed, flexible, or gradual quit date when taking Chantix. Chantix may cause mood changes, anger, anxiety, or even thoughts of suicide or murder. Tell your doctor immediately if this happens to you.

Sedative-Hypnotics – Benzodiazepines

C**lonazepam** (Klonopin)
A**lprazolam** (Xanax)
L**orazepam** (Ativan)
M**idazolam** (Versed*)

Indications: Anxiety, panic disorder, insomnia, sedation, anesthesia premedication seizures	Adverse drug reactions: Drowsiness, dizziness, confusion, CNS depression

• **Fig. 12.16** Sedative-Hypnotics—Benzodiazepines

Benzodiazepines

Benzodiazepines relieve anxiety, insomnia, and muscle spasms as their primary functionality but are also available for anesthesia premedication and seizures. Like the TCAs, benzodiazepines get their name from their chemical structure: a benzene ring and a diazepine ring combination. Because benzodiazepine has many syllables, most people call them benzos.

Examples include **clonazepam (Klonopin), alprazolam (Xanax), lorazepam (Ativan)**, and **midazolam (Versed*)**. By taking the first letters of each of those, one can spell the word CALM as a mnemonic, which is what benzodiazepines do. Benzodiazepines are notorious for causing drowsiness and dizziness. They may also cause confusion and CNS depression. Watch for combinations with opioids (Table 12.5, Fig. 12.16).

Note that benzodiazepines have similar generic suffixes: -azolam and -azepam. Benzos replaced barbiturates as a sleep aid because barbiturates can cause respiratory depression. A student remembered this by thinking of barbiturates (barbs) as literal barbs on razor wire fences that puncture lungs.

In looking at the specific medications, we want to first see how one might use a benzodiazepine for anxiety for example. First, a patient might try an SSRI, but if it does not work, then the prescriber might add a benzo after a month or month and a half. In situations where the person might make a presentation every other week or so, it would make little sense to put that patient on a daily medication when a single benzodiazepine dose would do (Fig. 12.17).

Midazolam (Versed*) is an IV benzodiazepine that has a special use in that it can cause anterograde amnesia. Just as your *ante*brachium is your forearm, and the *ante* is the money poker players put out before the dealer deals, *ante*rograde amnesia is the inability to form memories.

Benzodiazepines

Alprazolam (Xanax), diazepam (Valium), lorazepam (Ativan), and midazolam (Versed*) are benzodiazepines.

Indications: Alprazolam, diazepam, and lorazepam treat anxiety disorders. We can use midazolam to stop seizures and for sedation during procedures. Lorazepam injection and diazepam can treat seizures as well. Additionally, diazepam can treat alcohol withdrawal syndrome and muscle spasms.

Contraindications: Do not use benzodiazepines with acute narrow-angle glaucoma. Diazepam should not be used with untreated open-angle glaucoma. Alprazolam interacts with strong CYP3A4 inhibitors and midazolam with protease inhibitors. Be sure to look up which ages may receive which drug and where injections can be administered, as these vary among benzodiazepines. Do not use if allergic

to any component of the drug or another benzodiazepine. Diazepam and alprazolam should not be used with sleep apnea and lorazepam should be avoided during severe breathing problems unless it's for intubation.

Adverse effects: Drowsiness and sedation are common adverse effects. Midazolam especially may cause slowed breathing.

Patient education and care: Benzodiazepines can be habit forming. Therefore, be sure to take them as prescribed and not any longer than necessary. If you have taken them for a long time, do not stop abruptly. Talk to your doctor about how to slowly stop the drug. Use caution when taking benzodiazepines with opioids and look out for dangerously slowed breathing.

SCENARIO 12.5. THE NERVOUS PUBLIC SPEAKER

A businesswoman wants to calm her nerves before a presentation. She's currently on an SSRI medication, fluoxetine, for her depression, but has still experienced a few instances where her nerves made it impossible for her to present in front of others. Would alprazolam or midazolam be more appropriate for her to take?

Answer: As midazolam causes anterograde amnesia and is an IV form, this would be a poor choice. Rather, a tablet like alprazolam, which can be broken into parts for smaller doses, might take enough anxiety away to allow her to perform her job.

ADHD Medications

ADHD stimulants calm a patient who has a hyperactive mind and/or body without a sedative effect. In an ADHD brain, there is more activity in the prefrontal cortex than in a normal brain, causing difficulty with planning, problem solving, short-term memory, and, sometimes, behavior (Table 12.6, Fig. 12.18).

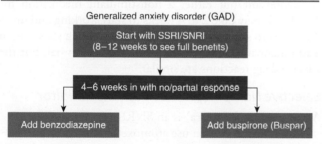

Generalized Anxiety Disorder – Treatment

• **Fig. 12.17** Treatment for Generalized Anxiety Disorder

TABLE 12.6 ADHD Medications—Classes, Dosages, and Adverse Effects

Generic (Brand)	Drug Class	Dosage	Adverse Effects
Methylphenidate (Ritalin, Concerta)	CNS stimulant	ER: Begin at 18–36 mg daily, may increase to max 72 mg daily	Decreased appetite, insomnia, irritability, headache
Dexmethylphenidate (Focalin)	CNS stimulant	ER: Begin at 10 mg daily, may increase to max 40 mg daily	Headache, decreased appetite, insomnia, anxiety
Dextroamphetamine and amphetamine (Adderall)	CNS stimulant	ER: Begin at 10–20 mg daily, may increase to max 40–60 mg daily	Decreased appetite, hypertension, headache, insomnia
Atomoxetine (Strattera)	Selective norepinephrine reuptake inhibitor	Begin at 40 mg daily, may increase to max 100 mg daily	Nausea, decreased appetite, headache, sweating, insomnia, erectile dysfunction

CNS, Central nervous system; *ER*, extended release.

ADHD – Overview

Attention Deficit Hyperactivity Disorder (ADHD)

Prefrontal Cortex
- Planning
- Problem solving
- Short-term memory
- Behavior

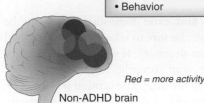
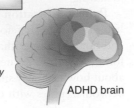

Red = more activity

Non-ADHD brain   ADHD brain

• **Fig. 12.18** Attention Deficit Hyperactivity Disorder (ADHD)—Overview

ADHD – Stimulants

Methylphenidate (Ritalin, Concerta) • 50:50 mix of levo- and dextro- isomers **Dexmethylphenidate (Focalin)** • All dextro- [active] isomer Available as immediate-release and extended-release versions	Adverse drug reactions • Weight loss • Growth suppression • Increased heart rate, BP • Psychosis • Withdrawal (if stopped)

• **Fig. 12.19** Attention Deficit Hyperactivity Disorder (ADHD)—Stimulants

Stimulant—Schedule II

Dexmethylphenidate (Focalin) and **methylphenidate (Concerta)** have the same root, **methylphenidate**. In chemistry, compounds direct plane-polarized light to either the left or the right. These terms are "d" or "(+)" for dextrorotatory compounds rotating plane-polarized light clockwise to the right. Or, one uses "l" or "(-)" for levorotatory compounds rotating plane-polarized light counterclockwise to the left. **Dexmethylphenidate** should be more effective, last longer, and have fewer side effects than methylphenidate because it is the sole active form (Fig. 12.19).

CNS Stimulant

Dextroamphetamine and amphetamine (Adderall), methylphenidate (Ritalin, Concerta), and dexmethylphenidate (Focalin) are CNS stimulants.

Indications: We can use these CNS stimulants for ADHD. Methylphenidate and dextroamphetamine and amphetamine can be used for narcolepsy as well.

Contraindications: These medications should not be used within 14 days of an MAOI or with hypersensitivity to any drug component. Some CNS stimulants should not be used with hypertension, heart disease, glaucoma, anxiety, or a history of drug abuse.

Adverse effects: Insomnia, headache, irritability, and decreased appetite are common adverse effects of CNS stimulants.

Patient education and care: This medication has the potential for abuse. Make sure to take it exactly as directed

ADHD – Nonstimulants

Atomoxetine (Strattera)

Selective norepinephrine reuptake inhibitor with no dopamine activity

2–4 weeks to see effects, up to 12 for full benefits

Less effective than stimulants but no abuse potential

Adverse drug reactions same as stimulants

• **Fig. 12.20** Attention Deficit Hyperactivity Disorder (ADHD)—Nonstimulants

and do not share your pills. Do not drink while on this medication.

Nonstimulant—Nonscheduled

Atomoxetine (Strattera) is a nonstimulant medication. Because there is no potential for abuse, it does not carry a Drug Enforcement Agency (DEA) schedule. It is *not* an SSRI, like **fluoxetine**, even though it ends in -oxetine. Side effects might include weight loss, growth suppression, increased blood pressure, psychosis very similar to schizophrenic symptoms, and withdrawal if stopped (Fig. 12.20).

Note that the -oxetine stem here is also not an SSRI antidepressant but rather a nonstimulant medication for ADHD. It may take 2 to 4 weeks to start working and up to 3 months to see the full benefit, which is much slower than a stimulant medicine. There is no abuse potential, but the adverse drug reactions are similar.

Selective Norepinephrine Reuptake Inhibitor

Atomoxetine (Strattera) is an SNRI.

Indications: We can use atomoxetine for ADHD.

Contraindications: Do not use atomoxetine within 14 days of an MAOI. It should also be avoided in anyone with heart disease, as it raises blood pressure.

Adverse effects: Dry mouth, decreased appetite, and headache are common adverse effects.

Patient education and care: Get up from sitting and reclining slowly to avoid dizziness. Talk to your doctor before using drugs that raise blood pressure, such as ibuprofen, cold medicine, and diet pills.

SCENARIO 12.6. THE NEW STUDENT

A student diagnosed with ADHD has previously been on a stimulant medication and is taking a break from the medicine while school is out. Her parents want her on a nonstimulant for the fall semester and it's the middle of summer. When should this student start taking atomoxetine?

Answer: Since this is a trial, it would likely need to start at least 2 to 4 weeks before school starts, but maybe a little sooner for the full effect.

TABLE 12.7 Bipolar Disorder Medications—Classes, Dosages, and Adverse Effects

Generic (Brand)	Drug Class	Dosage	Adverse Effects
Lithium (Lithobid)	Antimanic agent	Start at 600–900 mg daily in 2–3 divided doses May increase to 900 mg–1.8 g daily	Hypothyroidism
Risperidone (Risperdal)	Antimanic agent, second-generation antipsychotic	4–6 mg daily Begin at 1–3 mg/day and increase Max 8 mg daily	Sedation, drowsiness, hyperprolactinemia

Bipolar Disorder – Lithium

Lithium (Lithobid)

Mechanism for helping is unknown but possibly affects cell energy metabolism to protect neurons

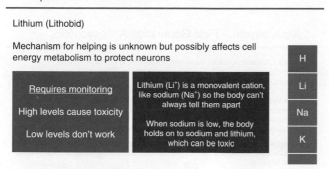

Requires monitoring

High levels cause toxicity

Low levels don't work

Lithium (Li⁺) is a monovalent cation, like sodium (Na⁺) so the body can't always tell them apart

When sodium is low, the body holds on to sodium and lithium, which can be toxic

H
Li
Na
K

• **Fig. 12.21** Bipolar Disorder—Lithium

Bipolar Disorder

Mood stabilizers such as **lithium** are especially likely to cause electrolyte imbalances. If you look at the periodic table, you see that lithium (Li) and sodium (Na) are in the same group (the alkali metals) and both have a +1 charge as an ion. Because of this similarity, what happens to sodium will happen to **lithium**, causing either a toxic or subtherapeutic state if too much **lithium** is retained or excreted, respectively. Other meds, like **risperidone**, can help control certain symptoms of the disease until the **lithium** level is correct (Table 12.7).

Simple Salt

Lithium (Lithobid) sits in the same group on the periodic table of elements as the Latin *Natrium* (Na), commonly known as the chemical element sodium. The body has trouble telling the difference between lithium and sodium, and too much or too little salt can wreak havoc on **lithium** levels (Fig. 12.21). A way to remember this is the saying, "Where the salt goeth, the **lithium** goeth."

Antimanic Agents

Lithium (Lithobid) is an antimanic agent.

Indications: We can use lithium for bipolar disorder.

Contraindications: Do not use lithium with diuretics, kidney disease, if severely dehydrated, or with low sodium.

Adverse effects: Hypothyroidism, or low thyroid hormone levels, is a common adverse effect of lithium.

Patient education and care: Too much lithium in your system can be fatal. Do not take more than prescribed and

get levels checked as advised by your doctor. Maintain hydration while taking lithium, especially if you have been sweating. Tell your doctor if you have fever, vomiting, or diarrhea. This can dangerously increase levels of lithium. Tell your doctor if you plan on decreasing salt in your diet.

SCENARIO 12.7. THE RUNNER

A patient on lithium states that he is a runner and is excited to complete a full marathon in a very warm state. However, you are concerned that he will sweat out a significant amount of sodium during the race. What will the body try to do to sodium during the race and what will happen to his lithium levels?

Answer: The body will try to conserve or hold on to sodium and at the same time hold on to the lithium, possibly creating a toxicity with this medication.

Schizophrenia

We break schizophrenia medication classification into typical or conventional (first-generation) or atypical (second-generation). We further divide the typical antipsychotics **chlorpromazine (Thorazine*)** and **haloperidol (Haldol)** into low potency and high potency, respectively. Atypical antipsychotics such as **quetiapine (Seroquel)** and **risperidone (Risperdal)** cause fewer extrapyramidal symptoms but have more negative metabolic effects such as weight gain, diabetes, and hyperlipidemia. Extrapyramidal symptoms are movement disorders associated with antipsychotics (Table 12.8, Fig. 12.22).

While these two antipsychotics have the same therapeutic effects, their side effect profiles are different. Low-potency drugs such as **chlorpromazine** cause more sedation but fewer extrapyramidal symptoms. High-potency drugs such as **haloperidol** cause more extrapyramidal symptoms but less sedation. We prescribe typical antipsychotics for symptoms such as delusions, hallucinations and paranoia.

There are four primary movement disorders in extrapyramidal symptoms (EPS).

1. Acute dystonia—spasms of the back, face, neck, and tongue
2. Parkinsonism—shares symptoms with Parkinson disease (impaired speech, muscle stiffness, slow movement, and visible tremors)
3. Akathisia—restlessness

TABLE 12.8   Drugs for Schizophrenia, Classes, Dosages, and Adverse Effects

Generic (Brand)	Drug Class	Dosage	Adverse Effects
Haloperidol	First-generation antipsychotic	Begin with 2–10 mg/day, then increase to usual dose of 2–20 mg/day	Fatigue, anxiety, constipation, extrapyramidal reaction
Chlorpromazine	First-generation antipsychotic	200–800 mg daily in 2–4 divided doses. Start with 30 mg daily and titrate to effect.	Constipation, dry mouth, fatigue, extrapyramidal reaction
Quetiapine (Seroquel)	Second-generation antipsychotic	Initial: 25 mg twice daily and increase to 400–800 mg/day. Lower doses are needed for acute therapy.	Dry mouth, weight gain, increased blood pressure, increased blood sugar, increased cholesterol

Neuropsych – Antipsychotics

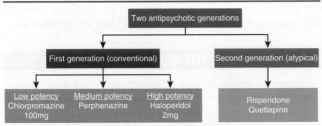

• **Fig. 12.22** Antipsychotics—Generations

4. Tardive dyskinesia—a late onset of involuntary facial and jaw movements that is often a permanent movement disorder

First-Generation Antipsychotic (FGA) Low Potency

Chlorpromazine (Thorazine*) was the first antipsychotic. While it carries side effects, it represented a new treatment option for schizophrenic patients. Generational classifications are especially important in antipsychotics because of differences in both side effects and effects on positive versus negative symptoms.

First-Generation Antipsychotic High Potency

Haloperidol (Haldol)—many think of the "halo" in *halo-**peridol** to remember that this is high potency (Fig. 12.23).

First-Generation Antipsychotics

Haloperidol and **chlorpromazine** are first-generation antipsychotics.

Indications: We can use haloperidol and chlorpromazine for schizophrenia, behavioral disorders, and hyperactivity. Haloperidol can also be used to manage tics in Tourette syndrome. Chlorpromazine can also be used for bipolar disorder, nausea and vomiting, intractable hiccups, as well as other indications.

Contraindications: Do not use haloperidol in a patient with Parkinson disease, dementia with Lewy bodies, with severe CNS depression, or coma. Do not use

Neuropsych – First-Generation Antipsychotics

Can block CNS acetylcholine, dopamine, histamine, and norepinephrine. Blocking dopamine can lead to extrapyramidal effects (EPS) which can be permanent. **EPS examples include:**

1. Acute dystonia – dys + tonia = bad + muscles (spasms back, face, neck, tongue)
2. Parkinsonism – looks like Parkinson disease, but shares symptoms
3. Akathisia – literally "dance" = restlessness. NOT akinesia, lack of movement
4. Tardive dyskinesia – late + bad + movement = choreoathetoid movements

Drug name	Potency	Sedation	EPS potential
Chlorpromazine (Thorazine*)	Low	High	Moderate
Haloperidol (Haldol)	High	Low	Very high

• **Fig. 12.23** First-Generation Antipsychotics

chlorpromazine in patients who are in a coma or using large doses of depressants, such as alcohol, opioids, and barbiturates.

Adverse reactions: Extrapyramidal side effects and parkinsonism are common adverse effects of first-generation antipsychotics.

Patient education and care: Do not drive until you know how these medications affect you. Get in contact with your physician immediately if you develop a fever and muscle stiffness or trouble controlling your movements.

Second-Generation Antipsychotics (SGA; Atypical Antipsychotics)

The improvement from the first generation to the second came in a lower incidence of extrapyramidal symptoms (EPS), but with added metabolic symptoms such as diabetes, dyslipidemia, and weight gain.

Risperidone (Risperdal)—note that the stem -peridol from **halo*peridol*** and the stem -peridone from **ris*peridone*** are similar. This can help you remember that both of these are antipsychotics. In this drug, there is a moderate blocking of dopamine and moderate incidence of EPS.

Que*tiapine* (Seroquel)—if you rearrange the first 5 letters in **quetiapine**, you get the word "quiet," as in quieting the voices. We can expect a low to moderate dopamine blockade and very low EPS (Fig. 12.24).

Second-Generation Antipsychotics

Risperidone (Risperdal) and quetiapine (Seroquel) are second-generation antipsychotics.

Indications: We can use risperidone and quetiapine to treat schizophrenia and bipolar disorder. Risperidone also treats irritability from autism and quetiapine also treats MDD.

Contraindications: Do not take quetiapine or risperidone if allergic to any component of the drug or similar drugs.

Adverse effects: Risperidone causes sedation and hyperprolactinemia. Dry mouth, weight gain, increased blood pressure, increased blood sugar, and increased cholesterol are common adverse effects of quetiapine.

Patient education and care: Quetiapine can cause suicidal thoughts, which should be reported to your doctor immediately. Do not drive until you know how you are affected by this drug.

SCENARIO 12.8. THE DIABETIC

A diabetic patient has difficulty controlling his blood sugar levels. He starts on a new medication for newly diagnosed schizophrenia, a concomitant condition. Do you expect the prescriber will give a first- or second-generation antipsychotic?

Answer: With the metabolic effects of the second-generation medicines, it's more likely that the prescriber will give a first-generation antipsychotic, which will have a minimal effect on the patient's blood sugar.

Neuropsych – Second-Generation Antipsychotics

Block dopamine, receptors and strongly block 5-hydroxytryptamine (5-HT, serotonin) receptors with less D_2 affinity; a lower EPS risk results. However, this generation is known for metabolic symptoms:
1) Diabetes
2) Dyslipidemia
3) Weight gain

Drug name	D_2 blockade	5-HT blockade	Sedation	*EPS*
Risperidone (Risperdal)	Moderate	High	Low	*Moderate*
Quetiapine (seroquel)	Low-moderate	High	Moderate	*Very low*

Both also produce histamine blockade

• **Fig. 12.24** Second-Generation Antipsychotics

Antiepileptics

The traditional antiepileptics **carbamazepine (Tegretol)**, **divalproex (Depakote)**, and **phenytoin (Dilantin)** have been around for a long time. Thus, we usually know what to expect with their use (Table 12.9).

We may have less experience with the newer antiepileptics, such as **gabapentin (Neurontin)** and **pregabalin (Lyrica)**, but they are often just as effective as the traditional drugs. Neurologists try various medications in a patient until one drug finally relieves the seizure symptoms.

Traditional Antiepileptics

Carbamazepine (Tegretol) works by inhibiting sodium channels and stopping action potential. With this drug, we are especially worried about bone marrow suppression, teratogenicity (damage to the fetus), and increased levels from grapefruit juice (Fig. 12.25).

Divalproex (Depakote) has "val" in its name. While you can find "val" in many medication names, it is helpful to think of the "val" in **di*val*proex** and its similarity with the "vul" in con*vul*sions. I know it's a stretch. One student thought of **divalproex** as a *pro* at *ex*tracting seizures. This drug works

Epilepsy – Carbamazepine

Carbamazepine (Tegretol)

- Inhibits sodium channels on hyperactive neurons
  - Prevents sodium from entering neuron, stopping action potential
- Serious drug reactions:

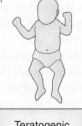
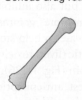

Bone marrow suppression	Teratogenic	Grapefruit juice increases levels

• **Fig. 12.25** Epilepsy—Carbamazepine

TABLE 12.9 Antiepileptics—Classes, Dosages, and Adverse Effects

Generic (Brand)	Drug Class	Dosage	Adverse Effects
Carbamazepine (Tegretol)	Anticonvulsant	2–3 mg/kg/day up to 400 mg daily	Dizziness, drowsiness nausea
Divalproex (Depakote)	Anticonvulsant, histone deacetylase inhibitor	10–15 mg/kg/day increased to response. Max 60 mg/kg/day.	Headache, drowsiness, dizziness, nausea
Phenytoin (Dilantin)	Anticonvulsant, hydantoin	Maintenance: 100 mg 3–4 times daily, adjust based on response and levels	Headache, anxiety, change in taste, nausea
Gabapentin (Neurontin)	Anticonvulsant, GABA analog	300–600 mg 3 times daily	Nausea, vomiting, diarrhea, dry mouth
Pregabalin (Lyrica)	Anticonvulsant, GABA analog	Initial: 150 mg in 2–3 divided doses, then increase to up to 600 mg daily	Dizziness, drowsiness, headache, fatigue

GABA, Gamma-amino-butyric-acid.

Epilepsy – Divalproex

Divalproex (Depakote)
- Works in three ways:
  1. Inhibits sodium channels on hyperactive neurons (like carbamazepine)
  2. Inhibits calcium influx into neurons
  3. Promotes GABA activity and release
- Serious adverse drug reactions:

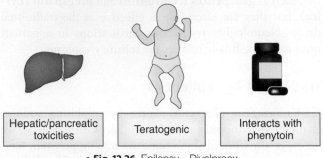

| Hepatic/pancreatic toxicities | Teratogenic | Interacts with phenytoin |

• **Fig. 12.26** Epilepsy—Divalproex

Epilepsy – Phenytoin

Phenytoin (Dilantin)

Inhibits sodium channels on hyperactive neurons
- Prevents sodium from entering neuron, stopping action potential
- Same as carbamazepine

Requires lots of monitoring
- Small dose increases can cause toxicities
- Small dose decreases can cause therapy failure

• **Fig. 12.27** Epilepsy—Phenytoin

on sodium channels such as carbamazepine but also inhibits calcium influx to the neurons. Finally, it promotes gamma-amino-butyric-acid (GABA) activity and release to help stop seizures. Some adverse reactions include hepatic (liver) toxicity, teratogenicity, and interactions with phenytoin (Fig. 12.26).

Pheny*toin* (Dilantin) is one of the best antiepileptics available but has a narrow therapeutic window. This means that a dose a little too high or a little too low can cause significant problems. Like carbamazepine, it works to inhibit sodium channels. Of the traditional antiepileptics, it is the least teratogenic, though there are newer antiepileptics with less teratogenicity risk (Fig. 12.27).

Newer Antiepileptics

*Gab*apentin (Neurontin) is an adjunct therapy for epilepsy, as is pregabalin, its metabolite. The "gab" stem is a little misleading. Neither *gab*apentin nor pre*gab*alin directly affect GABA receptors. However, both having the same stem helps set a memory device for the newer antiepileptics. Common adverse reactions we expect include drowsiness, blurry vision, and peripheral edema (Fig. 12.28).

Anticonvulsants

Carbamazepine (Tegretol), valproic acid (Depakote), phenytoin (Dilantin), and **gabapentin (Neurontin)** are antiepileptics.

Epilepsy – Gabapentin & Pregabalin

Gabapentin (Neurontin)
Pregabalin (Lyrica)

Pregabalin is a metabolite of gabapentin

Both used as adjunct therapies for epilepsies

Common adverse drug reactions are drowsiness, blurry vision, peripheral edema

• **Fig. 12.28** Epilepsy—Gabapentin and Pregabalin

Indications: We can use antiepileptics to treat seizures. Gabapentin can also treat nerve pain. Phenytoin can treat status epilepticus. Valproic acid can be used for bipolar disorder and to prevent migraines. Carbamazepine can also be used for nerve pain and bipolar disorder.

Contraindications: Do not use antiepileptics if allergic to any component of the drug or similar drugs. Be sure to check for interactions as certain antiepileptics should not be used with various medications. Valproic acid should not be used with mitochondrial disorders or liver disease. Do not use phenytoin injection with certain heart arrhythmias.

Adverse effects: Dizziness, drowsiness, headache, and nausea are common adverse effects of antiepileptics.

Patient education and care: Phenytoin and carbamazepine may cause hormonal birth control to be less effective. Use a backup method while on therapy. Watch out for liver problems with valproic acid. This might look like yellowing skin, dark urine, stomach pain, and light stool.

SCENARIO 12.9. PREGNANCY AND SEIZURES

A patient is newly diagnosed with seizures but has just learned she is pregnant. Which of carbamazepine, divalproex, or phenytoin should she take if all help the type of seizure she has?

Answer: On a spectrum of teratogenicity, or possible damage to the fetus, phenytoin is the least teratogenic and carbamazepine and divalproex are the most.

Parkinson Disease, Alzheimer Disease, and Motion Sickness

Parkinson Disease

The goal in treating Parkinson disease is to help the patient regain better movement and eliminate movement disorders. Common concerns in the Parkinson patient include postural instability, tremors, rigidity, bradykinesia, and feet shuffling (Fig. 12.29).

Ultimately, there is a deficiency of dopamine, which acts as an accelerator to movement. GABA works as the brake. However, with low dopamine and elevated acetylcholine, the system is like a stoplight that keeps switching back and forth between red and green without pausing at yellow (Fig. 12.30).

Levodopa/carbidopa (Sinemet) for Parkinson disease works to restore *dopa*mine, a neurotransmitter responsible for proper motor function that is seriously depleted by the disease.

Sele*giline* (Eldepryl) prevents monoamine oxidase B from breaking down the dopamine, retaining more to help the Parkinson patient.

Either way, more dopamine levels in the brain is the goal. However, there is a problem in that dopamine, as a neurotransmitter, cannot cross the blood-brain barrier . The solution is to give a precursor such as levodopa, which can cross the blood-brain barrier and then convert into dopamine in the brain (Fig. 12.31).

Even after getting levodopa to the brain, the problem is not yet solved. The body readily degrades levodopa in the periphery. To keep this from happening, carbidopa works as a decoy for the body to degrade while more levodopa makes it to the brain. **Carbidopa** doesn't actually have an antiparkinsonian effect, but it reduces the degradation of **levodopa** so that more is available to the patient from a smaller dose. Then, the increased dopamine can work optimally to improve motor function.

MAOI Anti-Parkinson Agent

Selegiline (Eldepryl) is an MAOI anti-Parkinson agent.

Parkinson Disease – Presentation

Low dopamine/high acetylcholine result in:

Postural impairment

Tremors

Overall rigidity of limbs and body

Bradykinesia & feet shuffling

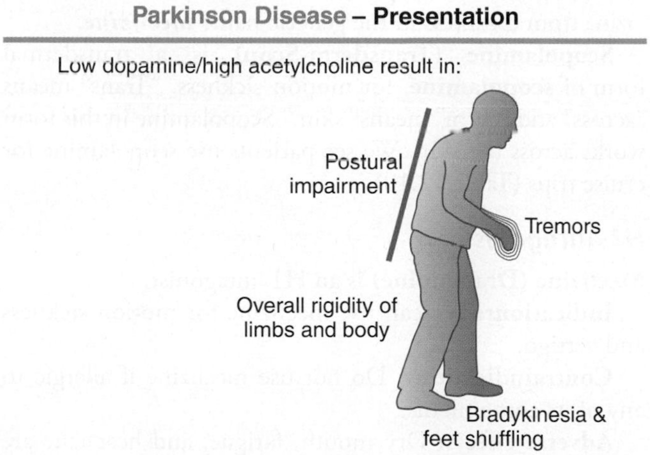

• **Fig. 12.29** Parkinson Disease—Presentation

Indications: We can use selegiline as an add-on to Sinemet to treat Parkinson disease. Selegiline transdermal patches can treat depression.

Contraindications: Selegiline interacts with multiple prescription and OTC medications. Be sure to check for interactions with the patient's full medication list.

Adverse effects: Nausea, dizziness, insomnia, and headache are the most common adverse effects of selegiline.

Patient education and care: Avoid foods such as cheese and red wine, which can cause very high blood pressure. Avoid alcohol while on this therapy. Rise slowly to avoid dizziness upon standing.

Anti-Parkinson Agent

Levodopa-carbidopa (Sinemet) is an anti-Parkinson agent.

Indications: We can use Sinemet for Parkinson disease.

Contraindications: Do not use Sinemet within 14 days of nonselective MAOIs. Do not use if allergic to any component of it.

Adverse reactions: Nightmares, fatigue, dry mouth, and insomnia are common adverse effects of Sinemet.

Patient education and care: You may feel Sinemet wearing off as it becomes time for your next dose. Let you doctor know if this bothers you. Rise slowly to prevent dizziness upon standing.

Alzheimer Disease

With Alzheimer disease especially, the patients *and* their caregivers desperately need your help. The patient has decreased acetylcholine levels and some hallmark anatomical issues, such as beta amyloid plaques and microtubules, that make it difficult for neurons to function properly (Fig. 12.32).

Parkinson Disease – Treatment

Goal: Restore dopamine levels in brain

Problem: Dopamine does not cross blood-brain barrier (BBB)

Solution: Give a dopamine precursor that does cross BBB

• **Fig. 12.31** Parkinson Disease (PD) —Treatment

Parkinson Disease – Pathology

Substantia nigra - gas and brake pedal for motor cortex of brain
Dopamine = accelerator
GABA = brake - inhibits smooth movement

Smooth movement

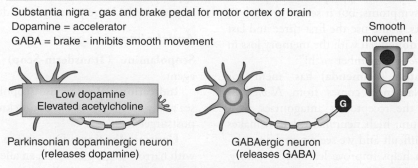

Low dopamine
Elevated acetylcholine

Parkinsonian dopaminergic neuron (releases dopamine)

GABAergic neuron (releases GABA)

• **Fig. 12.30** Parkinson Disease—Pathology

Alzheimer Disease – Pathology

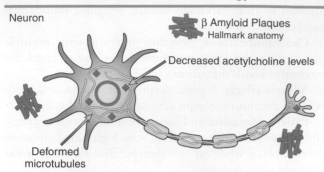

• **Fig. 12.32** Alzheimer Disease—Pathology

Alzheimer Disease – Donepezil

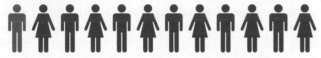

Donepezil (Aricept)

Mild-moderate symptoms
Cholinesterase inhibitor
• Prevents breakdown of acetylcholine, common neurotransmitter

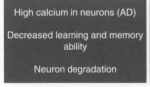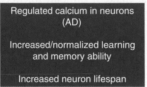

• **Fig. 12.33** Alzheimer Disease (AD)—Donepezil

Alzheimer Disease – Memantine

Memantine (Namenda)

NMDA receptor antagonist
• Regulates calcium levels in neurons by binding NMDA receptors

High calcium in neurons (AD)	Regulated calcium in neurons (AD)
Decreased learning and memory ability	Increased/normalized learning and memory ability
Neuron degradation	Increased neuron lifespan

• **Fig. 12.34** Alzheimer Disease (AD)—Memantine

Done*pezil* (**Aricept**) works to restore the neurotransmitter acetylcholine by reducing its breakdown by acetylcholinesterase (Fig. 12.33). Sometimes, we give a medicine that releases a neurotransmitter; in this case, we are preserving a neurotransmitter. Donepezil is appropriate for patients with mild to moderate symptoms, but it seems to work in only 1 out of 10 patients. Some use the first three and last three letters to associate **donepezil** with the memory loss in Alzheimer disease as "I *don*'t remember *zil*ch!"

The generic **memantine** (**Namenda**) has "mem" for *mem*ory. The brand **Namenda** comes from *N*-methyl-*D*-*a*spartate (**NMDA**), the receptor it antagonizes. This medicine regulates calcium; high neuronal calcium makes learning and memory difficult and we see neuron degradation. Regulated calcium helps improve learning, memory, and neuron lifespans (Fig. 12.34).

Acetylcholinesterase Inhibitor

Donepezil (Aricept) is an acetylcholinesterase inhibitor.

Indications: We can use donepezil for Alzheimer disease.

Contraindications: Do not use donepezil in anyone with an allergy to any component of the drug or drugs within the same class.

Adverse effects: Diarrhea, nausea, insomnia, and injury from faintingare common adverse effects of donepezil.

Patient education and care: Donepezil does not cure Alzheimer disease. Continue to see your doctor.

NMDA Antagonist

Memantine (Namenda) is an NMDA antagonist.

Indications: We can use memantine for moderate and severe Alzheimer disease.

Contraindications: Do not use memantine in anyone allergic to it or its components.

Adverse reactions: Dizziness, headache, diarrhea, and constipation are common adverse effects of memantine.

Patient education and care: Take with or without food.

Motion Sickness/Antivertigo

Meclizine (Dramamine) is an OTC antiemetic/motion sickness medicine. It also has a brand name **Antivert**, for *anti-vert*igo, which helps with memorization. You can see "izin" from d*izzin*ess in the generic name **mec***lizin*e.

Scopolamine (Transderm-Scop) is a transdermal form of **scopolamine**, for motion sickness. "Trans" means "across" and "derm" means "skin." Scopolamine in this form works across the skin. We see patients use scopolamine for cruise trips (Table 12.10).

H1 Antagonist

Meclizine (Dramamine) is an H1 antagonist.

Indications: We can use meclizine for motion sickness and vertigo.

Contraindications: Do not use meclizine if allergic to any of its components.

Adverse effects: Dry mouth, fatigue, and headache are common adverse effects of meclizine.

Patient education and care: Avoid driving until you know how meclizine affects you. Avoid alcohol during therapy. If you are over 65 years old, use meclizine with caution, as you may be more prone to its side effects.

Anticholinergic Agent

Scopolamine (Transderm-Scop) is an anticholinergic agent.

Indications: We can use scopolamine to prevent nausea and vomiting from motion sickness, postanesthesia, and postsurgery.

Contraindications: Do not use scopolamine in anyone with narrow-angle glaucoma, an allergy to any drug component, or an allergy to similar drugs.

TABLE 12.10 Medications for Parkinson Disease, Alzheimer Disease, and Motion Sickness—Classes, Dosages, and Adverse Effects

Generic (Brand)	Drug Class	Dosage	Adverse Effects
Carbidopa-levodopa (Sinemet)	Anti-Parkinson agent	Carbidopa 25 mg/levodopa 100 mg 3 times daily	Nightmares, fatigue, dry mouth, insomnia
Selegiline (Eldepryl)	Anti-Parkinson agent, MAOI	5 mg twice daily with breakfast and lunch along with carbidopa/levodopa	Nausea, dizziness, insomnia, headache
Donepezil (Aricept)	Acetylcholinesterase inhibitor (for Alzheimer)	5 mg daily, increase to 10 mg daily after 4–6 weeks Severe: 23 mg daily	Diarrhea, nausea, insomnia, injury from fainting
Memantadine (Namenda)	NMDA antagonist (for Alzheimer)	IR: 5 mg daily and titrate to 20 mg daily (> 5 mg in 2 divided doses) ER: 7 mg daily, and titrate to 28 mg daily	Dizziness, headache, diarrhea, constipation
Meclizine (Dramamine)	H1 antagonist (for motion sickness)	25–50 mg 1 hour before travel. May repeat in 24 hours.	Dry mouth, fatigue, headache
Scopolamine (Transderm Scop)	Anticholinergic agent (for motion sickness)	Apply 1 patch to hairless area 4 hours before event and every 3 days	Dry mouth, drowsiness, dizziness

ER, Extended release; *IR,* immediate release; *MAOI,* monoamine oxidase inhibitor; *NMDA,* N-methyl-D-aspartate.

Adverse effects: Dry mouth, drowsiness, and dizziness are common adverse effects of scopolamine.

Patient education and care: Do not drive until you know how scopolamine affects you. Avoid alcohol while using scopolamine. Use caution if you are over 65 years old, as you may be more prone to adverse effects.

SCENARIO 12.10. PARKINSON DISEASE SYMPTOMS

A caregiver believes a patient has Parkinson disease. What signs or symptoms might one expect from this patient?

Answer: A Parkinson patient might experience postural instability, tremors, rigidity, bradykinesia, and feet shuffling.

Summary

- Amide-type local anesthetics such as lidocaine are safer than ester types such as benzocaine because of allergenicity.
- Sedatives are meant to calm patients and hypnotics are meant to help a patient sleep. Often, the difference in effect comes from the dosage level. However, benzodiazepine-like drugs are often meant specifically for sleep.
- Antidepressants fall into five major categories: SSRIs, SNRIs, TCAs, MAOIs and atypical medications.
- We often name antidepressant classes by neurotransmitter (e.g., SSRIs such as fluoxetine), chemical shape (e.g., TCAs such as amitriptyline), or enzymatic effect (e.g., an MAOI such as isocarboxazid).
- Two primary therapeutic choices in smoking cessation are bupropion, an atypical antidepressant, and varenicline, a partial nicotinic receptor agonist.
- General therapeutic uses for benzodiazidines include treating anxiety, insomnia, and muscle spasms.

- We divide ADHD medications into two areas: DEA-controlled stimulants, such as methylphenidate, and nonstimulants, such as atomoxetine.
- Lithium is a simple salt that is often effective for bipolar disorder, but its similarity to sodium can lead to issues with salt intake.
- First-generation antipsychotics are often more likely to cause issues such as sedation and/or EPS. Second-generation antipsychotics have a lower incidence of EPS but a greater propensity for negative metabolic effects such as weight gain, diabetes, and hyperlipidemia.
- Traditional antiepileptics have a long and studied history of use with greater adverse effects, while newer antiepileptics have less data but fewer effects.
- Parkinson disease is a condition of low dopamine and elevated acetylcholine while Alzheimer disease patients have decreased acetylcholine levels. Treatments for both are meant to normalize the neurotransmitter levels.

Review Questions

1. A medication that ends in -caine is most likely a(n):
   a. Local anesthetic
   b. SSRI
   c. SNRI
   d. Benzodiazepine

2. Patients looking for medication over-the-counter to help them sleep might use:
   a. Acetaminophen/diphenhydramine
   b. Ramelteon
   c. Clonazepam
   d. Midazolam

3. In the morning, it would be appropriate for a patient to use which medication?
   a. Sertraline
   b. Ramelteon
   c. Zolpidem
   d. Eszopiclone

4. At night, one might expect which of the following medications to work as a "sleeping pill?"
   a. Escitalopram
   b. Zolpidem
   c. Citalopram
   d. Haloperidol

5. There are two primary medications to help patients quit smoking. One that may cause vivid dreams and works to block the reward smoking provides is:
   a. Varenicline
   b. Bupropion
   c. Lorazepam
   d. Citalopram

6. All of the following medicines would be appropriate if the patient were to get an SSRI for depression except:
   a. Atomoxetine
   b. Paroxetine
   c. Fluoxetine
   d. Citalopram

7. Which of the following represents a nonstimulant medication for ADHD?
   a. Atomoxetine
   b. Methylphenidate
   c. Dexmethylphenidate
   d. Midazolam

8. Which of the following represents a stimulant ADHD medication?
   a. Fluoxetine
   b. Methylphenidate
   c. Paroxetine
   d. Midazolam

9. While sodium is important in many drugs' mechanisms of action, dietary sodium is a special concern with which medication?
   a. Lithium
   b. Divalproex
   c. Phenytoin
   d. Carbamazepine

10. A medicine that does not directly affect the amount of dopamine in the brain but rather protects another medicine's path to the blood-brain barrier is:
    a. Carbidopa
    b. Citalopram
    c. Selegiline
    d. Levodopa

13

Cardiology

LEARNING OBJECTIVES

1. Discuss the management of cardiovascular conditions.
2. Describe the pathophysiology of common cardiovascular conditions.
3. Identify various medication classes in the therapeutic treatment of cardiovascular diseases.

4. Compare and contrast cardiovascular medicines.
5. Discuss the mechanisms of action, indications, drug interactions, and adverse effects of common cardiovascular medications.

Introduction

The word *cardiovascular* comes from "cardio," meaning heart, and "vascular," meaning vessels (in this case, arteries, veins, and capillaries that carry blood). The cardiovascular system, also called the circulatory system, is where the heart and vessels work together to perform many important tasks (Fig. 13.1). These include:

1. Transporting and distributing nutrients and oxygen to tissues.
2. Removing waste and products of metabolism.
3. Maintaining homeostasis or a balanced environment by managing the body's temperature, immune system, and communication through hormones.

Major Components of the Cardiovascular System

1. The heart—the pump that actively moves blood throughout the system
2. The blood—carries nutrients, including oxygen and waste.
3. The vessels—which we break into three categories:
   a. *Distribution vessels*—such as the high-pressure arteries that dole out blood to the various areas of the body
   b. *Exchange vessels*—the capillaries that move nutrients back and forth between tissues and the blood
   c. *Collection vessels*—veins that hold blood and return it to the heart (Fig. 13.2).

A common misconception is that arteries always carry oxygen and veins lack oxygen. However, this is not always true; the pulmonary artery has deoxygenated blood and the pulmonary vein has oxygenated blood. The better definition

is that an artery is a vessel that moves away from the heart and a vein is one that moves back to the heart.

The blood lands in various areas of the body, with the majority—over 80%—in the systemic circulation. The rest is in the pulmonary system, with the lungs (around 9%) and heart (around 7%). The blood contains four major components, including white blood cells that are important for the immune system, red blood cells for transport, platelets for clotting, and plasma.

Cardiac Output

An important calculation we should put to memory is that of cardiac output (Fig. 13.3). Knowing this equation helps us know what medicines will help or hurt a cardiac patient.

Cardiac Output (CO) = Heart Rate (HR) * Stroke Volume (SV)

One way to think about cardiac output is to think of blood flow from the heart. If output is too *low*, there is not enough blood flow to properly oxygenate the tissues, which can exacerbate cardiac disease. If output is too *high*, the heart may be trying to compensate for other issues.

Many medicines can raise or lower heart rate. We can see that if we raise heart rate on the right side of the equation, we will likely raise output on the left side. If we lower heart rate on the right side, we will likely lower output on the left. There are some exceptions in that if the heart beats so fast it cannot fill properly, as in an arrhythmia, the stroke volume is compromised and the output might actually go down.

Blood Pressure

One metric we often measure is blood pressure, using a pressure cuff (Fig. 13.4). The measurement of both systolic

---

* Brand discontinued, now available only as generic
† Naming conventions can vary between prescription and OTC formulations

Cardiovascular system – overview

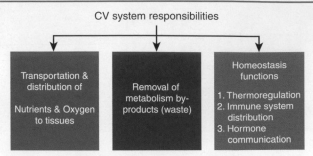

CV system responsibilities

| Transportation & distribution of Nutrients & Oxygen to tissues | Removal of metabolism by-products (waste) | Homeostasis functions 1. Thermoregulation 2. Immune system distribution 3. Hormone communication |

• **Fig. 13.1** Cardiovascular (CV) System Overview—CV System Responsibilities

Cardiovascular System – Overview

Made up of five different components

1. Pump (heart)
2. Blood
3. Distribution vessels (arteries)
4. Exchange vessels (capillaries)
5. Collection vessels (veins)

Lungs
4
5   Pulmonary circulation   3

1

5   3

Systemic circulation
4
Body

• **Fig. 13.2** Cardiovascular System Overview—5 components

Cardiovascular System – Cardiac Output

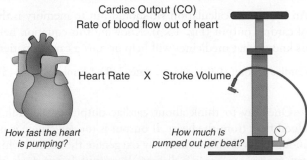

Cardiac Output (CO)
Rate of blood flow out of heart

Heart Rate   X   Stroke Volume

How fast the heart is pumping?   *How much is pumped out per beat?*

• **Fig. 13.3** Cardiovascular System—Cardiac Output

Cardiovascular System – Pressure

Arterial Pressure (Blood Pressure)
Pressure of the blood on the arterial walls

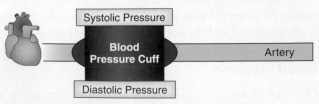

Systolic Pressure

Blood Pressure Cuff   Artery

Diastolic Pressure

• **Fig. 13.4** Cardiovascular System—Pressure

Kidneys – Tubule Transport System

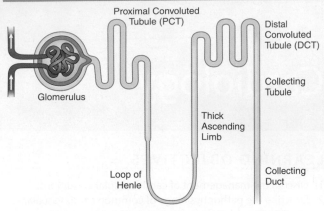

• **Fig. 13.5** Kidneys—Tubule Transport System (Part 1)

and diastolic pressures allows us to see how the cardiovascular system is working at a given time. Systolic pressure (the top number) measures the pressure during heart contraction. The diastolic blood pressure (the bottom number) measures the time between heart beats when the coronary arteries resupply the heart with blood.

SCENARIO 13.1. THE CARDIOVASCULAR SYSTEM

Your patient comes in for a cardiac stress test to see if he has heart failure. While doing the test, his heart rate increases. How will the increase in heart rate generally affect the patient's cardiac output?

Answer: The cardiac output will likely go up as the heart rate increases. What happens on the right of the CO = HR × SV calculation will usually happen on the left.

Diuretics

Diuretics are a class of medications that play a very important role in maintaining a hemodynamic balance in cardiovascular patients. First, however, let's discuss the kidneys and their three primary processes:

1. *Filtration*—provides a cleaning and filtering of extracellular fluids
2. *Reabsorption*—maintains acid-base balance and prevents electrolyte loss
3. *Active secretion*—removes wastes, in the process of urination

In the kidney, there are millions of nephrons, the kidney's base units. Inside the nephron, we have the glomerulus, a bed of capillaries, and afferent and efferent arterioles. Afferent is going in and efferent is going out. Compare efferent and the word "exit" to help you remember. The nephron's pressure is high at the glomerulus and lowers going through to the collecting duct. This fact matters because medicines work along this path, providing various levels of fluid loss or diuresis (Fig. 13.5).

The order of important structures in the nephron goes from the glomerulus to proximal convoluted tubule (PCT)

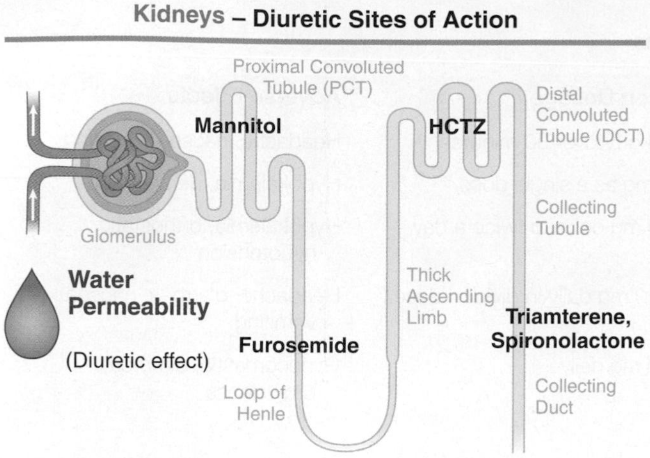

Kidneys – Diuretic Sites of Action

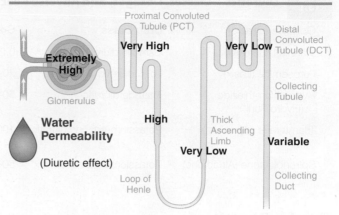

• **Fig. 13.6** Kidneys—Diuretic Sites of Action

Kidneys – Tubule Transport System

• **Fig. 13.7** Kidneys—Tubule Transport System (Part 2)

to the loop of Henle to the distal convoluted tubule (DCT) to the collecting duct.

The order of diuretics (Fig. 13.6) would then be:

1. Osmotic diuretics such as **mannitol (Osmitrol)** work by increasing osmotic pressure inside the lumen (tube) of the PCT. This action increases water diuresis and in turn, decreases blood volume and lowers blood pressure.
2. Loop diuretics such as **furosemide (Lasix)** inhibit sodium and chloride reabsorption in the ascending loop of Henle.
3. Thiazide diuretics such as **hydrochlorothiazide (Microzide*)** inhibit sodium and chloride resorption in the DCT.
4. Potassium-sparing diuretics such as **triamterene (Dyrenium)** and **spironolactone (Aldactone)** work at the collecting duct. They exchange sodium for potassium and inhibit potassium excretion, "sparing" potassium or keeping more of it in the body.

Picture a water slide. A lot of water flows at the top (the glomerulus). A trickle flows at the bottom (the collecting duct). Similarly, diuretics produce less diuresis as they continue down the water slide. The order from most to least diuresis is osmotic > loop > thiazide > potassium sparing (Fig. 13.7; Table 13.1).

Osmotic Diuretic

Mannitol (Osmitrol) is an osmotic diuretic that reduces intraocular and intracranial pressure, usually in an emergency. It acts on the PCT, preventing reabsorption of sodium and water, increasing urine volume. Adverse reactions can include dehydration, headache, potassium and sodium electrolyte imbalances, as well as nausea and vomiting. The brand name **Osmitrol** combines the class of medication, *osmo*tic, and adds that it helps con*trol* brain swelling.

Indications: Generally, we use osmotic diuretics for elevated cerebral or intraocular pressures, whether from trauma or disease. Also, they are used if the patient is in danger of acute renal failure.

Contraindications: Watch for patients who have conditions such as congestive heart failure (CHF), cranial hemorrhage, dehydration, or pulmonary congestion.

Adverse effects: Include nausea, vomiting, dry mouth, dehydration, tachycardia, and electrolyte imbalances.

Patient education and care: Watch for electrolyte and fluid imbalances by monitoring weight and intake and output ratios. In intravenous administration, watch for accidental extravasation or administration of the medicine in the surrounding tissues. Patients may need to increase their fluid intake to avoid dehydration and have ice chips to relieve immediate thirst.

Loop Diuretic

Furo*semide* (Lasix) is a loop diuretic named after the loop of Henle. It prevents sodium from being reabsorbed in the loop and the water follows the sodium's lead, staying in the tube and exiting as urine. Prescribers often use loop diuretics for edema. Hypokalemia (low potassium) and ototoxicity (damage to hearing) are potential side effects. The -semide stem indicates a furosemide-type loop diuretic. The brand name **Lasix** indicates it *la*sts *six* hours.

Indications: Most often used for hypertension and edema.

Contraindications: Watch for hypokalemia, anuria, and hypovolemia.

Adverse effects: May include diarrhea, nausea, ototoxicity presenting as tinnitus (ringing in the ears) or hearing loss, orthostatic hypotension, hyperglycemia, and electrolyte imbalances.

Patient education and care: Watch for electrolyte and fluid imbalances by monitoring weight and intake and output ratios and resulting blood pressure decrease. May need to add potassium supplementation but avoid taking at bedtime, as there is significant diuresis. Patients with diabetes mellitus may need to watch for hyperglycemia, an increase in blood sugar.

TABLE 13.1   **Diuretics—Classes, Dosages, and Adverse Reactions**

Generic (Brand)	Drug Class	Common Dosage	Adverse Effects
Mannitol (Osmitrol)	Osmotic diuretic	0.25 g/kg IV over 30 minutes	Headache, nausea, vomiting
Furosemide (Lasix)	Loop diuretic	20–80 mg as a single dose	Hypokalemia, dehydration
Hydrochlorothiazide (HydroDiuril*)	Thiazide diuretic	50–100 mg once to twice a day	Hypokalemia, orthostatic hypotension
Triamterene (Dyrenium)	Potassium-sparing diuretic	100–300 mg daily in divided doses	Headache, diarrhea, nausea, vomiting
Spironolactone (Aldactone)	Potassium-sparing diuretic	50–100 mg daily	Gynecomastia, diarrhea, drowsiness

Thiazide Diuretic

Hydrochloro*thiazide* (Microzide*)—Thiazide diuretics get their class name from the stem of generic drugs such as **hydrochlorothiazide**. Prescribers often abbreviate hydrochlorothiazide as HCTZ. Thiazides don't produce as much diuresis as loop diuretics, but are good for initial hypertension treatment. They work by preventing sodium reabsorption in the DCT. Water once again follows sodium, and urine volume increases. While the "hydro" in **hydrochlorothiazide** stands for the *hydro*gen atom, you can think of "hydro" as "water" for diuretic to remember its use.

    Indications: Most often used for hypertension and edema.

    Contraindications: Watch for hypokalemia and anuria.

    Adverse effects: May include diarrhea, nausea, orthostatic hypotension, and electrolyte imbalances.

    Patient education and care: Watch for electrolyte and fluid imbalances by monitoring weight and intake and output ratios and resulting blood pressure decrease. May need to add a potassium-sparing diuretic or combine in such a product, for example, hydrochlorothiazide/triamterene (Dyazide). The idea is to keep potassium levels in balance by adding one drug that reduces the potassium level and one drug that raises it. As with other diuretics, consider giving in the morning to avoid nighttime urination. Patients with diabetes mellitus may need to watch for hyperglycemia, an increase in blood sugar.

Potassium-Sparing Diuretic

Spironolactone (Aldactone) is one potassium-sparing diuretic, but this drug can cause gynecomastia, an enlargement of male breasts. **Spironolactone** blocks *aldo*sterone, an important steroid hormone in retaining sodium and water under hypotensive conditions.

    Indications: Most often used for hypertension, heart failure, hypokalemia (low potassium), and edema associated with CHF and nephrotic syndrome.

    Contraindications: With increased potassium comes the danger of other medications that raise potassium levels, including angiotensin-converting enzyme (ACE) inhibitors such as lisinopril or enalapril.

    Adverse effects: May include gynecomastia, a swelling of breast tissue in men, and irregular menses or amenorrhea in women as well as electrolyte imbalances.

    Patient education and care: Watch for electrolyte and fluid imbalances by monitoring weight and intake and output ratios. May need to watch diet for potassium-rich foods that may contribute to electrolyte imbalances.

Electrolyte Replenishment

Potassium chloride (K-Dur*) can supplement a patient when we cannot use a potassium-sparing diuretic or when a patient is on the more diuresis-producing loop diuretic. Normal potassium levels hover between 3.6 and 5.2 millimoles per liter (mmol/L). The "K" in the former branded drug name **K-Dur*** is potassium's chemical symbol, which is the first letter of Kalium. The "Dur" is for long *dur*ation, indicating that the supplement has a long-lasting effect.

SCENARIO 13.2. DIURETICS

Your patient with a past medical history of poorly controlled hypertension now presents with signs of ankle edema. The prescriber gives furosemide to treat the extra fluid. In what area of the nephron does furosemide work and what electrolyte imbalance worries us?

    Answer: Furosemide works in the loop of Henle and we worry about hypokalemia, a deficiency of potassium in the bloodstream. We would supplement with potassium chloride, if necessary.

Renin-Angiotensin-Aldosterone System

The renin-angiotensin-aldosterone system (RAAS) maintains fluid and salt levels in the body and, in turn, blood pressure (Figs. 13.8 and 13.9). The two main enzymes involved with the RAAS are renin and the ACE. The body releases renin as a response to low blood pressure and converts angiotensinogen into angiotensin I, the first step. The next step comes from the ACE, which converts angiotensin

RAAS – Overview

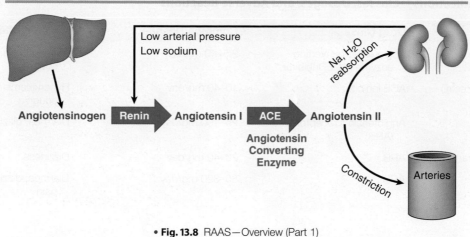

• **Fig. 13.8** RAAS—Overview (Part 1)

RAAS – Overview

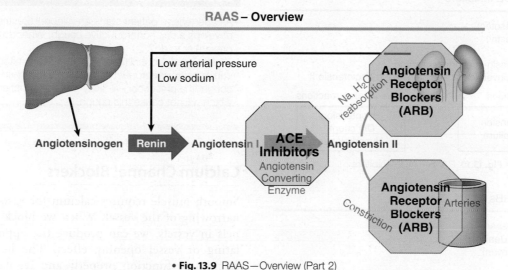

• **Fig. 13.9** RAAS—Overview (Part 2)

I to angiotensin II. Angiotensin II is important in blood pressure control because it can (1) promote sodium and water reabsorption and (2) maintain vasoconstriction. Both actions increase blood pressure. Therefore, we expect a patient with high blood pressure to get medicines that block areas of the RAAS system (Table 13.2).

Angiotensin-Converting Enzyme Inhibitors

Enala*pril* (Vasotec) is one ACE inhibitor medication sometimes referred to as a pril because of its medication stem. While a patient takes **enalapril** orally, **enalaprilat** is the injectable form and enalapril's active metabolite. **Lisinopril (Zestril)** is another medication in this class with the same stem.

ACE inhibitors (Fig. 13.10) block the action of ACE, stopping the conversion from angiotensin I to angiotensin II. This blocks fluid retention and vasoconstriction, resulting in lower blood pressure.

Indications: Most often used for hypertension and heart failure.

Contraindications: Patients with angioedema or patients with diabetes taking aliskiren.

Adverse effects: Side effects include hypotension, hyperkalemia, and a dry cough.

Patient education and care: A potassium-sparing diuretic can further aggravate hyperkalemia. If the patient has a dry cough secondary to the medicine, the prescriber will not treat it; rather the prescriber will give the patient an angiotensin II receptor blocker (ARB) that does not have that side effect. We will talk about this next.

Angiotensin II Receptor Blockers

Lo*sartan* (Cozaar) is an ARB. The -sartan suffix helps a person recognize other drugs in this class, such as **olme*sartan* (Benicar)** and **val*sartan* (Diovan)**.

ARBs prevent angiotensin II from binding to receptor sites on the kidneys and arteries, resulting in vasodilation and preventing sodium reabsorption (Fig. 13.11). As such, we can use these medicines for hypertension and heart failure. Note, however, that although similar in function,

TABLE 13.2	RAAS Medications—Classes, Dosages, and Adverse Reactions			
Generic (Brand)	Drug Class	Common Dosage	Adverse Effects	
Enalapril (Vasotec)	Angiotensin-converting enzyme (ACE) inhibitor	2.5–40 mg/day	Hyperkalemia, hypotension, cough	
Lisinopril (Prinivil, Zestril)	ACE inhibitor	10–40 mg/day	Hyperkalemia, hypotension, cough	
Losartan (Cozaar)	Angiotensin II receptor blocker (ARB)	25–100 mg/day	Diarrhea, dizziness, back pain	
Olmesartan (Benicar)	ARB	20–40 mg/day	Dizziness	
Valsartan (Diovan)	ARB	80–320 mg/day	Diarrhea, dizziness, abdominal pain	

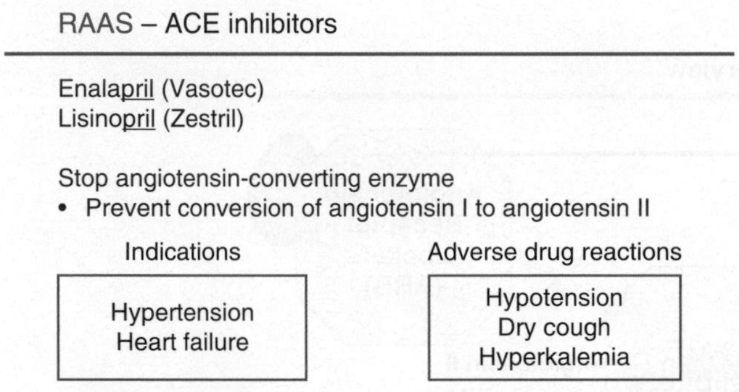

RAAS – ACE inhibitors

Enalapril (Vasotec)
Lisinopril (Zestril)

Stop angiotensin-converting enzyme
• Prevent conversion of angiotensin I to angiotensin II

Indications	Adverse drug reactions
Hypertension Heart failure	Hypotension Dry cough Hyperkalemia

• **Fig. 13.10** RAAS—ACE Inhibitors

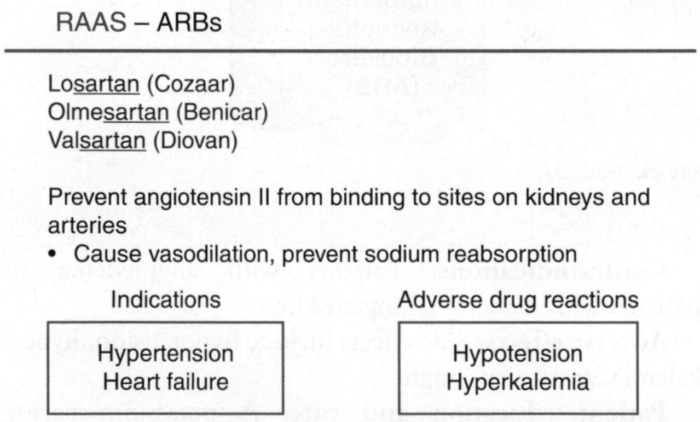

RAAS – ARBs

Losartan (Cozaar)
Olmesartan (Benicar)
Valsartan (Diovan)

Prevent angiotensin II from binding to sites on kidneys and arteries
• Cause vasodilation, prevent sodium reabsorption

Indications	Adverse drug reactions
Hypertension Heart failure	Hypotension Hyperkalemia

• **Fig. 13.11** RAAS—ARBs

the two drug classes should not be used together. They are not more effective as a combination and could have a bad effect on kidney function. Watch for hypotension and hyperkalemia.

Indications: Most often used for hypertension and heart failure.

Contraindications: Patients with diabetes taking aliskiren.

Adverse effects: Side effects include hypotension and hyperkalemia.

Patient education and care: Monitor the medication's effectiveness through blood pressure readings. Ensure that patients are on either an ACE inhibitor or ARB, not both.

SCENARIO 13.3. RAAS

A hypertensive patient starts on lisinopril (Zestril) and quickly develops a dry, nonproductive cough. What do you expect the prescriber to do?

Answer: Lisinopril (Zestril) is an ACE inhibitor that can cause a dry, nonproductive cough. Rather than treat the cough, the prescriber will likely switch the patient to an ARB, which will not cause this cough.

Calcium Channel Blockers

Smooth muscle requires calcium for vasoconstriction, a narrowing of the vessel. When we block calcium channels in vessels, we can produce the opposite, a vasodilating or vessel opening effect. The heart also needs calcium to function properly and regulate contraction timing. Some calcium channel blockers (CCBs) work to reduce arrhythmias. We then divide CCBs into two main classes: those that affect the heart and those that do not. These may not always be the first choice therapeutically due to adverse effects. These two CCB classes, the nondihydropyridines and dihydropyridines, vasodilate vessels (Table 13.3).

Nondihydropyridine CCBs

These CCBs blocks calcium channels in the heart and blood vessels, which can help patients with cardiac dysrhythmia, hypertension, and angina pectoris or chest pain (Fig. 13.12). Side effects include constipation and bradycardia (slow heart rate). Two nondihydropyridines are verapamil (Calan) and diltiazem (Cardizem).

Dil*tiazem* (Cardizem): The -tiazem stem identifies **diltiazem** as a nondihydropyridine. The brand name **Cardizem** adds the first five letters from *cardi*ac to the last three letters of the generic diltia*zem*.

Vera*pamil* (Calan): The -pamil stem identifies **diltiazem** as a nondihydropyridine. The brand name **Calan** takes

TABLE 13.3	**Calcium Channel Blocker Medication—Classes, Dosages, and Adverse Reactions**		
Generic (Brand)	Drug Class	Common Dosage	Adverse Effects
Diltiazem (Cardizem CD)	Nondihydropyridine calcium channel blocker	180–420 mg/day	Constipation, bradycardia, dizziness
Verapamil long-acting (Calan SR)	Nondihydropyridine calcium channel blocker	120–350 mg/day	Constipation, bradycardia, dizziness
Amlodipine (Norvasc)	Dihydropyridine calcium channel blocker	2.5–10 mg/day	Peripheral edema, headache
Nifedipine long-acting (Procardia XL)	Dihydropyridine calcium channel blocker	30–60 mg/day	Peripheral edema, headache

CCBs – Nondihydropyridines

Diltiazem (Cardizem)
Verapamil (Calan)

Block calcium channels in heart and blood vessels
• Used most commonly for dysrhythmias

Indications | Adverse drug reactions

Hypertension
Angina pectoris
Cardiac dysrhythmias

Constipation
Bradycardia

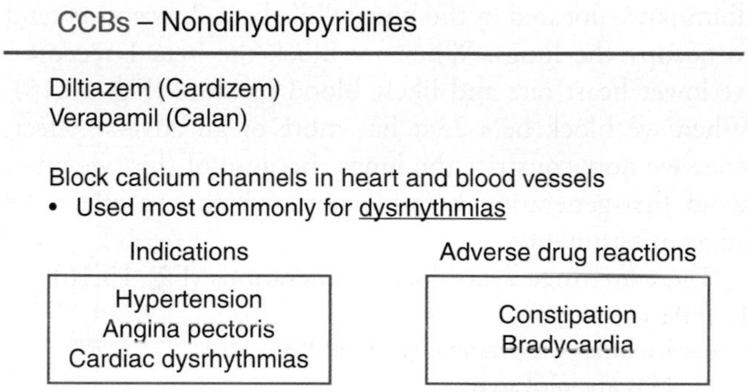

• **Fig. 13.12** CCBs—Nondihydropyridines

CCBs – Dihydropyridines

Amlodipine (Norvasc)
Nifedipine (Procardia)

Block calcium channels in blood vessels (no heart activity)
• Used most commonly for hypertension

Indications | Adverse drug reactions

Hypertension
Angina pectoris

Peripheral edema
Headache

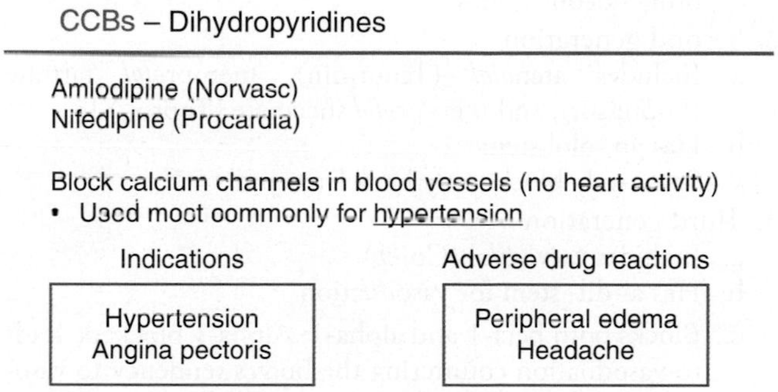

• **Fig. 13.13** CCBs—Dihydropyridines

three letters from the word *cal*cium and two from ch*an*nel blocker.

Indications: Most often used for hypertension, angina pectoris, and cardiac dysrhythmias.

Contraindications: Patients with hypotension, severe left ventricular dysfunction or hypersensitivity.

Adverse effects: Side effects include constipation and bradycardia.

Patient education and care: Patients may have significant constipation and should alert their provider.

Dihydropyridine CCBs

Dihydropyridines block calcium channels only in the blood vessels and have no cardiac activity. Thus, we cannot use them for dysrhythmias. Therefore, the most common use for these medications is to treat hypertension (Fig. 13.13).

Examples include amlo*dipine* (Norvasc) and nife*dipine* (Procardia). Adverse reactions include peripheral edema and headache.

Amlo*dipine* (Norvasc): The -dipine stem comes from *di*hydro*pyridine*. We can often look at this as a drug that produces a *dip in* blood pressure.

Nife*dipine* (Procardia XL): Procardia takes the "pro" from *pro*motes and "cardia" from *cardia*c. Thus, you can remember the brand **Procardia XL** as *pro*moting *cardia*c health.

Indications: Most often used for hypertension and angina pectoris.

Contraindications: Patients with cardiogenic shock and use with caution in patients with heart failure or who are post–myocardial infarction.

Adverse effects: Peripheral edema and headache.

Patient education and care: If a patient needs a low-dose CCB to prevent uterine contractions, **nifedipine (Procardia XL)**, a dihydropyridine, is a proper choice because it does not suppress the mother's and fetus's hearts as the nondihydropyridines would.

SCENARIO 13.4. CCBS

A patient is about to be discharged from the hospital with diltiazem for his atrial fibrillation, a dysrhythmia. Is this drug a dihydropyridine or nondihydropyridine? Does this treatment class make sense for a patient with a dysrhythmia?

Answer: Diltiazem is a nondihydropyridine CCB that acts in the heart and blood vessels. Therefore, this would be an appropriate treatment. If the patient had been taking a dihydropyridine such as nifedipine, that would have been an inappropriate treatment.

Alpha-Blockers and Beta-Blockers

Hypertension can lead to many other issues, such as myocardial infarction, heart failure, chest pain, and stroke. Several ways a person might start working on hypertension without medicine include weight loss, aerobic activity, diet, and moderation of alcohol use.

When treating hypertension with drug therapy, we generally start with ACE inhibitors or ARBs, CCBS, or thiazide diuretics (Fig. 13.14). Which drug we use varies by patient.

Some patient populations respond better to CCBs and thiazide diuretics; ACE inhibitors and ARBs work better for others. We might use a two-drug combination if one drug does not do the job. Alpha- or beta-blockers might be that addition (Table 13.4).

The first two letters of the Greek alphabet are alpha and beta—these are the names of where these medications work. An adrenergic alpha *agonist* works *like* adrenaline on the alpha receptor while an adrenergic alpha *antagonist* works in the *opposite* manner.

The prefix adren- refers to the *adren*al glands, which are *above* (ad) the *kidney* (renal) and secrete adrenaline. The suffix -ergic refers to "works like" in Greek. Therefore, these drugs work like **adrenaline** (also called **epinephrine**).

Alpha-Blockers

Instead of calling these drugs blood pressure pills or antihypertensives (its therapeutic class name), prescribers classify these drugs by receptor. **Doxazosin**, the alpha-blocker, has multiple uses, including for hypertension and benign prostatic hyperplasia (BPH). This is why classifying by the receptor name makes more sense than classifying this drug by therapeutic use.

Doxazosin (Cardura) can block alpha-1 receptors, cause vasodilation, and a reduction in blood pressure. Memorize the stem -azosin, which starts with the letter "a," as an alpha-blocker. However, we generally use alpha-blockers as an adjunct to other treatment.

Indications: Most often used as a hypertension add-on, for enlarged prostate, and pheochromocytoma.

Adverse effects: Dizziness, insomnia, nausea, and abdominal pain.

Patient education and care: The patient might encounter "first-dose syncope" or "first-dose effect" in which, upon standing, the blood pressure drops rapidly, causing dizziness or fainting. Therefore, patients should take the first dose at bedtime.

Beta-Blockers

There are two beta receptors important to beta-blocker pharmacology: beta-1 and beta-2. Beta-1 receptors are predominantly located in the heart while beta-2 receptors tend to occupy the lungs. When we block the beta-1 receptor, we lower heart rate and likely blood pressure (Fig. 13.15). When we block beta-2, it has more of an adverse effect, since we now constrict the lungs. Because of this, we often avoid first-generation beta-blockers, which can affect the lungs in asthmatics.

There are three beta-blocker generations (Fig. 13.16):
1. First generation
   a. Includes propran*olol* (Inderal LA)
   b. Has an -olol stem
   c. Nonselectively blocks beta-1 and beta-2 receptors
   d. Avoid using for asthma/COPD patients due to bronchoconstriction
2. Second generation
   a. Includes aten*olol* (Tenormin), metopr*olol* tartrate (Lopressor), and metopr*olol* succinate (Toprol XL)
   b. Has an -olol stem
   c. Selectively blocks only beta-1 receptors
3. Third generation
   a. Includes carve*dil*ol (Coreg)
   b. Has a -dil- stem for vaso*dil*ation
   c. Blocks both beta-1 and alpha-1: Alpha-1 blockade leads to vasodilation countering the body's tendency to vasoconstrict as a response to lower blood pressure

Practitioners rarely highlight the distinction in salts such as metoprolol tartrate and metoprolol succinate. However, in this case, metoprolol tartrate and succinate work for different lengths of time. The tartrate is short acting and the succinate is long acting, hence the XL (extra-long) ending for brand name Toprol XL.

Hypertension Treatment

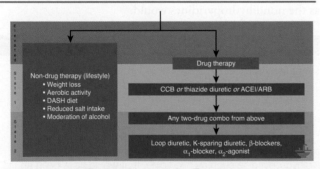

• **Fig. 13.14** Hypertension Treatment

TABLE 13.4	**Alpha- and Beta-Blockers—Classes, Dosages, and Adverse Reactions**		
Generic (Brand)	**Drug Class**	**Common Dosage**	**Adverse Effects**
Doxazosin (Cardura)	Alpha adrenergic blocker	1–16 mg/day	Hypotension
Propranolol (Inderal LA)	First-generation beta-blocker	4–160 mg/day	Bradycardia, dizziness, lethargy
Atenolol (Tenormin)	Second-generation beta-blocker	25–100 mg/day	Bradycardia, dizziness, lethargy
Metoprolol (Lopressor)	Second-generation beta-blocker	50–100 mg/day	Bradycardia, dizziness, lethargy
Carvedilol (Coreg)	Third-generation beta-blocker with alpha activity	12.5–50 mg/day	Bradycardia, dizziness, lethargy

Hypertension – β-Receptor Antagonists

AKA the β-blockers

Two different β receptors: β_1 and β_2

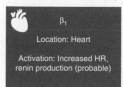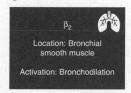

• **Fig. 13.15** Hypertension—Beta Receptor Antagonists

Hypertension – β-Receptor Antagonists

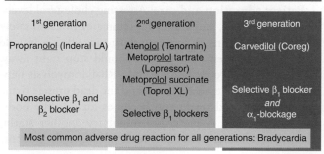

• **Fig. 13.16** Hypertension—Beta Receptor Antagonists, First to Third Generations

Indications: High blood pressure, angina, and migraine prophylaxis.

Contraindications: With first-generation beta-blockers, watch for asthmatics. The beta-2 blockade can cause bronchoconstriction.

Adverse effects: Dizziness, drowsiness, fatigue, and bradycardia.

Patient education and care: Beta-blockers can mask the signs and symptoms of hypoglycemia, such as tachycardia. Ensure that patients monitor blood sugars regularly.

SCENARIO 13.5. ALPHA-BLOCKERS AND BETA-BLOCKERS

An asthma patient presents to a clinic complaining of increased asthma attacks. Looking at the chart, you notice propranolol. Which generation is propranolol in and why is this a poor choice for this patient?

Answer: Propranolol is a first-generation beta-blocker that blocks beta-1 and beta-2 receptors. First-generation beta-blockers can cause increased asthma attacks and COPD worsening because of their constrictive effect on the lungs.

Antihyperlipidemics

Dyslipidemia is literally "bad" lipids or bad lipid levels (Table 13.5). With some lipids, we worry about having levels that are too high; with others, we worry about the levels being too low. "Bad cholesterol" is so named because it takes cholesterol to the tissues, increasing our levels. The "good

TABLE 13.5	Desirable Lipid Levels	
Lipid	**Desirable Level**
Total cholesterol	< 200 mg/dL
High-density lipoprotein cholesterol	Women: > 50 mg/dL Men: > 40 mg/dL
Low-density lipoprotein cholesterol	< 100 mg/dL
Triglycerides	< 150 mg/dL

Dyslipidemia – lipoproteins

Dyslipidemia: Abnormal levels of one or more lipoproteins

VLDL	LDL	HDL
Very-low-density lipoprotein	Low-density lipoprotein	High-density lipoprotein
Transports triglycerides from liver to tissues	Transports cholesterol from liver to tissues	Transports cholesterol from tissues back to liver
	"Bad cholesterol"	"Good cholesterol"

• **Fig. 13.17** Dyslipidemia—Lipoproteins

cholesterol" does the opposite, moving the cholesterol back to the liver for breakdown. Hyperlipidemia is the increase in levels of lipids such as cholesterol and triglycerides. Hypercholesterolemia is the specific increase in levels of cholesterol in the blood (Fig. 13.17).

The three main lipoproteins we are worried about are as follows:
1. Very-low-density lipoprotein (VLDL)
   a. These transport triglycerides from the liver to tissues.
   b. Can result in hypertriglyceridemia, a rise in triglycerides.
2. Low-density lipoprotein (LDL)
   a. Transports cholesterol from liver to tissues, creating higher levels.
   b. This is the so-called "bad cholesterol."
3. High-density lipoprotein (HDL)
   a. Transports cholesterol from tissues back to liver for breakdown, creating lower levels.
   b. This is the so-called "good cholesterol."

Hypercholesterolemia is "high" cholesterol, which impacts the arteries and is part of the atherosclerosis disease state (Fig. 13.18). This happens in four steps:
1. Normal artery—Blood flows smoothly
2. Fatty streak—Excess lipids form a fatty deposit
3. Fibrous cap—The fatty streak "heals" with fibrous tissue on top.
4. Cap rupture—The fibrous tissue breaks to create a blood clot (thrombus). This clot may lead to a stroke or heart attack.

Nondrug Therapy

Dietary changes such as reducing dietary fat may help with hypercholesterolemia. Additionally, the patient should consider a weight loss of 10% or more, controlling high blood pressure, and quitting smoking (Fig. 13.19).

HMG-CoA Reductase Inhibitors (Statins)

Often, we shorten the HMG-CoA reductase inhibitors drug class name to simply "statins," taking the last six letters of the medications in the class, such as atorvastatin and lovastatin (Table 13.6). HMG-CoA reductase, as the -ase implies, is an enzyme responsible for cholesterol formation in liver cells (hepatocytes). By blocking the enzyme, cholesterol production drops. The maximum LDL lowering happens after 4 to 6 weeks of treatment (Fig. 13.20).

One mnemonic is to use letters of the HMG-CoA class to memorize potential adverse effects: "H" for *h*epatotoxicity,

Hypercholesterolemia – Progression

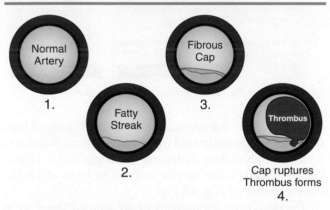

• **Fig. 13.18** Hypercholesterolemia—Progression

Hypercholesterolemia – treatment

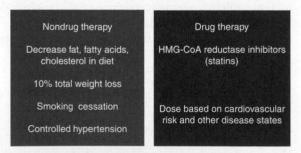

• **Fig. 13.19** Hypercholesterolemia—Treatment

"M" for *m*yositis, "G" for *g*estation, or that it cannot be used in pregnancy.

Ator*vastatin* (Lipitor) and rosu*vastatin* (Crestor) share the -vastatin ending. Be careful—some mistake nystatin (Mycostatin*), an antifungal, for being a cholesterol drug in this class because it ends in -statin. Watch out for this common mistake.

Indications: Dyslipidemia and the primary prevention of heart attack, stroke, and myocardial infarction.

Contraindications: Liver disease, pregnancy, and rhabdomyolysis. In addition, statins interact with grapefruit juice, which can increase their level in the body.

Adverse effects: Muscle pain, rhabdomyolysis, and tendon rupture.

Patient education and care: Assessing cholesterol levels, liver function tests, and kidney function are critical to safely administering statins. A common statin side effect is muscle pain. If this happens, the patient should stop right away. This can progress to rhabdomyolysis. Rhabdomyolysis happens when a muscle breaks down and the dead muscle tissue gets into the bloodstream and becomes toxic to the body. This can be fatal. A prescriber might try another statin, which might not have the same toxic effects on the patient.

Fibric Acid Derivatives

High triglyceride levels often correspond to coronary disease and plaques. While blood levels generally do not guide treatment for high cholesterol, we might treat with fibrates. We are especially concerned with a triglyceride level above 500 mg/dL (Fig. 13.21).

Fibric acid derivatives work by creating more enzyme to break down triglycerides—lipoprotein lipase. We then see a reduction in the VLDL levels. Some effects might include abnormal liver function tests, backache, and abdominal pain.

Feno*fibrate* (**Tricor**) has the stem -fibrate, a triglyceride-lowering fibric acid derivative.

Niacin

While niacin (nicotinic acid) is a B vitamin, it can help increase HDL cholesterol. As an over-the-counter vitamin, niacin is not as strictly regulated as traditional

TABLE 13.6	Antihyperlipidemic Medications—Classes, Dosages, and Adverse Reactions			
Generic (Brand)	Drug Class	Common Dosage	Adverse Effects
Atorvastatin (Lipitor)	HMG-CoA reductase inhibitor	10 mg/day	Abdominal pain, tendon rupture, muscle pain
Rosuvastatin (Crestor)	HMG-CoA reductase inhibitor	5–20 mg/day	Abdominal pain, tendon rupture, muscle pain
Fenofibrate (Tricor)	Fibrate	48–145 mg/day	Abdominal or back pain, abnormal liver function tests
Niacin (Niaspan)	Vitamin	300–600 mg/day	Flushing, dyspepsia

SCENARIO 13.6. ANTIHYPERLIPIDEMICS

When looking at atorvastatin (Lipitor) and fenofibrate (Tricor), we know they both affect an enzyme. Which affects lipoprotein lipase and which blocks HMG-CoA reductase?

Answer: Atorvastatin (Lipitor) is a statin medication that acts by blocking HMG-CoA reductase and fenofibrate (Tricor) affects lipoprotein lipase.

Hypercholesterolemia – Statins

Atorvastatin (Lipitor)
Rosuvastatin (Crestor)

HMG-CoA = enzyme responsible for creating cholesterol in hepatocytes
Statins inhibit HMG-CoA and decrease cholesterol production

Indications	Adverse drug reactions
Hypercholesterolemia Hypertriglyceridemia Mixed dyslipidemia	Muscle pain Rhabdomyolysis Tendon rupture

• **Fig. 13.20** Hypercholesterolemia—Statins

Hypertriglyceridemia – Fibrates

Fenofibrate (Tricor)

Cause creation of more lipoprotein lipase, which breaks down triglycerides in the liver
• VLDL levels decrease as there is less triglycerides for them to transport

Indications	Adverse drug reactions
Hypercholesterolemia Hypertriglyceridemia Mixed dyslipidemia	Abdominal pain Backache Abnormal liver function tests

• **Fig. 13.21** Hypertriglyceridemia—Fibrates

prescription medications as it falls under the category of dietary supplement.

Anticoagulants and Antiplatelets

Coagulation is the clotting of cells to protect the body from bleeding in lower pressure environments such as veins. Platelets form, much like leaves in a gutter, to prevent bleeding in higher-pressure vessels such as arteries. By blocking coagulation or platelets, we aim to reduce the risk of developing blood clots, but blocking too much increases the patient's risk of bleeding.

One key physiologic principle to understand is the coagulation cascade (Fig. 13.22). The coagulation cascade has various interactions between various proteins (factors) that initiate deposits of fibrin at the injury site. These factors have Roman numeral names in the order that they were discovered, not in what one would expect, an order of function. The coagulation cascade begins in one of two

Coagulation Cascade – Overview

Interaction between different proteins (factors) to cause fibrin to be deposited at tissue injury site

Proteins were named as roman numerals (Factor VI, etc.) and were numbered based on discovery, not function
• *Cascade does not follow numerical order*

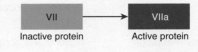

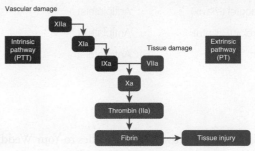

• **Fig. 13.22** Coagulation Cascade

paths. The intrinsic pathway recognizes vascular damage. The extrinsic pathway activation comes from tissue damage. Anticoagulants act on many factors in the pathway (Table 13.7).

Vitamin K Antagonists

The Wisconsin Alumni Research Foundation (WARF) first developed Vitamin K antagonists as a rodent poison, causing bleeding in the animals. However, later, the research helped make warfarin into a life-saving medicine that can be finely tuned for an individual patient at risk for a clot.

Warfarin (Coumadin*)— the -parin stem from the anticoagulants **heparin** and **enoxaparin** and the -farin stem of **warfarin** are similar. This reminds students they are all anticoagulants. You can associate bleeding, warfarin's primary side effect, with *warfare*.

Indications: Prophylaxis of deep venous thrombosis, pulmonary emboli, and emboli after myocardial infarction.

Contraindications: Active ulceration.

Adverse effects: Hemorrhage, skin necrosis, dermatitis, nausea, diarrhea, abdominal pain.

Patient education and care: It can take warfarin up to a week to work properly, and any changes in dose might take 1 to 2 weeks. Because of this and the narrow range that warfarin levels need to stay in, we monitor the drug levels carefully using the international normalized ratio (INR).

The INR will compare a healthy patient's coagulation time to that of the ill patient's time. A healthy patient's INR is 1.0, but with warfarin INRs, we would like them to be between 2.0 and 3.0 for many disease states. A low INR requires us to increase the warfarin dose, as the coagulation rate is not high enough. If the INR is too high, we decrease the dose; too much coagulation is a concern.

The warfarin tablets have color coding to help patients keep track of which dosages they should be taking using the

TABLE 13.7 Anticoagulants and Antiplatelets—Classes, Dosages, and Adverse Reactions

Generic (Brand)	Drug Class	Common Dosage	Adverse Effects
Warfarin (Coumadin*)	Oral anticoagulant	2–10 mg/day	Bleeding
Enoxaparin (Lovenox)	Parenteral anticoagulant	30 mg twice daily	Bleeding
Heparin	Parenteral anticoagulant	Various	Bleeding, heparin-induced thrombocytopenia
Dabigatran (Pradaxa)	Novel oral anticoagulant	Up to 150 mg twice daily	Bleeding, gastritis
Clopidogrel (Plavix)	Antiplatelet	75 mg/day	Bleeding, dyspnea
Ticagrelor (Brilinta)	Antiplatelet	90 mg twice daily	Bleeding, dyspnea
Aspirin	Antiplatelet	81–325 mg/day	Bleeding, gastrointestinal ulceration, dyspepsia

"Please Let Georgia Brown Bring Peaches to Your Wedding" mnemonic.

1 mg—Pink
2 mg—Lavender
2.5 mg—Green
3 mg—Brown
4 mg—Blue
5 mg—Peach
6 mg—Teal
7.5 mg—Yellow
10 mg—White

The brand and generic medications might be the same color but may not be the same shape.

Heparins

Heparins, like warfarin, require patient monitoring. Thus, this heparin can be used only in the hospital. However, the more expensive low-molecular-weight heparin (LMWH) **enoxaparin (Lovenox),** which does not require monitoring, can be used by the patient at home.

He*parin* and "bleedin'" have a bit of rhyme as a way to remember heparin's most common adverse effect.

Enoxaparin (Lovenox): Enoxa*parin* and **he***parin* share the -parin stem because they are related. Enoxaparin is also for bridge therapy when starting **warfarin** therapy.

Novel Oral Anticoagulants (NOACs)

Dabigatran (Pradaxa) is one newer anticoagulant class (Fig. 13.23). It works as an oral direct thrombin inhibitor, making the monitoring we do with warfarin unnecessary. While a warfarin patient might get INR checks every 1 to 3 months, dabigatran does not need that type of monitoring. Dabigatran is relatively expensive compared with warfarin and still can cause bleeding.

NOTE: Dabigatran (Pradaxa) has the -gatran stem to denote the difference between anticoagulants.

Antiplatelet Agents

Clopido*grel* **(Plavix)** inhibits glycoproteins IIb/IIIa, which act on platelets, grabbing even more platelet hands to form a clot. **Ticagrelor (Brilinta)** is similar in action to clopido-*grel* with a different side effect profile. **Aspirin** works similarly, leading to a reduced likelihood that platelets will stick together and clot.

Clopidogrel prevents the action and clot formation for antiplatelets, including preventing heart attacks and stroke. Like anticoagulants, a side effect can be bleeding.

The indication for aspirin changed recently. The guideline now is that prescribers should make recommendations for aspirin and that patients should not take it on their own.

SCENARIO 13.7. ANTICOAGULANTS AND ANTIPLATELETS

A patient on warfarin (Coumadin*) presents to the anticoagulation clinic for his weekly INR testing. Is warfarin (Coumadin) an inhibitor of direct thrombin or a vitamin K antagonist? What INR goal might you expect?

Answer: Warfarin (Coumadin*) acts as a vitamin K antagonist and the INR goal is likely between 2 and 3.

Angina Pectoris

We often see vasodilators when treating angina pectoris, a type of sternal chest pain often caused by atherosclerosis from coronary artery disease (CAD). It is often a supply and demand issue. In a healthy patient, oxygen supply is enough to meet the body's demands. However, in a patient with angina pectoris, oxygen supply cannot meet the demand. Thus, the two ways to help a patient are to either increase oxygen supply or reduce the oxygen demand.

There are three angina pectoris classifications:
1. Chronic stable angina or exertional angina: Often caused by CAD
2. Variant angina or vasospastic angina: Caused by coronary artery spasm

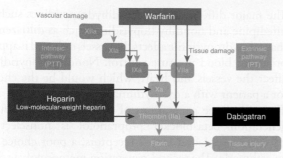

• **Fig. 13.23** Novel Oral Anticoagulants (NOACs)

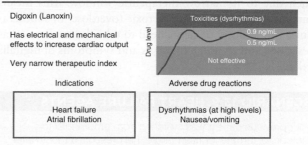

• **Fig. 13.24** Heart Failure—Cardiac Glycoside

3. Unstable angina: Caused by severe CAD with clots or blockages, which is a medical emergency

Beta-blockers are only for chronic stable angina and act by decreasing heart rate and contractility. Beta-blockers will not work for variant angina and vasospasms.

CCBs work for both chronic stable and variant angina.

Nitrates

These are a mainstay treatment. We give nitroglycerin (Nitrostat) for acute angina management. It has many forms, including sublingual tablets, oral sprays, and transdermal patches.

Nitroglycerin **(Nitrostat)** converts to nitric oxide, a vasodilator. Make sure the patient sits when taking the medication because it causes significant dizziness. With **Nitrostat**, think "*nitro*us" from sports cars—the patient and blood pressure drop "*stat*." Nitro- is this vasodilator's stem in the prefix position.

Indications: Anginal pain.

Contraindications: Watch for PDE-5 inhibitors such as sildenafil (Viagra). The combination can create dangerously low blood pressure.

Adverse effects: Severe hypotension.

Patient education and care: The patient should carry nitroglycerin at all times. The patient should be asked for the bottle at every visit to check the expiration date and remind the patient specifically how to take the medication.

SCENARIO 13.8. ANGINA PECTORIS

Your neighbor is mowing his lawn when he grabs at his chest and leans on his fence. He asks you to run inside and to grab his nitroglycerin (Nitrostat) tablets. What concerns you about his positioning?

Answer: Nitroglycerin (Nitrostat) is a nitrate for acute angina attacks. Because it causes a rapid decrease in blood pressure, the patient should not stand while taking the tablets.

Heart Failure Agents

Heart failure is when the heart "fails" to produce enough cardiac output. The heart still pumps, just not as well as it needs to.

Heart FAILURE – Cardiac Glycoside

In heart failure, the body tries to compensate for the heart's failings often by increasing the heart rate. This can actually have a negative effect on cardiac output as the heart lacks time to fill properly.

The heart failure treatment goal is to temper compensatory mechanisms and increase cardiac output. First-line heart failure treatment involves ACE inhibitors. For those who cannot tolerate ACE inhibitors, we should use ARBs.

Prescribers also give diuretics to reduce salt, water, and blood volume and the amount of work the heart has to do. A common side effect of diuretics is electrolyte imbalance, which can cause problems with digoxin.

Beta-blockers work to slow the heart rate, making it more efficient. Only certain beta-blockers, such as metoprolol succinate, are used—not tartrate and carvedilol. Common side effects include bradycardia and fatigue.

Prescribers might use digoxin (Lanoxin) in heart failure and dysrhythmias such as atrial fibrillation. Sometimes, you will hear arrhythmia for dysrhythmia. Technically, however, arrhythmia means no rhythm at all. Digoxin acts on the sodium/potassium pump in myocardial cells, resulting in more sodium in the cells. The body exchanges sodium for calcium, which then helps increase contraction strength. Digoxin acts electrically by delaying conduction velocity from the sinoatrial node (SA node) to the atrioventricular (AV node). This decreases heart rate and allows more time for heart-chamber filling between contractions.

A cardiac glycoside (Fig. 13.24), such as **digoxin (Lanoxin)**, increases the force or speed of contraction of the heart. We call this a positive inotropic effect. Also, an antidysrhythmic, **digoxin** changes the electrochemistry of the heart to prevent dysrhythmias.

Digoxin (Lanoxin) treats CHF by increasing the force of the heart's contractions. **Digoxin** is derived from the plant *Digitalis lanata*. In Latin, *digitalis* means something like hand or "digits," while *lanata* means "wooly" because the actual plant is fuzzy. Therefore, **digoxin** comes from the name *digitalis*, and brand name **Lanoxin** comes from *lanata*.

Indications: Atrial fibrillation, flutter, and CHF.

Contraindications: Hypersensitivity to digoxin.

Adverse effects: Dysrhythmias, bradycardia, heart block, dyspepsia, nausea, vomiting, digoxin toxicity effects such as visual disturbances.

Patient education and care: We do not use digoxin as much due to its narrow therapeutic window. This means that small dose changes can be toxic (overdose) or subtherapeutic (underdose). Patients need to take the medication as prescribed and to watch for signs and symptoms of digitalis toxicity.

SCENARIO 13.9. HEART FAILURE AGENTS

Your previous patient was switched from propranolol to metoprolol tartrate for heart failure. He presents a month later complaining of heart failure symptoms. Why might this patient be experiencing an exacerbation of symptoms?

Answer: Metoprolol tartrate is not approved for heart failure patients. Metoprolol succinate and carvedilol are appropriate treatments.

Summary

- The formula for cardiac output is Cardiac Output (CO) = Heart Rate (HR) * Stroke Volume (SV). Knowing how medicines affect cardiac output helps us understand how the medication can help or hurt the patient.
- Diuretics produce less diuresis as they continue down the water slide from osmotic to loop to thiazide and finally to potassium sparing. Loop and thiazide diuretics are likely to cause hypokalemia, and potassium-sparing diuretics can cause hyperkalemia.
- If an ACE inhibitor such as lisinopril causes a dry cough, the prescriber will likely replace it with an ARB rather than treat the cough.

- The major difference between dihydropyridines such as nifedipine and nondihydropyridines such as diltiazem is that a dihydropyridine affects the vessels only and is appropriate for blood pressure control. Nondihydropyridines affect the vessels and heart, which would be the choice for a patient with a dysrhythmia.
- There are three generations of beta-blockers. The first-generation beta-blocker propranolol is nonselective, affecting beta-1 and beta-2 receptors, a poor choice for an asthmatic. The second-generation metoprolol, a selective beta-blocker, affects only beta-1 receptors. The third-generation beta-blocker carvedilol affects both alpha receptors to vasodilate and beta receptors to reduce heart rate.
- Atorvastatin, an HMG-CoA reductase inhibitor, works well to reduce LDL, the "bad" cholesterol. Fenofibrate, a fibric acid derivative, primarily works on triglycerides.
- Anticoagulants such as warfarin and heparin work by affecting the coagulation cascade in vessels with slower moving blood flow. Antiplatelets such as clopidogrel and aspirin affect the arteries in areas of faster blood flow.
- Angina pectoris is a supply and demand issue in which the heart either does not get enough of an oxygen supply or has too much demand. Solutions target reducing demand or increasing oxygen supply.
- Compensatory measures meant to help a heart failure patient often exacerbate the issue. Treatments such as diuretics, beta-blockers, and ACE inhibitors are meant to reduce the work the heart has to do.

Review Questions

1. Which of the following medications is a thiazide diuretic?
   a. Hydrochlorothiazide (Microzide*)
   b. Furosemide (Lasix)
   c. Spironolactone (Aldactone)
   d. Amlodipine (Norvasc)
2. Which of the following diuretics can cause gynecomastia?
   a. Furosemide (Lasix)
   b. Spironolactone (Aldactone)
   c. Hydrochlorothiazide (Microzide*)
   d. Triamterene (Dyrenium)
3. What stem would you expect from an angiotensin II receptor blocker?
   a. -sartan
   b. -pril
   c. -dipine
   d. -olol
4. Which of the following medications is a dihydropyridine calcium channel blocker?
   a. Furosemide (Lasix)
   b. Diltiazem (Cardizem)

   c. Verapamil (Calan)
   d. Amlodipine (Norvasc)
5. Match the correct words for the following blanks: _____ affect the vessels only, while _____ affect the vessels and the heart.
   a. Nondihydropyridines, dihydropyridines
   b. Dihydropyridines, diuretics
   c. Dihydropyridines, nondihydropyridines
   d. Nondihydropyridines, diuretics
6. Which of the following medications is a second-generation long-acting beta-blocker?
   a. Propranolol
   b. Metoprolol tartrate
   c. Metoprolol succinate
   d. Carvedilol
7. Match the correct words for the following blanks: Fibrates help to treat high _____ levels, while HMG-CoA reductase inhibitors help to treat high _____ levels.
   a. Triglyceride, cholesterol
   b. Triglyceride, ergosterol
   c. Cholesterol, ergosterol
   d. Cholesterol, triglyceride

8. Which of the following is an antiplatelet drug that inhibits glycoproteins IIb/IIIa?
   a. Warfarin
   b. Dabigatran
   c. Clopidogrel
   d. Heparin
9. Which anticoagulant can be used at home but is a bit more expensive?
   a. Warfarin
   b. Aspirin
   c. Clopidogrel
   d. Enoxaparin
10. Blocking which receptor might be a concern when treating an asthmatic?
   a. Alpha-1
   b. Alpha-2
   c. Beta-1
   d. Beta-2

14

Endocrine

LEARNING OBJECTIVES

1. Discuss the management of endocrine conditions.
2. Describe the pathophysiology of common endocrine conditions.
3. Identify various medication classes in the therapeutic treatment of endocrine diseases.
4. Compare and contrast endocrine medicines.
5. Discuss the mechanisms of action, indications, drug interactions, and adverse effects of common endocrine medications.

Diabetic Agents

Endocrine conditions such as diabetes mellitus (DM) often have two sides to them. In the case of diabetes, it is a condition of hyperglycemia, too much blood sugar. The other side is hypoglycemia, or low blood sugar. The same is true of hyperthyroid, too much thyroid hormone, versus hypothyroid, too little. With DM pathophysiology, we can divide it into three types (Fig. 14.1):

1. Type I DM
   a. Historically known as juvenile-onset diabetes.
   b. The immune system destroys insulin-producing cells in the pancreas and the body cannot produce insulin.
   c. Treatment requires insulin.
2. Type II DM
   a. Historically known as adult-onset diabetes.
   b. Insulin is produced but not well utilized.
   c. Treatment starts with oral medications but may include insulin in severe cases.
3. Gestational DM
   a. Similar to Type II diabetes.
   b. Occurs during pregnancy; continues shortly after delivery.
   c. Treatment similar to Type II diabetes.

All DM types have excess blood glucose, and treatment is working towards moving that glucose either to the cells or out of the body. There are various organs involved in regulating blood glucose, primarily the liver, pancreas, small intestine, and circulatory system (Fig. 14.2). Five ways that medications can target organs are as follows (Fig. 14.3):

- Stopping intestinal absorption of glucose
- Stopping liver glucose production
- Increasing insulin sensitivity
- Increasing insulin production from the pancreas
- Providing outside insulin

---

* Brand discontinued, now available only as generic
† Naming conventions can vary between prescription and OTC formulations

In the pancreas, the islets of Langerhans and the beta cells that reside there produce and release insulin (Fig. 14.4). These cells are destroyed if a patient is a Type I diabetic, necessitating outside insulin. In Type II diabetics, a patient can use medications and may not need insulin.

SCENARIO 14.1. DIABETIC AGENTS

A patient recently diagnosed with diabetes starts on metformin. He mentions that his doctor said his pancreas works well, but his body can't use the insulin that it makes. What type of diabetes does this patient most likely have?

Answer: As this patient's pancreas works well and produces insulin, he is most likely a Type II diabetic. When the patient is female, gestational diabetes is a possibility.

Oral Diabetes Agents

Depending on a patient's individual circumstances, there are various medicines that can help lower blood sugar (Table 14.1). Many generic and brand name oral medications have "gl" or "glu" for glucose in their names. Four of these drugs are **metformin (*Glu*cophage)**, ***gl*ipizide (*Glu*cotrol)**, **glyburide (DiaBeta)**, and **sita*gl*iptin (Januvia)**.

Biguanides

Metformin (Glucophage) is a biguanide and a mainstay Type II DM treatment (Fig. 14.5). It works by (1) decreasing intestinal glucose absorption, (2) decreasing liver glucose production, and (3) increasing insulin sensitivity. Common gastrointestinal (GI) side effects include nausea/vomiting and diarrhea. It is important that a patient begins at a lower dose when starting on metformin. Sometimes, the body will acclimate to the GI effects, but a large initial dose makes that more difficult. One rare side effect of metformin is lactic acidosis; we are especially concerned about patients with poor renal function.

Diabetes Mellitus (DM) – Pathology

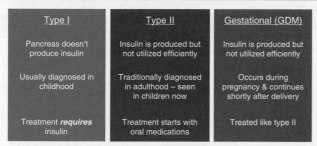

Type I	Type II	Gestational (GDM)
Pancreas doesn't produce insulin	Insulin is produced but not utilized efficiently	Insulin is produced but not utilized efficiently
Usually diagnosed in childhood	Traditionally diagnosed in adulthood – seen in children now	Occurs during pregnancy & continues shortly after delivery
Treatment **requires** insulin	Treatment starts with oral medications	Treated like type II

• **Fig. 14.1** Diabetes Mellitus (DM)—Pathology (Part 1)

DM – Pathology

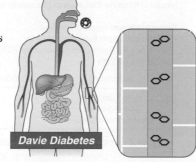

Multiple organs are involved in regulating insulin and glucose levels
• Liver
• Pancreas
• Small intestine
• Circulatory system

Davie Diabetes

• **Fig. 14.2** Diabetes Mellitus—Pathology (Part 2)

DM – Pathology

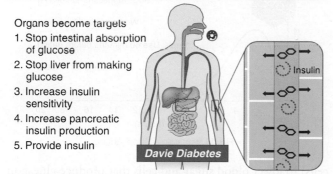

Organs become targets
1. Stop intestinal absorption of glucose
2. Stop liver from making glucose
3. Increase insulin sensitivity
4. Increase pancreatic insulin production
5. Provide insulin

Insulin

Davie Diabetes

• **Fig. 14.3** Diabetes Mellitus—Pathology (Part 3)

Met*formin* (Glucophage) has the -formin stem to identify the drug class. Phagocytosis is cellular eating. Think of the brand name **Glucophage** as the medicine performing glucose eating.

Sulfonylureas

Glyburide (DiaBeta*) and **glipizide (Glucotrol)** are sulfonylureas that stimulate the pancreas to increase insulin production (Fig. 14.6). We see these medications for Type II and gestational DM. A concern is hypoglycemia, or too little blood sugar. Ensure that patients take it with a meal, and use with caution for the elderly, who have a significant fall risk.

DM – Pancreatic Beta Cells

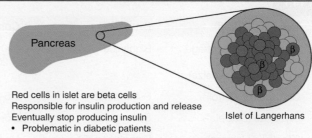

Red cells in islet are beta cells
Responsible for insulin production and release
Eventually stop producing insulin
• Problematic in diabetic patients

Islet of Langerhans

• **Fig. 14.4** Diabetes Mellitus—Pancreatic Beta Cells

Gli*pizide* (Glucotrol) has a gli- prefix stem that indicates it is a sulfonylurea antidiabetic medicine. The gly- stem in **gly*buride* (DiaBeta*)** is an old one, but we still have some prescribers using the medicine. The former brand name **DiaBeta** combines the "dia" from *dia*betic, and the "Beta" from the beta cells that release insulin.

Dipeptidyl Peptidase-4 Inhibitors

Dipeptidyl Peptidase-4 (DPP-4) inhibitors such as **sita-gliptin (Januvia)** act on the pancreas to increase insulin production (Fig. 14.7). They are more expensive than other choices but may have fewer side effects, such as headache. Rarely, they will cause pancreatitis.

Sita*gliptin* (Januvia) has the -gliptin stem. Some students associate it with the Lipton brand of iced tea and the sugar some people put into iced tea.

Patient education and care: Proper diet and weight management, if necessary, should remain part of a plan for a patient with diabetes. Oral drugs that reduce blood sugar can have a high incidence of hypoglycemia (glipizide, glyburide). Therefore, patients need to monitor their blood sugars regularly and be aware of possible signs/symptoms. Drugs such as metformin can upset the stomach if taken at a high milligram dose too quickly. Starting low and going slow makes it more likely a patient will stay on the medication. Excellent communication with a provider is key.

SCENARIO 14.2. ORAL DIABETES AGENTS

A patient takes a metformin/glyburide combination. How does glyburide's mechanism of action complement the mechanisms of action of metformin?

Answer: Metformin works by (1) decreasing intestinal glucose absorption, (2) lowering liver glucose production, and (3) increasing insulin sensitivity. Glyburide is a sulfonylurea that stimulates the pancreas to increase insulin production, a fourth mechanism

Insulins

Insulin is a hormone that causes cells to take up glucose, reducing the amount in the bloodstream (Fig. 14.8). Since Type I diabetics cannot produce insulin, they must use insulin as a treatment. Some Type II diabetics use insulin

TABLE 14.1 Oral Diabetes Medications

Generic (Brand)	Drug Class	Common Dosage	Adverse Effects
Metformin (Glucophage, Glucophage XR, Fortamet, Glumetza)	Biguanide	500 mg/day with a meal, up to 2000 mg	Nausea, vomiting, diarrhea, loose stools, lactic acidosis (rare)
Glipizide (Glucotrol)	Sulfonylurea	2.5–5 mg/day with breakfast	Hypoglycemia, nausea, vomiting
Glyburide (DiaBeta*)	Sulfonylurea	2.5–5 mg/day with breakfast	Hypoglycemia, nausea, vomiting
Sitagliptin (Januvia)	Dipeptidyl peptidase-4 (DPP-4) inhibitor	Up to 150 mg twice daily	Headaches, pancreatitis (rare)

Oral Meds for DM – Biguanides

Metformin (Glucophage)

Work on three of the targets
1. Stop intestinal absorption of glucose
2. Stop liver from making glucose
3. Increase insulin sensitivity

Indications	Adverse Drug Reactions
Type II diabetes Gestational diabetes	Nausea/vomiting Diarrhea/loose stools Lactic acidosis (rare)

• **Fig. 14.5** Oral Meds for Diabetes Mellitus—Biguanides

Oral Meds for DM – Sulfonylureas

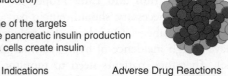

Glyburide (DiaBeta*)
Glipizide (Glucotrol)

Work on one of the targets
1. Increase pancreatic insulin production
   • Beta cells create insulin

Indications	Adverse Drug Reactions
Type II diabetes Gestational diabetes (last-line)	Hypoglycemia Nausea/vomiting

• **Fig. 14.6** Oral Meds for Diabetes Mellitus—Sulfonylureas

Oral Meds for DM – DPP4 inhibitors

Sitagliptin (Januvia)

Dipeptidyl peptidase IV (DPP4) inhibitors

Work on one of the targets
1. Increase pancreatic insulin production

Indications	Adverse Drug Reactions
Type II diabetes	Nothing seen commonly, pancreatitis (rare)

• **Fig. 14.7** Oral Meds for Diabetes Mellitus—DPP4 Inhibitors

if their condition is severe. Usually, we see insulin in Type II diabetics after oral medications fail to help them reach their targets. Insulin comes from the Latin word *insula*, which means *island*—referring to the islets of Langerhans in the pancreas, which have cells that produce insulin (beta

Injectable Meds for DM – Insulins

Insulin : Hormone that causes glucose to be taken up by cells

Several different types of insulins
• Difference is how long they work for
• Two types available over-the-counter (OTC)
   • Others Rx only

Indications	Adverse Drug Reactions
Type I diabetes Type II diabetes Gestational diabetes	Hypoglycemia

• **Fig. 14.8** Injectable Meds for Diabetes Mellitus—Insulins

Insulin – Short Acting

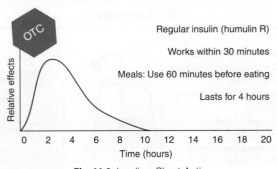

Regular insulin (humulin R)

Works within 30 minutes

Meals: Use 60 minutes before eating

Lasts for 4 hours

• **Fig. 14.9** Insulin—Short Acting

cells) to lower blood sugar and cells that produce glucagon (alpha cells), which tell the body to raise blood glucose levels.

Insulins have become very expensive, and while two are technically over-the-counter (OTC), drugstore personnel store them in the pharmacy refrigerator. This helps prevent theft and allows the pharmacy staff to control the temperature and ensure a consistent temperature while the insulin is there. One way to remember that insulins should be refrigerated is that the insulin vial's box forms a refrigerator shape.

There are many insulin types (insulin lispro and insulin glargine); two are OTC (regular insulin, NPH insulin). The difference is generally between onset and duration of action.

Insulin OTC

Regular insulin (Humulin R) is short-acting (Fig. 14.9). Be careful not to confuse short-acting with rapid-acting,

Insulin – Intermediate Acting

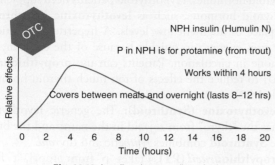

• **Fig. 14.10** Insulin—Intermediate Acting

Insulin – Rapid Acting

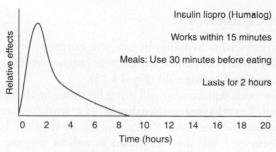

• **Fig. 14.11** Insulin—Rapid Acting

which has an even quicker onset. Medical insulin used to come from pigs or cows, but with advances in science, we now synthesize a human form. Hence, the brand name Humulin, a combination of human + insulin.

NPH insulin (Humulin N)—The NPH in **NPH insulin** represents *n*eutral *p*rotamine *H*agedorn, or how Hagedorn, the inventor, altered the insulin chemically (Fig. 14.10). The letter N and "intermediate" start with similar sounds to help you connect them.

Prescription Insulins

Insulin lispro (Humalog) is a rapid-acting insulin that one must take near mealtime (Fig. 14.11). The brand **Humalog** comes from *huma*n insulin ana*log*.

Insulin glargine (Basaglar, Lantus, Toujeo) lasts a very long time. While there are multiple brand names, using "lazy Lantus" seems to be a good way to remember that it is a 24-hour drug (Fig. 14.12).

Summary List (Fig. 14.13):
1. Rapid-acting insulin
   a. Insulin lispro (Humalog)
   b. Works within 15 minutes, lasts for 2 hours
   c. Taken 30 minutes before meals
2. Short-acting insulin
   a. Regular insulin (Humulin R)
   b. Works within 30 minutes, lasts for 4 hours
   c. Taken 60 minutes before meals
3. Intermediate-acting insulin
   a. NPH insulin (Humulin N)
   b. Works within 4 hours, lasts 8 to 12 hours

Insulin – Long Acting

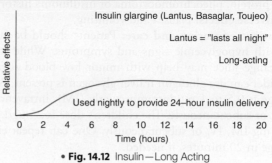

• **Fig. 14.12** Insulin—Long Acting

Insulin – Comparison

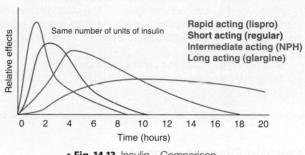

• **Fig. 14.13** Insulin—Comparison

   c. Covers between meals and overnight
4. Long-acting insulin
   a. Insulin glargine (Lantus, Basaglar, Toujeo)
   b. Lasts 24 hours
   c. Given nightly to provide 24-hour insulin delivery

Indications: Insulin is for insulin-dependent DM, non–insulin-dependent DM, and ketoacidosis.

Contraindications: Hypersensitivity to any components.

Adverse effects: Hypoglycemia and the signs and symptoms associated with it, such as tachycardia, tremors, and lethargy.

Patient education and care: Familiarity with the length of onset and peak duration as well as the medication's role. For example, a rapid-acting insulin would counteract the glucose spike during a meal. However, a longer-acting insulin covers the entire day. Proper diet and weight management along with regular testing are essential. Storage requirements such as refrigeration and expiration dates are also important. Educate the patient on the signs and symptoms of both hypoglycemia and hyperglycemia along with next steps for each condition.

Hypoglycemia

Glucagon (GlucaGen) helps a patient whose blood sugar has fallen dangerously low. One way to help remember that this medication is different from antidiabetics is to think of using glucagon when the *gluc*ose is *gone*.

Indications: Hyperglycemic agents increase the blood glucose level when hypoglycemia occurs.

Contraindications: Patients with an allergy to beef or pork protein, pheochromocytoma or insulinoma history.

Adverse effects: Nausea and vomiting.

Patient education and care: Patients should be familiar with hypoglycemic signs and symptoms. While candy or orange juice may help with minor low blood sugar, a provider can use glucagon if liver glycogen is present. Adult dosage is 0.5 to 1 mg intramuscularly (IM), intravenously (IV), or subcutaneously. The children's dose is 25 µg/kg up to 1 mg IM, IV, or subcutaneously. One can repeat either dosage in 20 minutes, if needed.

SCENARIO 14.3. INSULINS

A child complains of increased thirst and fatigue and the parents report a new bedwetting issue. The diagnosis returns as Type I diabetes. The parents ask if the child can use tablets instead of having to be poked with a needle. How do you respond?

Answer: Type I diabetics cannot produce insulin. Unfortunately, the oral medications would not help a child with this condition.

Thyroid Disorder Agents

The thyroid organ has a unique butterfly shape and produces hormones, signaling molecules produced by glands, to regulate heart rate, metabolism, and growth (Fig. 14.14). In healthy individuals, the thyroid produces the correct amount of thyroid hormones. Hypothyroid patients need supplemental thyroid hormone, such as **levothyroxine (Synthroid)**, to replace or augment low levels. A hyperthyroid patient's body uses energy too quickly because of the extra thyroid hormone in circulation. Patients can use **propylthiouracil (PTU)** to reduce the effects of too much thyroid hormone (Table 14.2).

Levothyroxine (Synthroid): The generic **levothyroxine** has the "thyro" from *thyro*id in the name and the brand name **Synthroid** combines *synth*etic and thy*roid*.

Propylthiouracil (PTU) takes "p" from *p*ropyl, "t" from "*t*hio," and "u" from *u*racil in the generic **propyl*t*hio*u*racil**. Although "thio" means there is a sulfur atom in the molecule, you can think of it as *t*hyroid lowering.

Hypothyroidism

In patients with hypothyroidism, the hormone levels are too low. Thus, the patient experiences fatigue, weight gain, shakiness, and feeling cold (Fig. 14.15).

Hormone replacement will bring hormone levels back to normal. **Levothyroxine (Synthroid)** is a synthetic version of the thyroid hormone. Prescribers adjust the dose based on hormone levels that are drawn as well as symptomatic improvement (Fig. 14.16).

Indications: Replacement treatment for cretinism, hypothyroidism, and myxedema.

Contraindications: Adrenal insufficiency, acute myocardial infarction (MI), thyrotoxicosis.

Adverse effects: Side effects would resemble a hypo- or hyperthyroid patient based on a dosage too high or low.

Patient education and care: Treatment can take up to 6 to 8 weeks for full effect. The tablets are color coded to reduce confusion regarding the correct dosage, as shown in Table 14.3.

Hyperthyroidism

In patients with hyperthyroidism, the hormone levels are too high. The patient experiences a lack of sleep, weight loss, sweating, and jitteriness (Fig. 14.17).

One treatment for hyperthyroidism is PTU, which stops the production of new thyroid hormones (Fig. 14.18).

Indications: Hyperthyroidism, thyroid storm, thyrotoxic crisis.

Contraindications: Hypersensitivity.

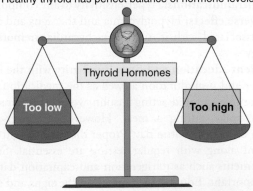

Thyroid Disorders – Pathology

Thyroid = butterfly-shaped organ on the trachea
Healthy thyroid has perfect balance of hormone levels

Thyroid Hormones

Too low   Too high

• **Fig. 14.14** Thyroid Disorders—Pathology

TABLE 14.2   Oral Thyroid Medications

Generic (Brand)	Drug Class	Common Dosage	Adverse Effects
Levothyroxine (Synthroid, Levoxyl)	For hypothyroidism	50–100 µg/day, titrating to effect	Hyperthyroidism signs and symptoms
Propylthiouracil (PTU)	For hyperthyroidism	100–150 mg/day	Hypothyroidism signs and symptoms

Adverse effects: Rash, itching, hives, alopecia, agranulocytosis (decrease in white blood cells).

Patient education and care: Monitor blood pressure, pulse, and blood work. The medication dose also lends to lab-drawn hormone levels and symptomatic improvement.

SCENARIO 14.4. THYROID DISORDER AGENTS

If a patient's record shows that he is on propylthiouracil, would you expect the diagnosis to be hyper- or hypothyroidism?
   Answer: PTU works for patients experiencing hyperthyroidism.

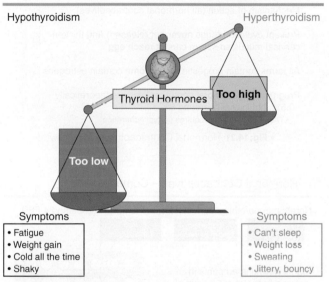

Thyroid Disorders – Pathology

Hypothyroidism / Hyperthyroidism

Thyroid Hormones — Too high / Too low

Symptoms
• Fatigue
• Weight gain
• Cold all the time
• Shaky

Symptoms
• Can't sleep
• Weight loss
• Sweating
• Jittery, bouncy

• **Fig. 14.15** Thyroid Disorders—Pathology of Hypothyroidism

---

Hypothyroidism – Hormone Replacement

Levothyroxine (Synthroid)

Synthetic version of thyroid hormone, thyroxine

Dose modified based on symptoms and hormone levels
• Takes 6–8 weeks to see full effects

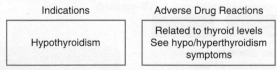

Indications	Adverse Drug Reactions
Hypothyroidism	Related to thyroid levels See hypo/hyperthyroidism symptoms

• **Fig. 14.16** Hypothyroidism—Hormone Replacement

TABLE 14.3 Levothyroxine Color Coding

Dose	Color	Dose	Color	Dose	Color
25 µg	Orange	50 µg	White	75 µg	Violet
88 µg	Olive	100 µg	Yellow	112 µg	Rose
125 µg	Brown	137 µg	Turquoise	150 µg	Blue
175 µg	Lilac	200 µg	Pink	300 µg	Green

Sex Hormones and Contraceptives

Testosterone

Testosterone is an androgen steroid hormone that naturally comes from the male testes. Prescribers can give it to patients with low testosterone levels or those going through gender conversion therapy. Testosterone as AndroGel is a synthetic gel that is identical to endogenous testosterone (Fig. 14.19).

   Testo*ster*one (AndroGel 1%) has the -ster- steroid stem. Andro- is the Greek prefix for male and -gel is the vehicle in the brand name.

   Indication: Testosterone replacement therapy in men with congenital or acquired primary hypogonadism.

   Adverse effects: Side effects can include acne breakout, an enlarged prostate, and breast development in male patients, known as gynecomastia.

   Patient education and care: An important caution is to cover the area so that one does not transfer the hormone to children.

Contraceptives Introduction

Hormonal contraceptives take the hormone cycle into account (Fig. 14.20). They work to prevent ovulation or the release of an egg, and thicken cervical mucus so that sperm cannot reach the egg. All hormonal birth control forms contain progestins, and some contain estrogens (Fig. 14.21). The theoretical effectiveness is about a 0.5% pregnancy rate. While we can see this rate in hormonal implants that are much less susceptible to human error regarding missed doses, the pill has an estimated pregnancy rate of around 8%.

Combined Oral Contraceptives

Norethindrone/ethinyl *estr*adiol/ferrous fumarate (Loestrin 24 Fe*) is a combination medicine in which we see the estrogen stem estr- (Fig. 14.22). This birth control pill includes an iron supplement. Some elements on the Periodic Table of Elements have the first letters of the element's name, such as Li for lithium and Ca for calcium. However, other elements, such as iron, refer to their Latin origins. The Fe represents ferrum, the Latin word for iron. This pill was designed to release hormones for 24 out of 28 days and reduce the length of menstruation.

Thyroid Disorders – **Pathology**

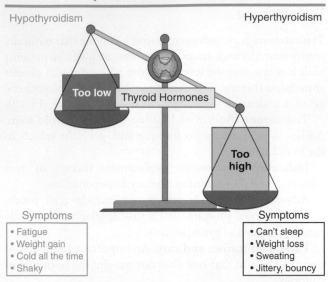

• **Fig. 14.17** Thyroid Disorders—Pathology of Hyperthyroidism

Hyperthyroidism – Antithyroid Agents

Propylthiouracil (PTU)

Stops production of new thyroid hormones

Dose modified based on symptoms and hormone levels
• Takes 6–8 weeks to see full effects

Indications	Adverse Drug Reactions
Hyperthyroidism	Related to thyroid levels See hypo/hyperthyroidism symptoms

• **Fig. 14.18** Hyperthyroidism—Antithyroid Agents

Sex Hormones – Testosterone

Testosterone (AndroGel)
• Transdermal gel

Synthetically made, but identical to endogenous testosterone

Application areas should be covered to prevent transfer to children

Indications	Adverse Drug Reactions
Low testosterone levels	Acne Prostate enlargement Gynecomastia (rare)

• **Fig. 14.19** Sex Hormones—Testosterone

Nor*gest*imate/ethinyl *estr*adiol (Tri-Sprintec) is a combination oral contraceptive that again has both the estrogen stem estr- and progestin stem -gest- (Fig. 14.23). This regimen has two different hormones and three different hormone levels, each given for 7 days, totaling 21 days. The last 7 days of placebo at the end allow a patient to take it every day and not have to remember to take a week off and then come back again.

Hormonal Contraceptives – Cycle Overview

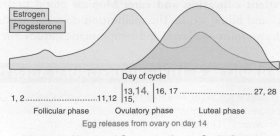

• **Fig. 14.20** Hormonal Contraceptives—Cycle Overview

Hormonal Contraceptives – Overview

Mechanism of action (all hormonal contraceptives):

Prevent ovulation (eggs never get released) and thicken cervical mucus so sperm cannot reach egg

All forms contain progestins, only some contain estrogens

Pregnancy rates of oral contraceptives are theoretically ~0.5%, but in reality around 8%
• Theoretical number requires <u>perfect</u> adherence

• **Fig. 14.21** Hormonal Contraceptives—Overview

Hormonal Contraceptives – Combined

Norethindrone/ethinyl estradiol/ferrous fumarate (Loestrin 24 FE*)

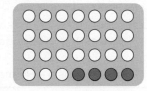

Same hormone amounts in active pills for 24 of 28 days of cycle to reduce length of menstruation

• **Fig. 14.22** Hormonal Contraceptives—Combined (Part 1)

Hormonal Contraceptives – Combined

Norgestimate/ethinyl estradiol (Tri-sprintec)

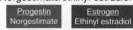
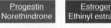

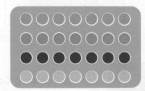

Three different hormone amounts over 21 days, each 7 days long
• More estrogen at beginning
• More progestin at end
• Last week is placebo
Why do this?

• **Fig. 14.23** Hormonal Contraceptives—Combined (Part 2)

The Patch and Ring

Norel*gest*romin/ethinyl *estr*adiol (Xulane) also has the -gest- and -estr- stems from the progestin and estrogen hormones, respectively (Fig. 14.24). Think of the "Norel" in **Norelgestromin** as "not oral" to remember that this is

Hormonal Contraceptives – Combined

Norelgestromin/ethinyl estradiol transdermal patch (Xulane)

Progestin	Estrogen
Norelgestromin	Ethinyl estradiol

Patch applied to torso, back, or buttock once per week for 3 weeks then 1 week off

Stays on all week long, even when showering/bathing

Actual failure rate: 8%

• **Fig. 14.24** Hormonal Contraceptives—Combined (Part 3)

Hormonal Contraceptives – Combined

Etonogestrel/ethinyl estradiol vaginal ring (NuvaRing)

Progestin	Estrogen
Etonogestrel	Ethinyl estradiol

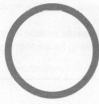

Flexible polymer ring that releases hormones slowly

Ring inserted vaginally for 21 days, removed for 7 days, then new one inserted

Actual failure rate: 8%

• **Fig. 14.25** Hormonal Contraceptives—Combined (Part 4)

Hormonal Contraception – Emergency

Levonorgestrel oral tablet (Plan B One-Step)

Progestin
Levonogestrel

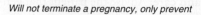

Progestin-only contraceptive

Effective up to 72 hours after unprotected sex

Will not terminate a pregnancy, only prevent

• **Fig. 14.26** Hormonal Contraception—Emergency

a patch. A transdermal patch can be applied to the torso, back, or buttock once per week for 3 weeks, with 1 week off. This patch should stay on even when showering or bathing. The failure rate is about 8%, similar to oral birth control.

Etonogestrel/ethinyl *est*radiol (NuvaRing)—in this case, think of the "Etono" in ***Etono*gestrel** as "Eat, oh no" to remember that it is not an oral dosage form (Fig. 14.25). This vaginal ring has a flexible polymer that slowly releases the dose. One inserts it for 3 weeks and then removes it for 1 week. Actual failure rate for this dosage form is also 8%.

Emergency Contraception

Levonor*gest*rel (Plan B One-Step) has the progestin -gest-stem (Fig. 14.26). It can cause nausea; sipping a flat (non-carbonated) soda may serve as a remedy for this discomfort. The name **Plan B One-Step** comes from the revised dosage form. A past form took two steps or doses.

Patient education and care: While the prior forms prevent pregnancy and are prescribed, one OTC option

Contraceptives – IUDs

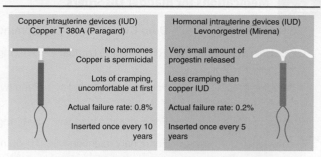

• **Fig. 14.27** Contraceptives—Intrauterine Devices

is the emergency contraceptive pill levonorgestrel (Plan B One-Step). It is a one-time dose to prevent pregnancy after unprotected sex. A patient must take it within 72 hours of unprotected sex for maximum efficacy. This pill does not terminate an existing pregnancy; it can only prevent one from happening.

Other Birth Control Forms

A hormonal intrauterine device (IUD) is available that contains **levonorgestrel (Mirena)**. It releases small doses of progestins directly into the uterus. A **copper IUD (ParaGard)** allows copper to act as a spermicidal agent. This prevents sperm from reaching the egg (Fig. 14.27).

Patient education and care: With Mirena, a prescriber inserts the device every 5 years. This device has a failure rate of 0.2%. Side effects are minimal. With ParaGard, this option can cause cramping and discomfort initially. Generally, a prescriber would insert this device every 10 years; its failure rate is near 0.8%.

SCENARIO 14.5. SEX HORMONES AND CONTRACEPTION

A female patient has questions about her new IUD and how it works. You see that she is going to use ParaGard. Is that a hormonal IUD or a copper IUD?

Answer: ParaGard is a copper IUD. The copper acts to kill sperm.

Bladder Disorders

We generally group bladder disorders into one of two categories: either a patient has an overactive bladder (OAB) or struggles with urinary retention. The goal is to "dry up" the bladder or allow the patient to urinate more comfortably (Table 14.4).

Overactive Bladder

OAB is a sudden urge to empty the bladder even when it might not be full. This is usually because the nerves, bladder muscle, and brain mistake how much urine is in the bladder

TABLE 14.4	Medications for Bladder Disorders			
Generic (Brand)	Drug Class	Common Dosage	Adverse Effects
Oxybutynin (Oxytrol, Ditropan*)	For overactive bladder	5–10 mg/day	Dry mouth, dizziness, constipation, urinary tract infections
Tolterodine (Detrol LA)	For overactive bladder	2 mg twice daily	Headache, dry mouth, dizziness, constipation, angioedema
Solifenacin (VESIcare)	For overactive bladder	5–10 mg/day	Dry mouth, constipation
Bethanechol (Urecholine)	For urinary retention	10–50 mg up to 3 times daily	Lacrimation, diarrhea, cramping

Overactive Bladder (OAB) - Pathology

Disconnect between nerves, bladder muscle, and brain about urine quantity

Sudden urge to empty bladder even when it is not full

Most commonly seen in older adults, but can occur in anyone, male or female

Medications focus on "drying" things up

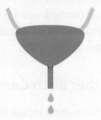

• **Fig. 14.28** Overactive Bladder (OAB)—Pathology

OAB – Antimuscarinics

Oxybutynin (Oxytrol, Ditropan)
Solifenacin (Vesicare)
Tolterodine (Detrol)

Relax smooth muscle of bladder (detrusor), allowing more urine to fill in bladder before needing to be emptied

Indications	Adverse Drug Reactions
Overactive bladder	Drowsiness Confusion Dry mouth Urinary retention

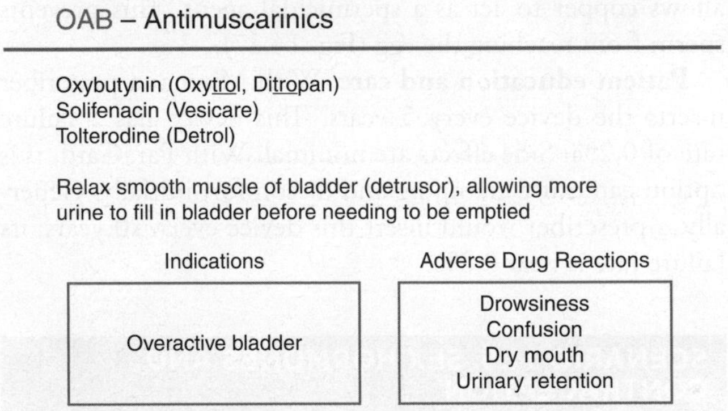

• **Fig. 14.29** Overactive Bladder—Antimuscarinics

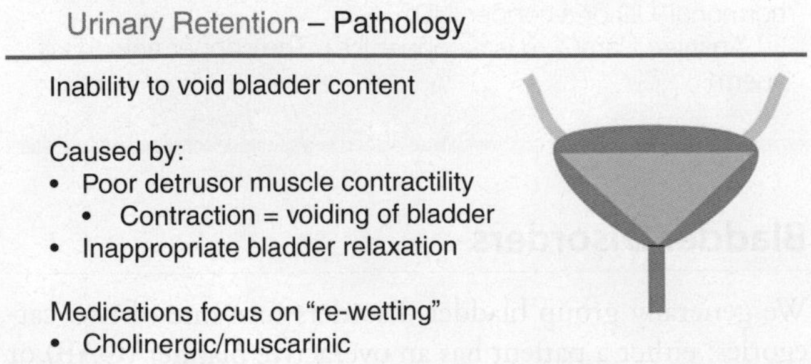

Urinary Retention – Pathology

Inability to void bladder content

Caused by:
• Poor detrusor muscle contractility
  • Contraction = voiding of bladder
• Inappropriate bladder relaxation

Medications focus on "re-wetting"
• Cholinergic/muscarinic

• **Fig. 14.30** Urinary Retention—Pathology

(Fig. 14.28). While this is a common condition for older adults, it can occur in any male or female patient.

Antimuscarinic medicines such as **oxybutynin (Oxytrol, Ditropan*)**, **tolterodine (Detrol)**, and **solifenacin (VESIcare)** are OAB mainstays (Fig. 14.29). These medications relax the bladder's smooth muscle wall. The generic **oxybutynin** brand names **Ditropan*** and

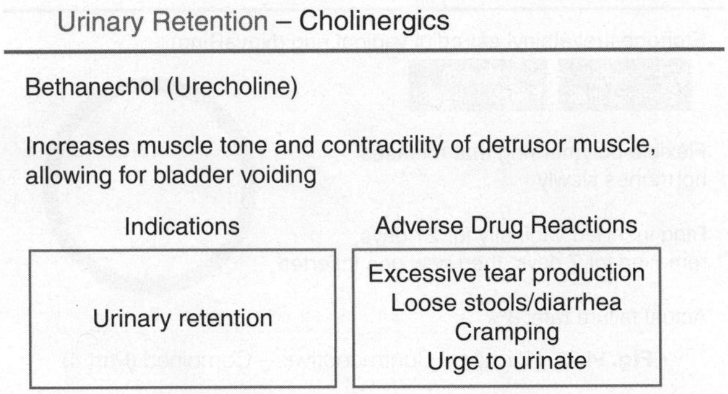

Urinary Retention – Cholinergics

Bethanechol (Urecholine)

Increases muscle tone and contractility of detrusor muscle, allowing for bladder voiding

Indications	Adverse Drug Reactions
Urinary retention	Excessive tear production Loose stools/diarrhea Cramping Urge to urinate

• **Fig. 14.31** Urinary Retention—Cholinergics

Oxytrol OTC have the "tro" from control for con*tro*lling an OAB. **Tolterodine (Detrol)** has the "tro" from con*trol* in the name as well. **Detrol** helps control the *detr*usor muscle, keeping urine in. **Solifenacin (VESIcare)** is a once-daily dose; therefore, think about urine that needs to be "fenced in."

Patient education and care: Advise the patient that general anticholinergic effects such as drowsiness, confusion, dry mouth, and urinary retention can happen. To combat dry mouth, candy or ice chips can help.

Urinary Retention

Urinary retention happens when a patient cannot completely void bladder contents (Fig. 14.30). The etiology comes from poor detrusor muscle contractility or inappropriate relaxation of the bladder. Medications are cholinergic/muscarinic, the opposite of OAB medications.

Bethanechol (Urecholine*) is a primary treatment for urinary retention (Fig. 14.31). It increases muscle tone and detrusor muscle contractility. This helps the bladder void more completely. The "chol" in **bethane*chol*** helps you remember that it is cholinergic. The former brand name **Urecholine** implies how it affects *uri*nation through *cho*-*line*rgic effects.

Patient education and care: Advise patients to expect the opposite of anticholinergic effects present in medications for OAB. Patients on bethanechol can expect excessive lacrimation (tears), loose stools/diarrhea, and cramping.

Benign Prostate Hyperplasia

Benign prostate hyperplasia (BPH) is a prostate growth that squeezes the urethra, inhibiting urine flow (Fig. 14.32). The urination urge remains, but the blockage impedes the actual ability to go. Two drug classes focus on two different treatment paths (Table 14.5).
1. Increasing the diameter of the urethra with alpha-blockers
2. Shrinking the prostate with 5-alpha reductase inhibitors

Alpha-1 Blockers

Alpha-1 blockers such as **tamsulosin (Flomax)** and **alfuzosin (Uroxatral)** can increase the diameter of the urethra and provide relatively quick relief, which increases urine flow (Fig. 14.33). Adverse reactions might include dizziness, orthostatic hypotension, and headaches that can be very severe, especially with the first dose. Patient education should also include that the patient should not chew extended-release preparations, but rather swallow the capsule or tablet whole.

Tamsulosin (Flomax) has the -osin ending, which is not an actual stem but rather a way to connect tamsulosin and alfuzosin as similar. **Flomax** allows for *max*imum urinary *flo*w, the goal of BPH treatment.

Alfuzosin (Uroxatral) is another option for BPH. The brand name **Uroxatral** sounds a little like *uri*ne con*tral*.

5-Alpha Reductase Inhibitors

5-Alpha reductase inhibitors such as **dutasteride (Avodart)** and **finasteride (Proscar)** work to decrease hormone production that helps the prostate grow, allowing for increased urine flow (Fig. 14.34). This may take a significant amount of time. Side effects can include decreased libido and erectile dysfunction (ED).

Dutasteride (Avodart) has the -steride stem, which is similar to the "ster" in steroid to help you remember that it is for men with a prostate concern.

Finasteride (Proscar, Propecia) has two brand names for two very different purposes. Proscar is for prostate care. Propecia alludes to hair growth, the reverse of alopecia (hair loss).

Patient education and care: The speed at which alpha-blockers work (quickly) and 5-alpha reductase inhibitors (slowly) may necessitate a combination treatment. Finasteride is contraindicated in women who are looking to become pregnant or who are pregnant.

Benign Prostate Hyperplasia (BPH) – Pathology

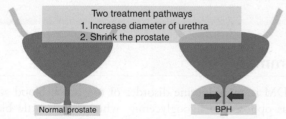

Growth of prostate that squeezes onto urethra and inhibits urine flow
Urge to urinate is still there, but flow is blocked

Two treatment pathways
1. Increase diameter of urethra
2. Shrink the prostate

Normal prostate   BPH

• **Fig. 14.32** Benign Prostate Hyperplasia—Pathology

TABLE 14.5	Medications for Benign Prostatic Hyperplasia and Erectile Dysfunction		
Generic (Brand)	Drug class	Common dosage	Adverse Effects
Alfuzosin (Uroxatral)	Alpha-1 blocker	10 mg/day	Dizziness, headache, orthostatic hypotension
Tamsulosin (Flomax)	Alpha-1 blocker	0.4 mg once daily	Dizziness, headache, orthostatic hypotension
Dutasteride (Avodart)	5-Alpha reductase inhibitor	0.5 mg daily	Decreased libido, erectile dysfunction
Finasteride (Proscar)	5-Alpha reductase inhibitor	5 mg daily	Decreased libido, erectile dysfunction
Sildenafil (Viagra)	Phosphodiesterase-5 (PDE-5) inhibitor	25–50 mg as a single dose 30 minutes to 4 hours before intercourse	Headache, heartburn, rarely priapism
Tadalafil (Cialis)	PDE-5 inhibitor	2.5, 5, or 10 mg as a single dose	Headache, myopathy, flushing, rarely priapism

BPH – Alpha-1 Blockers

Tamsulosin (Flomax)
Alfuzosin (Uroxatral)

Cause relaxation of prostate, increasing urine flow
• Increases urethra diameter

Indications	Adverse Drug Reactions
Benign prostate hyperplasia	All uncommon: Dizziness Headache Orthostatic hypotension

• **Fig. 14.33** Benign Prostate Hyperplasia—Alpha-1 Blockers

BPH – 5-Alpha Reductase Inhibitors

Dutasteride (Avodart)
Finasteride (Proscar)

Decrease hormone production the prostate uses to grow
• Eventually leads to prostate shrinkage

Indications	Adverse Drug Reactions
Benign prostate hyperplasia	Decreased libido Erectile dysfunction

• **Fig. 14.34** Benign Prostate Hyperplasia—5-Alpha Reductase Inhibitors

Erectile Dysfunction (ED) – Pathology

Inability to attain or maintain an erection

Most men with ED have some underlying microvascular disorder
• Hypertension
• Coronary artery disease
• Peripheral artery disease
• Diabetes mellitus (Type I or II)

Treatment involves increasing blood flow to the penis

• **Fig. 14.35** Erectile Dysfunction (ED)—Pathology

Erectile Dysfunction

A male has ED if he is unable to attain or maintain an erection (Fig. 14.35). Most men with ED will have an underlying microvascular disease. These include coronary artery disease (CAD), hypertension, or DM. Treatment focuses on increasing penile blood flow. We try not to use the old term "impotence" because of the harshness of the word and implication that the patient is being judged as "impotent."

Phosphodiesterase-5 (PDE-5) inhibitors are currently the primary ED treatment (Fig. 14.36). They increase penile blood flow through nitric oxide–induced vasodilation.

Silden*afil* (Viagra) has the -afil stem indicating that it is a PDE-5 inhibitor. **Viagra** brings *via*ble *g*rowth—an erection. This medicine has the shorter of the two medications' half-lives.

ED – Phosphodiesterase-5 (PDE-5) Inhibitors

Sildenafil (Viagra) – taken 1 hour before needed
Tadalafil (Cialis) – taken 1 hour before needed, lasts 72 hours

Increase penile blood flow through nitric oxide-induced vasodilation

Indications	Adverse Drug Reactions
Erectile dysfunction	Headache Flushing Hypotension

• **Fig. 14.36** Erectile Dysfunction—Phosphodiesterase-5 (PDE-5) Inhibitors

Tadal*afil* (Cialis) also has the -afil suffix and is commonly called the "weekend pill" because it, unlike **sildenafil**, lasts the weekend. This is due to its long half-life, a measure of how long the body will take to reduce the amount in the body by half.

Patient education and care: Adverse reactions include headache, flushing, and hypotension. PDE-5 inhibitors have a dangerous interaction with nitrates. The combination can lead to fatal hypotension. As such, do not combine PDE-5 inhibitors and nitrates.

SCENARIO 14.8. ERECTILE DYSFUNCTION

An elderly male with a history of angina pectoris presents a new prescription for sildenafil (Viagra). Why should you be concerned?

Answer: Sildenafil is a PDE-5 inhibitor, which interacts with nitrates. A patient with a history of angina likely takes nitrates as a vasodilator, which will cause a dangerous interaction with the PDE-5 inhibitor.

Summary

• DM is an endocrine disorder of too much blood sugar as opposed to hypoglycemia, which is too little blood sugar. The three types of diabetes are Type I, Type II, and gestational.
• Oral diabetic medications such as the biguanide metformin affect organ use and production of glucose. Metformin, for example, affects intestinal glucose absorption, liver glucose production, and insulin sensitivity.
• There are four primary insulin types that include two by prescription (insulin lispro and insulin glargine) and two OTC (regular and NPH). Insulin differences usually have to do with onset and duration of action.
• Hypothyroid patients need a supplemental thyroid hormone such as levothyroxine. Patients who are hyperthyroid will need a medication to reduce thyroid hormone levels, such as PTU.
• While there are many different hormonal forms for birth control, we usually see the estrogen stem estr- and progestin stem -gest- in pharmacologic names. Birth control pills can include an iron supplement.

- Anticholinergic medications for OAB, such as oxybutynin, are "drying" in their therapeutic effect and side effects. Medications for urinary retention, such as bethanechol, are "wetting."
- BPH is a prostate growth with two primary treatment options: (1) increase the diameter of the urethra with alpha-1 blockers such as tamsulosin or (2) shrink the prostate with 5-alpha reductase inhibitors such as finasteride.
- Treatments for ED include PDE-5 inhibitors such as sildenafil and tadalafil. These medications can cause a dangerous hypotensive state when combined with nitrates.

Review Questions

1. Which antidiabetic medicine is most likely to cause lactic acidosis?
   a. Insulin glargine (Lantus)
   b. NPH insulin (Humulin N)
   c. Metformin (Glucophage)
   d. Glyburide (DiaBeta*)
2. With regard to time courses of insulins, insulin lispro should be given ____ minutes before a meal, and will start working in ____ minutes
   a. 30, 15
   b. 15, 30
   c. 30, 60
   d. 60, 30
3. Which of the following insulins is short acting?
   a. Regular insulin (Humulin R)
   b. Insulin lispro (Humalog)
   c. NPH insulin (Humulin N)
   d. Insulin glargine (Lantus)
4. A medication for hypothyroidism is ____, while a medication for hyperthyroidism is ____.
   a. Insulin glargine (Lantus), metformin (Glucophage)
   b. Metformin (Glucophage), insulin glargine (Lantus)
   c. Levothyroxine (Synthroid), propylthiouracil (PTU)
   d. Propylthiouracil (PTU), levothyroxine (Synthroid)
5. Which additional instructions would you give a patient who was recently started on AndroGel?
   a. "Take this medication with food."
   b. "Cover the application area to avoid transfer to children."
   c. "This medication contains estrogen and progestin."
   d. "This is an oral medication that should be taken with water."
6. Which of the following birth control medications is a flexible polymer vaginal ring that is inserted for 3 weeks, and then removed for 1 week?
   a. Etonogestrel/ethinyl estradiol (NuvaRing)
   b. Levonorgestrel (Mirena)
   c. Norelgestromin/ethinyl estradiol (Ortho Evra*)
   d. Levonorgestrel (Plan B One-Step)
7. One would expect an anticholinergic such as oxybutynin (Ditropan*) to cause ____.
   a. Dry mouth
   b. Lacrimation
   c. Diarrhea
   d. Urinary incontinence
8. Which of the following medications for urinary retention might cause excessive tear production, loose stools/diarrhea, and cramping?
   a. Tamsulosin (Flomax)
   b. Tolterodine (Detrol)
   c. Bethanechol (Urecholine*)
   d. Sildenafil (Viagra)
9. Which of the following medications acts by decreasing hormone production of the prostate?
   a. Solifenacin (VESIcare)
   b. Finasteride (Proscar)
   b. Tamsulosin (Flomax)
   c. Alfuzosin (Uroxatral)
10. A dangerous interaction exists between sildenafil (Viagra) and which medication?
    a. Nitroglycerin, a nitrate
    b. Amlodipine, a calcium channel blocker
    c. Lisinopril, an ACE inhibitor
    d. Valsartan, an ARB

15

Pediatric Pharmacology

Pharmacology for Pediatric Patients

In this section, we will discuss pediatric patients, who range from newborns to adolescents. We are differentiating them from neonates, who are less than 4 weeks old. Children of all ages differ from adult patients in many ways, including those disease states that affect them and their medication dosing regimens. There is a reason that most pediatric over-the-counter medications list age and weight guidelines for dosing on their packaging. Most parents can accurately tell a person their child's age, but not their weight, which changes more often. However, weight is often a better way to dose medications for pediatric patients.

With a wide range of patient sizes, the dosing will also have a much larger scale. Dosing for pediatric patients must be individualized as much as possible. Unlike an adult, who can take a couple of ibuprofen for a headache, we often dose pediatric patients by weight and require some calculations to get the dosage just right. While this creates more precision, we sometimes sacrifice accuracy. Having to provide calculations creates opportunities for mistakes when choosing the correct dose. Children are also more vulnerable to medication errors because there is limited data published on medication use in pediatrics.

While there is extensive data on adult dosages, we cannot perform the same kinds of clinical trials on children because of ethical concerns about testing on children. As such, not as many drugs are explicitly labeled for use in children. There is also potential for an administration error by the parent or patient, who may or may not have functional health literacy. To minimize errors, we often provide marked syringes for oral liquids and counseling with demonstrations and teach-back to assess the parent or caregiver's understanding.

When determining the correct course of action, *The Harriet Lane Handbook* is a trusted resource for treating various pediatric diseases, as are the *Pediatric Dosage Handbook*, *Pediatric Drug Formulations*, Children's Hospital of Philadelphia: Extemporaneous Formulations for Oral Administration, and *Allen's Compounded Formulations*.

Calculations

Be sure to look up pediatric dosing in a trusted source. Do not rely on the following formulas for all medications, as they can vary based on many different factors!

Weight-Based Dosing

Weight-based dosing is the most common way to calculate dosing for pediatric patients, though there are other methods. The formulas are often given as the amount of drug needed per kilogram of the patient's body mass. If the child's weight is recorded in pounds, then it must be converted to kilograms before calculating the dosing. Each kilogram equals 2.2 pounds.

Example: Calculate the amount of amoxicillin needed for a 20-pound (lb) child. The weight-based dosing for amoxicillin is 25 to 50 mg/kg/day in 3 divided doses. That means 8.3 to 16.7 mg/kg/dose:

$$\text{Weight in kg} = 20 \text{ lb}/2.2 \text{ lb/kg} = 9.1 \text{ kg}$$

$$\text{Dose} = 8.3 \text{ mg/kg} \times 9.1 \text{ kg} = 75.5 \text{ mg/dose}$$

$$= 16.7 \text{ mg/kg} \times 9.1 \text{ kg} = 152 \text{ mg/dose}$$

$$\text{Dose} = 75.5 \text{ to } 152 \text{ mg/dose}$$

Now, since we cannot be that specific with dosing, we are going to see a dosage that is very near to those numbers at 75 to 150 mg per dose, or since the suspension comes as 250 mg/5 mL, the prescriber will indicate that the patient should take 1.5 to 3 mL of suspension per dose.

---

* Brand discontinued, now available only as generic
† Naming conventions can vary between prescription and OTC formulations

Clark's Rule

One formula to calculate pediatric dosing is Clark's rule. This formula is:

Dose = (Adult dose) × (Child's weight in lb/150).

Example: A 20-lb child is ordered a medication for which the adult dose is 500 mg.

Dose = (500 mg) × (20 lb/150 lb) = 66.7 mg

You can see how this is not as precise as using the weight but is somewhat close.

Young's Rule

Young's rule is based on age. The formula is:

Dose = (Adult dose) × (Age/Age + 12)

Example: A 5-year-old child is receiving a medication for which the adult dose is 500 mg.

Dose = (500 mg) × (5/[5 + 12]) = 147 mg

It is up to the prescriber to determine which formula is the best course of action for the dosage.

SCENARIO 15.1. DOSING DILEMMA

Shelby is a tall 11-year-old patient in your hospital. She is larger than most children her age, weighing 150 lbs. She is running a fever for which the doctor orders acetaminophen. The weight-based pediatric dose for acetaminophen is 10 to 15 mg/kg/dose every 4 to 6 hours, with a maximum of 4000 mg/day. How much acetaminophen should you give Shelby for each dose?

Answer: Shelby should receive acetaminophen 500 to 650 mg every 4 to 6 hours, the same as adult dosing.

When calculating a weight-based dose, you will get an answer that is well above the maximum daily dose of 4000 mg/day—10 to 15 mg/kg/dose would give 681 to 1022 mg/dose. If given every 4 hours, or six times that day, any dose in this range would exceed the maximum daily dose of 4000 mg/day. It is important to make sure that a weight-based dose does not exceed a maximum dose, as this could result in an overdose and serious harm to the patient.

Treatment and Prevention of Common Disease States

Fever

Fever occurs when the body raises its temperature through physiologic processes to fight infection. Normal body temperature is 37°C (98.6°F). A fever of concern depends on the child's age and the method of temperature measurement.

For infants under 3 months old, a fever of concern is anything above 38°C (100.4°F) taken rectally. For children 3 to 36 months old, a fever is 38°C to 39°C (100.4°F–102.2°F), and a fever of concern is above 39°C (102.2°F) taken rectally. For children over 36 months old and adults, a fever is 37.8°C to 39.4°C (100°F–103°F), and a fever of concern is anything above 39.5°C (103.1°F).

For infants under 3 months of age who have a fever, consult a doctor. This high temperature may be a sign of a severe infection. Do not treat with medication at home unless told by your provider, as the fever may be the only sign of infection. For infants and children over 3 months of age, treat a fever if the child is uncomfortable or the fever is exceedingly high. Get medical help for a fever of concern. Again, the provider is the best resource here.

The two main pharmaceutical treatments in pediatrics for fever are acetaminophen (Tylenol) and ibuprofen (Advil, Motrin*). Do not use aspirin in children and adolescents as this can cause a severe reaction called Reye syndrome, especially if they have a viral infection. Other nonpharmaceutical treatments include hydration and cold compresses.

Acetaminophen's weight-based dosing is 10 to 15 mg/kg/dose every 4 to 6 hours as needed. Do not exceed five doses per day, 1 g/dose, 75 mg/kg/day, or 4 g/day.

Ibuprofen's weight-based dosing is 5 to 10 mg/kg/dose every 6 to 8 hours as needed. Do not exceed 600 mg/dose, 40 mg/kg/day, or 2.4 g/day. Do not use ibuprofen in infants under 6 months old. Alternating medications is not recommended, as it is easy to confuse doses.

Acute Otitis Media

Acute otitis media, otherwise known as a middle ear infection, commonly affects young children. Viruses or bacteria may cause acute otitis media. This possible cause of the disease is why, with shared decision making, we may wait 48 to 72 hours from symptom onset before initiating antibiotic therapy.

We would start immediate antibiotic therapy if the patient is under 2 years old and both ears are affected, or their ears are running. Pain should be managed with acetaminophen or ibuprofen. Vaccination with Prevnar 13 and the annual influenza vaccine may help to prevent some acute otitis media infections.

First-line antibiotics are amoxicillin (Amoxil*), amoxicillin-clavulanate (Augmentin), or second- or third-generation cephalosporins. Clindamycin is an option for patients with penicillin and cephalosporin allergies or who have experienced treatment failure.

SCENARIO 15.2. THE EARACHE

Justin is 18 months old and has been tugging on his ears and crying more than usual. The pediatrician finds evidence of bilateral acute otitis media (double ear infection). He has no known drug allergies. What should be done for Justin?

Answer: We should choose immediate antibiotic therapy for Justin rather than watch and wait since he is under 2 years old and his acute otitis media is bilateral. As first-line treatment, we can choose amoxicillin. If this fails to treat the infection, we can try amoxicillin and clavulanate (Augmentin), second- or third-generation cephalosporin, or clindamycin.

Pharyngitis

Pharyngitis, or sore throat, may be caused by viruses or bacteria. The most common bacterium that causes pharyngitis is Group A beta-hemolytic streptococcus (GAS). This disease is otherwise known as strep throat and mostly affects school-aged children and adolescents.

It is essential to treat Group A strep with antibiotics to prevent it from progressing to rheumatic fever or glomerulonephritis, which are significantly more dangerous. Antibiotics commonly used are amoxicillin, penicillin V, or benzathine penicillin G injection. For those with penicillin allergies, we can use cephalexin, cefadroxil, clindamycin, azithromycin, or erythromycin.

Immunizations

Vaccines play an essential part in making children healthier and protecting them from disease. Vaccines have decreased the incidence and spread of conditions that can make a patient acutely ill and that may have lasting effects on one's health, including death. Vaccines have even eliminated smallpox. It is vital for enough members of a population to be vaccinated or immune to a disease to protect those who cannot receive the vaccine themselves. This concept is called *herd immunity*.

It is recommended that each child receive vaccinations as recommended based on their age. The recommended vaccine time frame and catch-up schedule are on the websites of the Centers for Disease Control and Prevention (CDC) and American Academy of Pediatrics. The vaccinations typically received in early childhood are hepatitis B, rotavirus, DTaP, Hib, PCV13, inactivated polio, MMR, varicella, possibly hepatitis A, and two doses of an annual influenza vaccine. They recommend older children receive Tdap, HPV, meningitis, and a yearly influenza vaccine. Particularly vulnerable patients may require additional vaccinations as well.

Summary

- Pediatric patients present unique challenges in medicine.
- Medications for pediatric patients are often calculated based on weight, but it is essential not to exceed the maximum dose.
- There are intricacies in each common disease state that lead to different criteria in the use of antibiotics.
- It is essential to follow the CDC's vaccination schedule to keep individual children and our population healthy.

Review Questions

1. Which is *not* a way of preventing administration errors in pediatric populations?
   a. Counsel caregivers using demonstrations
   b. Utilize dose-marked oral syringes
   c. Tell the caregiver to look it up
   d. Have the caregiver teach back to you

2. What is the most common way to calculate the dose of medication for a child?
   a. Weight-based dosing
   b. Take until the effect is reached
   c. Half the adult dose
   d. Same as the adult dose

3. While calculating weight-based dosing in mg/kg, what conversion often needs to happen?
   a. Kilograms to grams
   b. Pounds to kilograms
   c. Pounds to ounces
   d. Kilograms to pounds

4. Brian is 6 years old and weighs 45 lb. He needs a dose of ibuprofen (7.5 mg/kg) for his fever. What is the dosage?
   a. 95 mg
   b. 124 mg
   c. 153 mg
   d. 200 mg

5. Which should not be used for children with a fever?
   a. Acetaminophen
   b. Ibuprofen
   c. Hydration
   d. Aspirin

6. Which is a trusted source for treating pediatric patients?
   a. The red book
   b. *The Harriet Lane Handbook*
   c. The orange book
   d. The purple book

7. Which patient with acute otitis media is a candidate for a wait and watch?
   a. 18 months old with otorrhea
   b. 10 months old with bilateral acute otitis media
   c. 36 months old with unilateral acute otitis media
   d. 36 months old with otorrhea

8. A patient has failed amoxicillin therapy for acute otitis media. What should you try next?
   a. Acetaminophen
   b. Amoxicillin and clavulanate (14:1)
   c. Erythromycin
   d. Sulfamethoxazole-trimethoprim

9. How can you treat a patient with strep pharyngitis with a penicillin allergy?
   a. Azithromycin
   b. Penicillin V
   c. Amoxicillin
   d. Wait and watch

10. Which is a reason to keep a child (or adult) up-to-date on vaccines?
    a. Prevent disease that could harm the patient
    b. Prevent disease outbreaks in the community
    c. Herd immunity
    d. All of the above

16

Geriatric Pharmacology

LEARNING OBJECTIVES

1. Describe the process of aging and the geriatric population's medication use
2. Contrast pharmacokinetic parameters in the geriatric population.
3. Identify drugs and diseases of particular significance in the geriatric population.
4. Describe tactics to recognize and improve breaks in drug compliance in the elderly.

The Process of Aging

Before we begin, it makes sense to provide a delineation between adult and geriatric. While a person who is older than 65 years can feel or be physically healthier than someone who is younger than 65 years, having an age cutoff helps us group these patients who often have similar health challenges. The rate at which someone ages varies greatly depending on conditions the person can and cannot control. While individuals can commit to nutrition and exercise, genetics and diseases may affect them in ways beyond their control. In this chapter, we will focus on how these differences between the adult and geriatric population affect and are affected by medication therapy.

Geriatric Population's Medication Use

An increased life expectancy has allowed the population over 65 years to expand rapidly. The data show that, at least in the United States, this trend will likely continue. Newer drugs and treatments provide a foundation for living longer; however, these medications, especially the newer ones, can be prohibitively expensive. The geriatric population often uses a disproportionate number of prescriptions and, as they get older, their drug lists often lengthen (Fig. 16.1). Also, one condition can make another worse. For example, it is common to see patients who have high blood pressure also combating arthritis or asthma. As the number of drugs increase, so does the potential for medications to interact with each other.

Pharmacokinetic Changes and Aging

What happens to our organs and their efficiency as we age? Once an adult reaches the 30-year-old mark, there tends to be a regular drop in the ability of the cardiovascular system

to keep up with the demands of the body. This not only affects the heart, which feeds itself oxygenated blood, but also the liver, which is responsible for a significant portion of drug metabolism, and the kidneys, which often take on drug excretion. What happens when the body cannot metabolize or excrete a drug as quickly? The body has more drug around, and the drug produces toxic effects if there is no dosage reduction (Table 16.1). As we learn about how aging can affect pharmacokinetics, we will look specifically at the four arms of pharmacokinetics we touched on earlier in the book as they relate to the over-65 population: absorption, distribution, metabolism, and excretion.

Absorption

The primary response to increasing age is having a delayed drug action. When the medication enters the body, the small intestine generally takes the role of absorption. However, in the geriatric population, there is less blood flow to the gastrointestinal tract and less intestinal motion. As such, the drug absorbs slower and acts slower. This can be especially important if an antibiotic, for example, cannot reach a high enough peak to eliminate a bacterial infection.

Distribution

As slower absorption delays drug onset, the geriatric population also has to contend with the way the body distributes the drug. In general, we expect the need for lower doses because of changes in muscle mass and water. In the geriatric population, muscle often decreases, as does the total body water. This creates a situation in which the same drug a person took as an adult has a greater concentration as that patient ages.

A medication that is water soluble now has less water in which to dissolve. Since the body fat percentage also increases in the elderly, a lipid-soluble drug will now spread out more rather than quickly reaching the organs to metabolize and excrete them. This results in a longer duration of

---

* Brand discontinued, now available only as generic
† Naming conventions can vary between prescription and OTC formulations

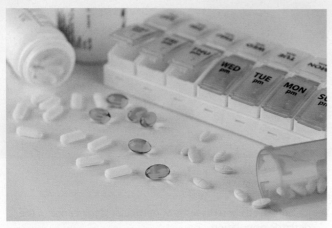

• **Fig. 16.1** Weekly Pill Box (©istock #160301690)

TABLE 16.1	Pharmacokinetic Changes in the Geriatric Population	
Pharmacokinetic Element	**Geriatric Population Characteristics**	
Absorption	Reduced gastrointestinal blood flow results in slower medication onset.	
Distribution	Reduced total body water, lean muscle mass, and plasma proteins lead to increased medication concentrations.	
Metabolism	Decreased metabolism leads to increased levels of medication.	
Excretion	Reduced kidney blood flow leads to reduced excretion and greater drug levels.	

action from the subsequent increase in half-life, the time it takes a drug to decrease by half. Another issue is the concentration of albumin, a protein in the plasma, which also lessens as patients get older. Drugs often bind to proteins such as albumin; with fewer proteins to latch on to, the drug can increase its effect. All together, these issues will generally necessitate a lower dosage.

Metabolism

In older patients, metabolism slows, increasing the time it takes the body to break down the drug and ultimately excrete it. While there are medications that induce (speed up) and inhibit (slow down) metabolism, their impact will be on a very different baseline in the geriatric population. Overall, however, if a drug remains in the body longer, the duration of action increases.

Excretion

The greatest concern with excretion comes from the reduced blood flow moving to the kidneys. With less blood flow, the process of excretion slows down, keeping more drug in the body. We use a few methods to determine the rate at which this slowing happens.

The glomerular filtration rate (GFR) provides an estimate of how much blood goes through the glomeruli per unit of time. The glomerulus is part of the nephron, the basic unit of the kidney. To dose medications, we want to know the creatinine clearance rate. This rate represents the amount of creatinine (a result of muscle breakdown) that the kidneys excrete per unit time. For example, the creatinine clearance in healthy men is about 120 mL/minute and 95 mL/minute in women.

SCENARIO 16.1. PHARMACOKINETICS

Mrs. Meyers, a 75-year-old female, is asking about diazepam, a benzodiazepine for anxiety. Her friend told her that it works longer than her current medication, alprazolam (Xanax). You know that it is a highly lipophilic (fat-loving) drug, highly protein bound, and is metabolized slowly in the elderly. Would this be a good choice for Mrs. Meyers?

Answer: No, diazepam should be avoided in the elderly. Its lipophilicity, high protein binding, and decreased metabolism lead to high concentrations of the drug. Mrs. Meyers should not be switched.

Drugs and Disease

While some of the factors involved in disease are beyond one's control, proper nutrition can go a long way to stave off infection and reduce the need for medications. Whether a patient is focusing on nutrition because of a condition such as diabetes or high cholesterol or for general well-being, the advantages of good nutrition are clear. Unfortunately, the geriatric population may encounter many disease states as they grow older, including sustained hypertension, diabetes, and coronary artery diseases, that all reduce the proper function of other organs (Fig. 16.2).

As we discussed earlier, if the liver and kidneys experience reduced blood flow, the metabolism and excretion of drugs suffer, which increases the risk of toxicity. This means that we must be especially aware of medications and the diseases that they impact, whether as a primary or secondary effect. In Table 16.2, we see how many drug classes can negatively impact an already established pathophysiologic state.

SCENARIO 16.2. DRUGS AND DISEASE

Mr. Johnson is 68 years old and has a past medical history of hypertension. He has nasal congestion and a cough due to a cold. He took pseudoephedrine (Sudafed) and Robitussin DM+ (guaifenasin/dextromethorphan) about 1 hour ago. His blood pressure is currently 170/96. What drug-disease interaction may be happening?

Answer: Pseudoephedrine is likely raising his blood pressure. Pseudoephedrine should be avoided in those with hypertension.

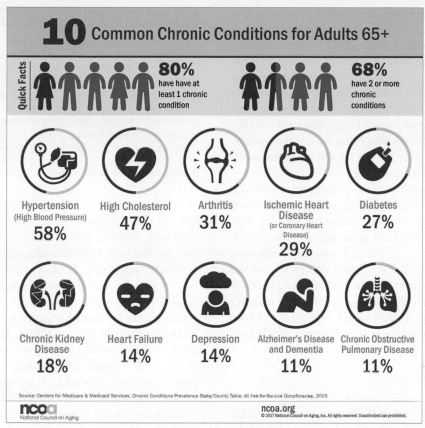

• **Fig. 16.2** 10 Common Chronic Conditions for Adults 65+ (from © National Council on Aging. https://www.ncoa.org/article/the-top-10-most-common-chronic-conditions-in-older-adults)

TABLE 16.2 Common Conditions, Drug Classes, Examples, and Dangerous Combination Results

Condition	Drug Class	Drug Example	Result
Hypertension	NSAIDs	Ibuprofen, naproxen	Increased salt/water retention, increasing blood pressure
Heart failure	Beta-blockers/nondihydropyridine calcium channel blockers	Propranolol/diltiazem and verapamil	Hypotension, reducing blood pressure dangerously
Low potassium with digoxin	Hypokalemic diuretics	Hydrochlorothiazide, furosemide	Cardiac arrhythmias
Asthma	First-generation beta-blockers	Propranolol	Bronchoconstriction
Renal failure	NSAIDs	Ibuprofen, naproxen	Decreased renal function
Benign prostatic hyperplasia	Anticholinergics	Diphenhydramine	Urinary retention
Diabetes	Beta-blockers	Propranolol	Masking signs and symptoms of hypoglycemia

NSAIDs, Nonsteroidal antiinflammatory drugs.

Drug Compliance

With a heightened sensitivity to certain medications, it is especially important that the elderly take medications properly. However, a lack of help, confusion, or disorientation might make this difficult and cause noncompliance, or a failure to take the medication when and/or how it is supposed to be taken. Also, it is not unusual to have a significant number of medications, which vary in the dosing schedule. One of the most important tactics to discuss with patients is how they will take their medications and who might help them ensure the proper use. As the number of medications increases, patients can also become overwhelmed with differing dosages and schedules. While many might feel they are able to handle the medication regimen, training is critically important, especially as it relates to devices. An arthritic patient will likely struggle to work with medications that require a significant level of dexterity, such as an injection or inhaler. Also, presbyopia, farsightedness that often happens starting in middle age, may require larger type or the ability to enlarge the type electronically. Recognizing the options that might be more suitable for the patient's abilities without embarrassing the individual is key.

While many are familiar with polypharmacy, which means both "many prescriptions" and getting prescriptions from many places, another issue is the prescribing cascade. When a patient complains of an adverse effect—say, constipation—a prescriber might add another medication to combat that ill effect. What helps is deprescribing, the follow-up with the patient to make sure that once a medication is no longer necessary, it is removed from the patient's regimen. Often, it takes an extra level of patience. However, the outcome, a better patient experience and health, is critical.

Beers Criteria

We learned in this chapter about the many ways in which a medication may be inappropriate for an older adult.

> ### SCENARIO 16.3. DRUG COMPLIANCE
>
> Mrs. Jones finds that she has trouble remembering if she took her medications. She also has trouble opening the childproof caps on her medication vials due to arthritis in her hands. What can be done to help Mrs. Jones?
>
>   Answer: Mrs. Jones can receive easy-open caps that are not childproof as long as she is able to keep her medications away from children. She can start using a pill box to remember whether she took her medication that day as long as she is able to keep track of the day of the week.

Due to the numerous drugs that should be avoided or used with caution, it is difficult to know whether you are making the best recommendation for your older patient without a reference. Luckily, there is the Beers Criteria for Potentially Inappropriate Medication Use in Older Adults. It is reviewed every 3 years by the American Geriatrics Society for any changes in evidence that might lead to changes in the Beers Criteria. Each table contains the drug, risk rationale, recommendation, quality of evidence, and strength of evidence. The recommendations cover common concerns of using medications in older adults, including drug-disease interactions, drug-drug interactions, age-related recommendations, and renal dose adjustments.

Summary

- We use age 65 years as a cutoff for differentiating between adult and geriatric. Those over 65 years may have multiple health conditions requiring multiple medications. As the number of medications increases, the potential for interactions increases.
- As we age, the pharmacokinetics—that is, the absorption, distribution, metabolism, and excretion of drugs—changes. This requires us to put extra consideration into which drug and which dose to use in an older patient. Generally, absorption is decreased, distribution is increased, metabolism is decreased, and excretion is decreased as we age.
- Certain disease states that are more common in older adults may be made worse by certain medications. When

selecting medications, drug-disease interactions must be accounted for, especially in older populations.
- Compliance may be reduced among the elderly due to declines in cognition, dexterity, and eyesight. It is important to select regimens that are within the patient's abilities. Reducing unnecessary medications and deprescribing is helpful in reducing polypharmacy and prescribing cascade.
- The Beers Criteria is a resource that summarizes medications to avoid or use with caution in older patients based on age, disease states, other drugs that they may be taking, and renal function.

Review Questions

1. What is the cutoff age that we consider geriatric?
   a. 42
   b. 54
   c. 65
   d. 72
2. What generally happens to absorption of drugs as we age?
   a. Increases
   b. Decreases
   c. Stays the same
   d. Fluctuates

3. What happens to the body composition of an older adult?
   a. Increase in body fat
   b. Increase in muscle mass
   c. Increase in total body water
   d. Increase in plasma proteins
4. What would happen to the concentration of a water-soluble drug in a geriatric patient compared to a younger adult?
   a. Decreases
   b. Increases
   c. Stays the same
   d. Fluctuates

5. In a geriatric patient, what generally happens to the concentration of highly protein bound drugs?
   a. Similar to younger adults
   b. Decreases
   c. Increases
   d. Fluctuates

6. What happens to the concentration of a drug that is metabolized by the liver in a geriatric patient compared to a younger adult?
   a. Increases
   b. Decreases
   c. Stays the same
   d. Fluctuates

7. What typically happens to the excretion rate of a drug in a geriatric patient?
   a. Fluctuates
   b. Stays the same
   c. Increases
   d. Decreases

8. For patients with diabetes, what do they need to be aware of while taking a beta-blocker?
   a. Masking signs and symptoms of hypoglycemia
   b. Urinary retention
   c. Increase in blood pressure
   d. Decreased renal function

9. Why should someone with renal failure avoid nonsteroidal antiinflammatory drugs?
   a. They cause photosensitivity.
   b. They cause hypoglycemia.
   c. They cause hypotension.
   d. They decrease renal function.

10. How can we improve polypharmacy and prescribing cascade?
    a. Leaving the regimen as is
    b. Adding more medications
    c. Deprescribing
    d. Cognitive behavioral therapy

17

Local and General Anesthetics

LEARNING OBJECTIVES

1. Describe the mechanism of action of local anesthetics.
2. Contrast local and general anesthetics.
3. Recognize the drug classes commonly used as anesthetics.

4. Identify the routes of administration of various anesthetics.
5. Recall adverse effects often seen in the use of anesthetics.

Local Anesthesia

Mechanism of Action

Before we can look at how to stop the pain, we must know what causes pain in the first place. For the body to sense pain after it has sustained damage, the primary afferent nociceptor, a sensory receptor for pain feelings, signals the spinal cord. Electrical impulses cause nerves to release the neurotransmitter glutamate, which triggers a second afferent neuron to send the message of pain to the brain. The electrical signals are dependent on sodium ions going into the neuron through a gated channel (Fig. 17.1).

Local anesthetics work by inhibiting these fast voltage-gated sodium channels of sensory neurons. This blockade causes numbness or an inability to sense feeling. The local anesthetics have a high affinity (or attraction) for the sodium channels when the channels are open and activated or refractory when they cannot be activated. The local anesthetic causes the channel's stabilization in a position in which the neuron cannot be activated (Fig. 17.2).

Amides Versus Esters

Amide local anesthetics contain an amide group in the drug's structure. Some examples of amide local anesthetics are lidocaine, prilocaine, ropivacaine, bupivacaine, etidocaine, and mepivacaine. Ester local anesthetics contain an ester group. Some examples are procaine, tetracaine, and chloroprocaine. There are more allergic reactions to esters than amides due to the para-aminobenzoic acid (PABA) metabolite of the ester local anesthetics; thus, we usually lean toward those medications in our therapy choices (Fig. 17.3).

Onset and Duration of Action

How long it takes for a local anesthetic to work depends on the rate of diffusion and lipophilicity. Diffusion will go more quickly if there are more uncharged, unionized molecules. The more basic the environment is, the more un-ionized these molecules will be, and the more local anesthetic will cross the barrier. Unfortunately, inflamed skin is more acidic, meaning that a smaller amount of drug will penetrate, making it more challenging to treat.

How do we know how much lipophilicity a drug has? We can represent this property by the partition coefficient (PC). If the PC is higher, the drug is more potent, and the prescriber would need to give less of this drug to exert an effect than a drug with a lower PC. Prilocaine and tetracaine provide good examples. Tetracaine has a higher PC, giving it more potency. It takes about four times as much procaine as tetracaine to get the same effect. Also, with higher lipophilicity, we expect to see a significantly longer half-life. The same is true of local anesthetics that have higher binding rates to proteins and other body tissues.

Adding a vasoconstrictor such as epinephrine may increase the duration of action. By squeezing the blood vessel and making it smaller, this action decreases blood flow to the site, allowing the drug to stay for a more extended amount of time before being cleared by the body. This benefit is why it is common to see the combination of a local anesthetic and vasoconstrictor. However, with patients with a cardiac history, we would have to be especially careful because a vasoconstrictor can raise blood pressure if we use too much.

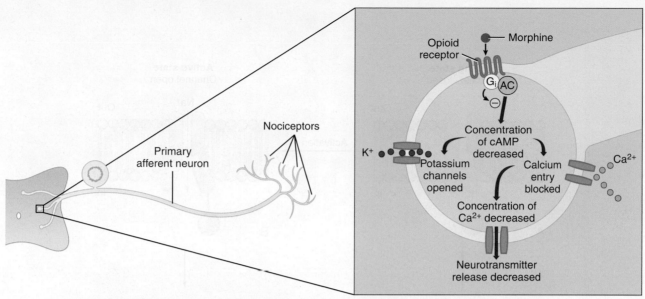

• **Fig. 17.1** Mechanisms of Opioid Action in the Spinal Cord. Morphine and other opioid agonists activate presynaptic μ, δ, or κ opioid receptors on primary afferent neurons. These receptors are coupled negatively to adenylate cyclase (AC) via G proteins (G αi). Inhibition of cyclic adenosine monophosphate (cAMP) formation leads to opening of potassium channels and closing of calcium channels. G βγ subunits may also participate in the modulation of ion channels. Potassium efflux causes membrane hyperpolarization. The closing of calcium channels inhibits the release of neurotransmitters, such as substance P. (From Brenner G, Stevens C. *Brenner and Stevens' Pharmacology*, ed 5, Philadelphia: Elsevier, 2018; Fig. 23.1.)

Route of Administration

There are many routes of administration for local anesthetics. One can use a local anesthetic topically, subcutaneously, in the epidural space or the subarachnoid space. Because of the dangers of the epidural space in the outermost part of the spinal canal and the subarachnoid space near the spine, only those specially trained to administer medication in the epidural or subarachnoid space should do so. This administration is typically done using ultrasound to ensure that the medicine goes where the prescriber intends. Not all local anesthetics have an indication for each administration route; thus, it is vital to choose the correct route when administering them (Fig. 17.4).

Adverse Effects and Special Considerations

When we give local anesthetics, we need to look at the side effects that the medications may cause. Cardiac effects are possible adverse effects of local anesthetics. For example, in cases in which the body absorbs a large dose systemically, the mitochondrial refractory period decreases, causing the inhibition of some fast sodium channels of the heart. This action may cause fatal arrhythmias, severe dysfunction of the heart rhythm. One way to avoid this side effect is by limiting the amount of local anesthetic that the patient receives. Note that even if the local anesthetic is topical, the body can still absorb it.

Local anesthetics can also cause central nervous system (CNS) effects in high systemic doses. The first signs might include a metallic taste, ringing in the ears, dizziness, and disorientation. These more benign symptoms might progress to

seizures caused by the higher selectivity for inhibitory neurons. The selectivity causes the unchecked firing of excitatory neurons, which may eventually result in a coma.

Allergic or hypersensitivity reactions can occur with any local anesthetic. However, this effect is more common with ester local anesthetics. An ester is a chemical part of a molecule that we can contrast against an amide. The body excretes amides through the kidney unchanged, while the breakdown of esters can often happen in the body. This enzymatic breakdown results in PABA production as a metabolite, which is responsible for more hypersensitivity reactions.

Generally, pregnant patients should avoid local anesthetics, but if a prescriber must use one, the preference is for lidocaine. Note that when a patient has poor renal clearance, it is essential to avoid amide local anesthetics, as decreased clearance will result in accumulation and toxicity. In this case, if a local anesthetic must be used in renal failure, an ester would be safer for the patient.

SCENARIO 17.1. THE EPIDURAL ALLERGY

Mrs. Singer needs an epidural for analgesia but has a history of reacting to ester local anesthetics. The doctor has a choice between bupivacaine, chloroprocaine, and lidocaine. Which local anesthetic can she safely choose for Mrs. Singer?

Answer: The physician can safely choose bupivacaine or lidocaine, as these are amide local anesthetics. Chloroprocaine would not be a safe choice because it is an ester local anesthetic, to which Mrs. Singer has an allergy.

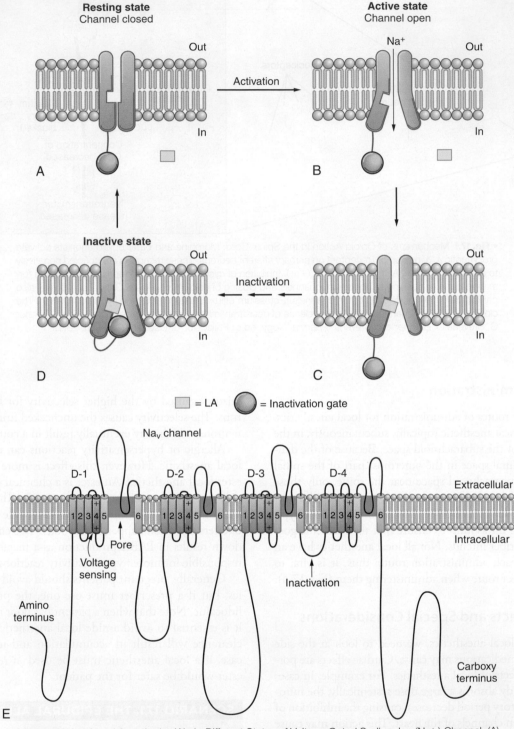

• **Fig. 17.2** How Local Anesthetics Work: Different States of Voltage-Gated Sodium Ion (Na⁺) Channel. (A) Channels in the resting state. Activation leads to opening of the resting (closed) channel (A) to allow the passage of Na⁺ in the activated (open) state (B). The inactivation gate closes the channel pore from the intracellular side and the channel inactivates (D). Local anesthetics *(LA)* preferentially bind to the activated and inactivated states (C and D). The local anesthetic binding site is in the pore of the channel (C and D). (E) Schematic structure of voltage-gated sodium ion (Na⁺) channel α-subunit. It contains four homologous domains, each with six α-helical transmembrane segments. The intracellular loops that connect S5 and S6 of each of the four domains (P loops) are positioned extracellularly and extend inward to form the narrowest point of the channel pore and provide its ion selectivity. (From Hemmings H, Egan, T. *Pharmacology and Physiology for Anesthesia*. Philadelphia: Elsevier, 2019; Figs. 20.5 and 20.6.)

	Structure	pKa	Ionization at pH 7.4 (%)	Partition coefficient	Protein bound (%)
Ester type					
Procaine	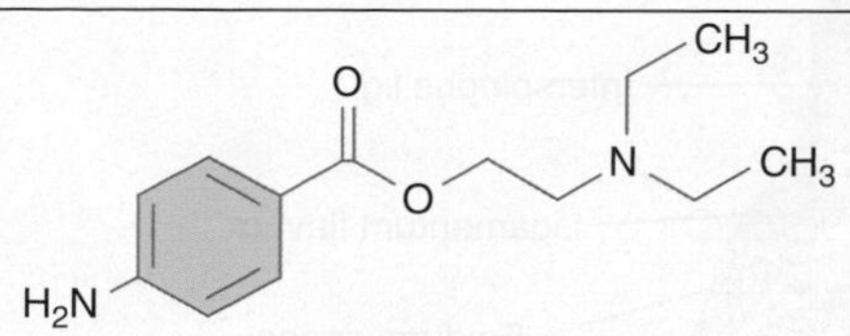	8.9	97	100	6
Tetracaine	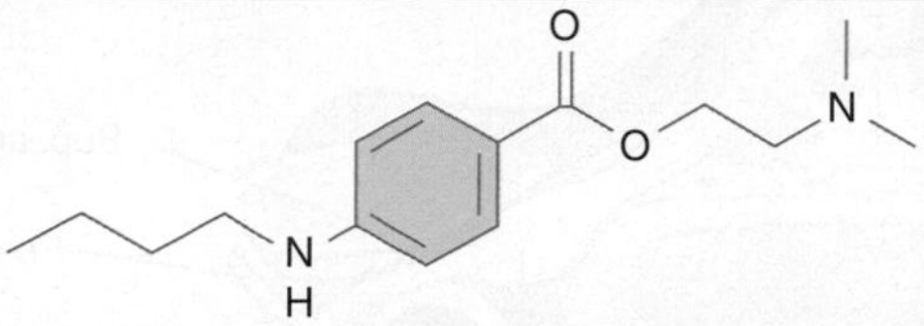	8.5	93	5822	76
Chloroprocaine	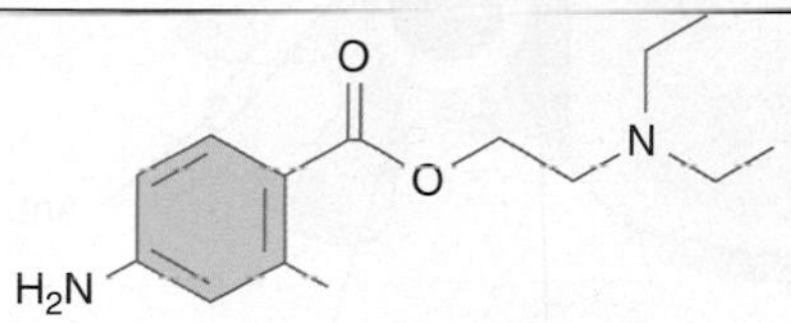	9.1	95	810	N/A
Amide type					
Lidocaine	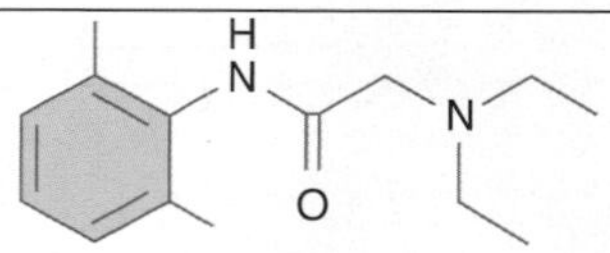	7.9	76	366	65
Prilocaine	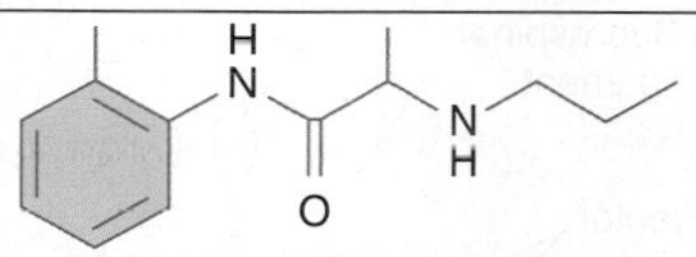	7.9	76	129	55
Ropivacaine	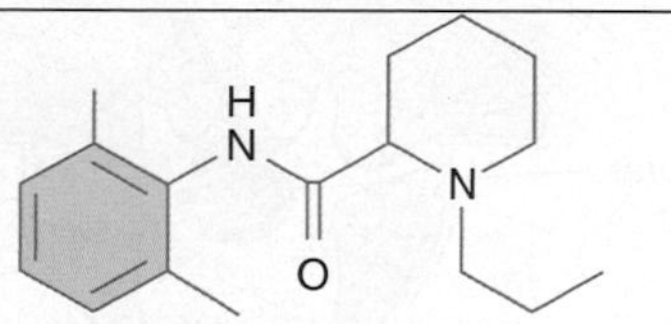	8.1	83	775	94

• **Fig. 17.3** Amides Versus Esters. (Modified from Hemmings H, Egan T. *Pharmacology and Physiology for Anesthesia*. Philadelphia: Elsevier, 2019.)

General Anesthesia

General anesthetics work by inducing unconsciousness, which provides two benefits: (1) the painful stimuli will not elicit a response and (2) it will not trigger memories. There are four stages of anesthesia.

Stage One: Analgesia, consisting of analgesia, amnesia, and euphoria.

Stage Two: Excitement, which is characterized as excitement, delirium, and combativeness. This stage is purposefully progressed through rapidly for the safety of everyone involved.

Stage Three: Surgical anesthesia, in which procedures are performed. Unconsciousness, decreased eye movement, and regular breathing characterize this stage. We must be careful not to progress to stage four.

Stage Four: Medullary depression, which may cause a patient to experience no eye movement and respiratory and/or cardiac arrest.

Route of Administration

We have many ways to provide a general anesthetic regimen. These administration routes include inhalation, intravenous,

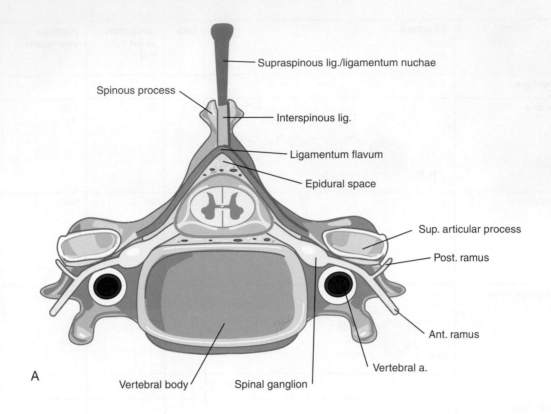

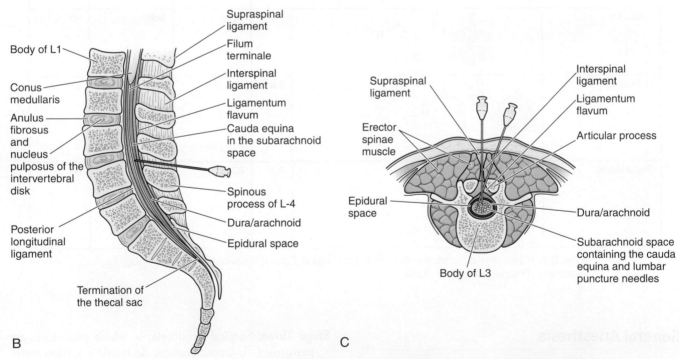

• **Fig. 17.4** (A) Epidural Administration From Waldman, S.: *Pain Management*, ed 2, Philadelphia, 2011, Saunders. Fig. 153.1 (B) Midsagittal section through the lumbar spinal column with a spinal puncture needle in place between the spinous processes of L3 and L4. Note the slightly ascending direction of the needle. The needle has pierced three ligaments and the dura/arachnoid and is in the subarachnoid space. (From Lachman E: Anatomy as applied to clinical medicine, *New Physician* 17:145, 1968.) (C) Horizontal section through the body of L3. Note the two puncture needles in the subarachnoid space. The medial needle is in the midline. The lateral needle exemplifies the lateral approach, which avoids the occasionally calcified supraspinal ligament. Note the lateral needle piercing the intrinsic musculature of the back and only one ligament, the ligamentum flavum. (From Lachman E: Anatomy as applied to clinical medicine, *New Physician* 17:145, 1968.)

oral, and topical. We will talk specifically about inhaled and intravenous anesthetics and their benefits.

When using an inhaled oral anesthetic, the depth of sedation depends on the drug concentration in the brain. The inhaled anesthetics move down the concentration gradient from the lung alveoli to the blood and into the brain. There is insufficient partial pressure in the blood for the drug to move into the brain until the blood saturates with gas.

Intravenous anesthetics have a very rapid onset and similar quick recovery. For this reason, these anesthetics often induce or start the sedation before the use of an inhaled anesthetic. They may also be used alone for procedures that do not take a lot of time. There are many intravenous anesthetics with diverse drug characteristics to choose from. They may provide deep sedation while allowing patients to breathe on their own and respond to verbal commands.

Medication Classes

Halogenated hydrocarbons are the commonly used general anesthetics. The hydrocarbon offers the necessary sedation while the halogen reduces the flammability of the agent.

Nonbarbiturates can induce anesthesia—in other words, to have a patient "put under." The commonly used nonbarbiturates are propofol, ketamine, etomidate, dexmedetomidine, droperidol, and some opioids.

Nonanesthetic Effects

CNS effects are pervasive with general anesthesia. These include nausea, vomiting, and confusion after the anesthetic wears off. It is critical to ensure that the patient has a support team even after the procedure for safety. Some agents may cause a decrease in heart rate, cardiac output, and blood pressure. Patients can commonly experience muscle weakness soon after general anesthetics have worn off.

It is vital to assess hepatic and renal function to adjust doses of general anesthetics accordingly. Some agents are metabolized by the liver, causing toxicity to occur if the liver does not function as well. Many are eliminated through the kidney and may cause an overdose if the dose is not decreased appropriately. The anesthetics themselves may potentially cause kidney damage due to hypotension.

Adjuncts

An adjunct is a medication we can add to reduce or prevent specific adverse effects. As we have seen throughout this chapter, there are many adverse effects of general anesthetics. As such, there are other medications to stop them or decrease their severity. Anticholinergics can decrease vomiting and other secretions. Antiarrhythmics can prevent cardiac problems due to the anesthetic. Some additional medications are for different aspects of the procedure. For example, analgesics can provide pain control and antibiotics can prevent infection. Antianxiety medicine may alleviate the stress that the patient may be feeling due to the procedure.

SCENARIO 17.2. GENERAL ANESTHESIA

Mr. Fields, a patient with decreased renal function, is scheduled to have surgery today. What should we do with the dose of his general anesthetic?

Answer: We should decrease the dose of his general anesthetic. General anesthetics typically eliminate through the kidney. Since his renal function is reduced, he will retain the drug longer, which could cause an overdose.

Summary

- Local anesthetics block pain signals by inhibiting sodium channels. They can be administered topically, subcutaneously, in the epidural space, and in the subarachnoid space.
- The onset of local anesthetics is influenced by lipophilicity and the rate of diffusion. Duration is influenced by binding to tissues and can be prolonged by vasoconstriction.
- Local anesthetics may cause various adverse effects that may be minimized by limiting the dose and avoiding systemic exposure.

- General anesthetics can induce unconsciousness and prevent memory formation. The third stage of anesthesia is where procedures are performed.
- General anesthetics are typically halogenated hydrocarbons. Induction agents used to put patients under are usually nonbarbiturates.
- General anesthetics may cause CNS, cardiac, and muscular side effects. Adjunct medications may minimize side effects or have value for other surgical reasons.

Review Questions

1. Which stage of anesthesia should be avoided?
   - **a.** 1
   - **b.** 2
   - **c.** 3
   - **d.** 4

2. In which stage of anesthesia does a surgeon commence the work?
   - **a.** 1
   - **b.** 2
   - **c.** 3
   - **d.** 4

3. Which stage of anesthesia may cause aggression and delirium?
   a. 1
   b. 2
   c. 3
   d. 4

4. What do we give as an adjunct to prevent vomiting?
   a. Anticholinergics
   b. Antianxiety medications
   c. Antiarrhythmics
   d. Antibiotics

5. A drug that has a high blood-gas partition coefficient will have a _____ onset.
   a. Slow
   b. Fast
   c. Moderate
   d. All of the above

6. Which channels do local anesthetics target?
   a. Potassium
   b. Chloride
   c. Sodium
   d. Fluoride

7. Which type of local anesthetic is most likely to cause hypersensitivity reactions?
   a. Hydroxide
   b. Ester
   c. Amide
   d. Carboxylic

8. What influences the onset of action of a local anesthetic?
   a. Salinity and rate of elimination
   b. Salinity and rate of diffusion
   c. Lipophilicity and rate of elimination
   d. Lipophilicity and rate of diffusion

9. Which is not a route of administration of local anesthetics?
   a. Oral
   b. Topical
   c. Epidural
   d. Subarachnoid

10. Which is not an adverse effect of local anesthetics?
   a. Metallic taste, dizziness
   b. Reproductive effects
   c. Arrhythmias
   d. Hypersensitivity

18

Alcohol and Drugs of Abuse

LEARNING OBJECTIVES

1. Describe the pathology of alcohol use disorder, tobacco use disorder, and the abuse of prescription and illegal drugs.
2. Contrast the withdrawal symptoms of various substances of abuse.

3. Recall the available treatments for alcohol use disorder, tobacco use disorder, and the abuse of prescription and illegal drugs.

Introduction

Substance use disorder, or addiction, occurs when a person cannot control the use of a substance despite the harm that it can cause. This damage may occur with the abuse of legal substances such as nicotine in tobacco, alcohol, and certain prescription drugs. It may also happen with illegal substances such as methamphetamine and hallucinogens, among others. Drugs of abuse often work on the reward pathway in the brain to create a feeling of euphoria, defined as well-being or elation. To create dependence, these substances may influence brain chemistry so that the body relies on the substance to feel normal. This reliance leads to withdrawal when the substance is abruptly discontinued. Withdrawal may be anywhere from uncomfortable to life-threatening. In this chapter, we will discuss the management of various substance use disorders.

Alcohol Use Disorder

Alcohol use disorder is common in the United States, affecting 14.4 million adults as of 2018. Alcohol has the potential for abuse due to the release of dopamine, a neurotransmitter, in the brain's reward center. We can recognize alcohol use disorder when a person is unable to limit alcoholic beverage intake; is unsuccessful in cutting back on drinking despite trying; continues drinking despite the physical, social, and interpersonal problems that it causes; and develops a tolerance to alcohol. Excessive alcohol use can cause liver disease, heart disease, and problems with digestion, vision, sexual function, and menstruation. Something to keep in mind is that some medications may interact with alcohol.

---

* Brand discontinued, now available only as generic
† Naming conventions can vary between prescription and OTC formulations

Withdrawal Symptoms

When stopping chronic alcohol use, one can experience withdrawal. After 6 hours, we may see the milder symptoms of anxiety, hands shaking, headache, nausea, and vomiting. The withdrawal becomes more severe after 12 to 24 hours, with hand tremors and disorientation. After 48 hours, withdrawal may become severe, with seizures, hallucinations, delirium tremens, and high blood pressure.

Treatments

Behavioral therapy to treat alcohol use disorder may take a few different forms. Individual counseling is one option. There are also group therapy options, such as Alcoholics Anonymous (AA).

Disulfiram (Antabuse*), naltrexone, and acamprosate (Campral*) are prescription medications for the treatment of alcohol use disorder. Disulfiram (Antabuse*) deters one from drinking by reacting with any alcohol to cause an unpleasant reaction. Naltrexone may be given as a monthly injection that blocks the euphoria, making alcohol less rewarding. Acamprosate decreases the severity of withdrawal symptoms.

SCENARIO 18.1. ALCOHOL USE DISORDER

Mrs. Charles confides in you that she is trying to stop drinking, but it is not going well. She is attending AA meetings but has had a few relapses because the cravings were too intense. She asks you if there is anything that she can take to decrease her withdrawal symptoms.

Answer: Mrs. Charles may be a good candidate for acamprosate. Acamprosate will likely decrease the severity of her cravings. Don't forget to congratulate Mrs. Charles on her progress and encourage her to keep trying!

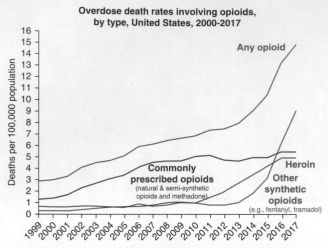

Overdose death rates involving opioids, by type, United States, 2000-2017

Any opioid

Commonly prescribed opioids
(natural & semi-synthetic opioids and methadone)

Heroin

Other synthetic opioids
(e.g., fentanyl, tramadol)

• **Fig. 18.1** Overdose Death Rates Involving Opioids, by Type, United States, 2000–2017 (From National Vital Statistics System, Centers for Disease Control and Prevention, US Department of Health and Human Services: Mortality, CDC WONDER, 2018. https://www.cdc.gov/drugoverdose/data/analysis.html)

Tobacco Use Disorder

In tobacco use disorder, a person cannot stop smoking, continues to smoke despite health problems, or gives up social activities that interfere with tobacco use. Nicotine is the addictive substance in tobacco that works by activating the reward pathway in the brain. Cigarette smoking is the leading cause of preventable disease and death in the United States. It causes about 1 in 5 deaths, an estimated 480,000 deaths per year. Some diseases caused by smoking include lung cancer, lung disease (chronic obstructive pulmonary disease [COPD]), heart disease, infertility, gum disease, and multiple other cancers. For this reason, it is essential to discuss quitting at every encounter with a patient who smokes.

Withdrawal Symptoms

One problem that makes quitting difficult is withdrawal symptoms. These typically manifest as intense nicotine cravings, anxiety, restlessness, hunger, and irritability. Nicotine withdrawal is highly unpleasant, making quitting difficult. Luckily, there are options to minimize withdrawal symptoms, increasing the chances of successfully quitting.

Treatment

Behavioral therapy may be used to aid in smoking cessation. Prescription medications such as varenicline (Chantix) or bupropion (Zyban*) are options that may increase the chances of success. Nicotine replacement therapy (NRT) is available as a prescription or over-the-counter in the form of patches, gum, and lozenges. At this time, it is not recommended to use vaping as nicotine replacement, as this has not been shown to aid smoking cessation successfully and carries its own risks.

Prescription Medication Misuse

Some prescription medications have the potential for abuse. These medications are especially important to take as prescribed, although this may not always prevent addiction. Here, we will discuss opioids, benzodiazepines, and anticonvulsants.

Opioids

Opioids work by blocking pain signals. They also release dopamine throughout the body, causing euphoria, and even taking them as prescribed may still cause addiction. The most common examples of prescription opioids are hydrocodone, oxycodone, fentanyl, morphine, and codeine. People taking an opioid should experience pain relief as well as relaxation and happiness. The opioid may also cause drowsiness, constipation, and slowed breathing. This slowed breath is what causes an opioid overdose to be so dangerous, possibly leading to death. This is why it is vital for anyone at risk of an overdose to have naloxone (Narcan) available and for others around them to know how to use it. Naloxone is an opioid antagonist that can reverse the overdose if given quickly enough. Depending on the formulation, it may be administered as an intramuscular injection or intranasal spray.

Withdrawal Symptoms

Opioid withdrawal typically involves severe cravings, diarrhea, vomiting, muscle and bone pain, cold flashes, trouble sleeping, and involuntary leg movements. We can use buprenorphine and methadone to decrease cravings and other symptoms of withdrawal.

Around 80% of people who use heroin have misused opioids first. In Fig. 18.1, you can see that as prescription opioid–related deaths increased, so did heroin-related deaths. Heroin overdose can be treated similarly to prescription opioid overdose, with naloxone (Narcan). Heroin withdrawal can also be treated similarly to that of prescription opioids, with buprenorphine or methadone.

Other Central Nervous System Depressants

Benzodiazepines are medications prescribed for anxiety disorders, among other indications, that have the potential for abuse (Fig. 18.2). Some common examples are diazepam

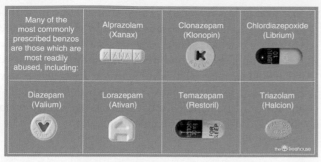

• **Fig. 18.2** Commonly Prescribed Benzodiapines (From https://www.labroots.com/trending/drug-discovery-and-development/13570/increasing-misuse-prescription-drugs)

(Valium), alprazolam (Xanax), clonazepam (Klonopin), triazolam (Halcion), and lorazepam (Ativan). Withdrawal can be severe and possibly life-threatening. An individual becoming addicted to a benzodiazepine would need to come off the medication slowly in a medically supervised detoxification. In the case of an overdose, we can use flumazenil.

Nonsedative hypnotics with the potential for abuse include zolpidem, eszopiclone, and zaleplon. Barbiturates, such as phenobarbital for epilepsy and other indications, also have the potential for abuse. Like benzodiazepines, in the case of addiction, these medications must be gradually tapered in a medically supervised setting to avoid life-threatening withdrawal symptoms.

SCENARIO 18.3. PRESCRIPTION DRUGS

Mr. James has started craving oxycodone and experiencing vomiting and inability to sleep when he does not take it. What is happening to Mr. James and what can be done about it?

Answer: Mr. James is experiencing opioid withdrawal. Buprenorphine or methadone may be used to decrease his cravings and other withdrawal symptoms.

Misuse of Other Substances

Marijuana

When a person uses marijuana, tetrahydrocannabinol (THC) binds to the cannabinoid receptors in the brain to activate the reward pathway. Marijuana use may cause short-term memory loss, difficulty problem solving, increased heart rate, and may permanently decrease IQ. A person addicted to marijuana may experience withdrawal

symptoms such as irritability, anxiety, depression, and flu-like symptoms upon abrupt discontinuation. To help a patient who uses marijuana, we must understand the reason for its use. Some patients may be self-medicating for depression or anxiety. If so, it is crucial to treat these underlying conditions properly. Cognitive behavioral therapy may help discontinue use.

It is important to note that, like prescription drugs, marijuana has some therapeutic uses in medicine. It may be used to stimulate the appetite in those with cancer and eating disorders, among other reasons for appetite loss. It may also be used to relieve nausea, glaucoma, chronic pain, and epilepsy.

Methamphetamines

Methamphetamines cause a significant surge of dopamine in the reward center of the brain. They may be addictive with a single use. Signs of methamphetamine use include hyperactivity, paranoia, aggression, weight loss, skin sores, infection, tooth decay, heart attack, and stroke. An overdose of methamphetamine can be lethal. Mild to moderate dependence may be treated in the outpatient setting. Severe dependence must be treated in an inpatient rehabilitation program. Both settings involve counseling.

Hallucinogens

Hallucinogens cause hallucinations, intense experiences, and increased heart rate. They may be stored in the body and released at a later date to cause flashbacks. While some hallucinogens, such as lysergic acid diethylamide (LSD), do not have addictive potential, phencyclidine (PCP, commonly known as "angel dust") can be addictive. There is not currently a well-known treatment for PCP addiction.

SCENARIO 18.4. ILLEGAL DRUGS

Ms. Reid lives in a state where marijuana is wholly illegal. She confides in you that she uses marijuana for her anxiety and has found that she is having trouble quitting marijuana. What can you suggest to Ms. Reid so that she receives safe treatment for her anxiety without the risk of legal repercussions?

Answer: Ms. Reid should receive proper treatment for her anxiety disorder, including medications indicated for that purpose. Cognitive behavioral therapy will likely help her to manage her disease and help her stop using marijuana.

Summary

• Alcohol use disorder is somewhat common in the United States and may result in severe, life-threatening withdrawal. We may treat alcohol use disorder with a combination of behavioral therapy and possibly prescription medications, such as disulfiram, naltrexone, or acamprosate.

• Tobacco use disorder is common in the United States and is responsible for many preventable deaths. Those with tobacco use disorder may increase their chance of quitting with varenicline, bupropion, or nicotine replacement therapy.

- Some prescription medications—such as opioids, benzodiazepines, and some antiepileptics—have the potential for abuse and addiction, even if taken as prescribed. The overdose of these substances can be fatal. Naloxone should be used to treat opioid overdose and flumazenil for benzodiazepine overdose. Opioid withdrawal is uncomfortable and can be managed with buprenorphine or methadone. Benzodiazepine withdrawal can be life-threatening and should be slow and medically supervised.

- Marijuana's legality varies among states, while methamphetamine and hallucinogens are illegal throughout the United States. Marijuana dependence is managed by treating underlying conditions and through cognitive behavioral therapy. Methamphetamine dependence may be managed in the outpatient setting if mild to moderate but must be handled inpatient if severe. There is no established treatment for hallucinogen use.

Review Questions

1. Which neurotransmitter is responsible for dependence?
   a. Serotonin
   b. Adrenaline
   c. Acetylcholine
   d. Dopamine
2. What are signs of severe alcohol withdrawal?
   a. Seizures, delirium tremens
   b. Cravings, hands that shake
   c. Nausea, vomiting
   d. Trouble sleeping, irritability
3. Which medication is used to create an unpleasant reaction to alcohol, deterring its use?
   a. Acamprosate
   b. Disulfiram
   c. Buprenorphine
   d. Naltrexone
4. Which medication blocks the euphoria caused by alcohol, making it less rewarding?
   a. Naltrexone
   b. Disulfiram
   c. Acamprosate
   d. Buprenorphine
5. Which is a partial nicotine agonist for smoking cessation?
   a. Bupropion
   b. Nicotine replacement therapy
   c. Varenicline
   d. Acamprosate
6. Which dosage form is not included in nicotine replacement therapy?
   a. Patch
   b. Gum
   c. Lozenge
   d. Injection
7. What is a contraindication to using bupropion as a smoking cessation aid?
   a. History of depression
   b. History of seizures
   c. History of arrhythmias
   d. History of lung disease
8. What is used to reverse an opioid overdose?
   a. Buprenorphine
   b. Flumazenil
   c. Naltrexone
   d. Naloxone
9. In a patient with benzodiazepine dependence, how should the medication be discontinued?
   a. Slowly, with medical supervision
   b. Slowly, at home
   c. Quickly, with medical supervision
   d. Quickly, at home
10. Which helps discontinue illegal drug use?
   a. Quitting cold turkey
   b. Replacing with another drug
   c. Cognitive behavioral therapy
   d. Continuing the drug

Top 200 Prescription Drugs

		Drugs by Brand, Generic, Classification, Indication		
	Brand Name	Generic Name	Drug Classification*	Indication or Use
1	Abilify	aripiprazole	Antipsychotic	Schizophrenia
2	Accupril	quinapril	ACE inhibitor	Hypertension
3	Actos	pioglitazone hydrochloride	Thiazolidinedione	Type 2 diabetes mellitus
4	Adderall XR	amphetamine/ dextroamphetamine	CNS stimulant	ADHD
5	Adipex	phentermine	CNS stimulant	Obesity
6	Advair Diskus	fluticasone propionate/ salmeterol xinafoate	Beta-2 agonist/ corticosteroid	Asthma, COPD
7		sodium chloride	Electrolyte	Supplement
8	Aldactone	spironolactone	Potassium-sparing diuretic	Hypertension, edema, hypokalemia
9	Alphagan P	brimonidine tartrate	Alpha-agonist	Glaucoma
10	Altace	ramipril	ACE inhibitor	Hypertension
11	Amaryl	glimepiride	Sulfonylurea	Type 2 diabetes mellitus
12	Ambien	zolpidem tartrate	Gamma-aminobutyric acid agonist	Insomnia
13	Amoxil	amoxicillin	Penicillin antibiotic	Bacterial infection
14	Androgel	testosterone topical	Androgen	Hypogonadism
15	Apresoline	hydralazine hydrochloride	Vasodilator	Hypertension
16	Aricept	donepezil hydrochloride	Acetylcholinesterase inhibitor	Alzheimer's disease
17	Arimidex	anastrozole	Hormonal oncologic	Cancer
18	Armour Thyroid	thyroid	Thyroid hormone	Hypothyroidism
19	Asacol	mesalamine	Inflammatory bowel disease	Ulcerative colitis
20	Asmanex Twisthaler	mometasone	Corticosteroid	Asthma
21	Aspir-Low, Ecotrin	aspirin	NSAID	Analgesic, stroke prevention
22	Ativan	lorazepam	Benzodiazepine	Anxiety
23	Atrovent	ipratropium	Anticholinergic	COPD
24	Augmentin	amoxicillin/clavulanate potassium	Penicillin/beta-lactamase combination antibiotic	Bacterial infection
25	Bactrim or Septra	sulfamethoxazole/ trimethoprim	Sulfa antibiotic	Bacterial infection
26	Beconase AQ	beclomethasone	Corticosteroid	Allergic rhinitis
27	Benadryl	diphenhydramine hydrochloride	H_1 antagonist	Allergies
28	Benicar	olmesartan medoxomil	ARB	Hypertension
29	Buspar	buspirone hydrochloride	$5\text{-}HT_{1a}$ receptor partial antagonist	Anxiety

Continued

	Brand Name	Generic Name	Drug Classification*	Indication or Use
			Drugs by Brand, Generic, Classification, Indication	
30	Bystolic	nebivolol hydrochloride	Beta-blocker	Hypertension
31	Calan	verapamil hydrochloride	Nondihydropyridine CCB	Hypertension
32	Calcium	calcium	Vitamin	Calcium deficiency
33	Cardizem	diltiazem hydrochloride	Nondihydropyridine CCB	Hypertension
34	Cardura	doxazosin mesylate	Alpha-1 blocker	Hypertension
35	Catapres-TTS	clonidine	Alpha-agonist	Hypertension
36	Celebrex	celecoxib	NSAID, COX-2 inhibitor	Inflammation
37	Celexa	citalopram	SSRI	Depression
38	Cheratussin AC	guaifenesin/codeine	Antitussive/expectorant combination	Cough suppressant and expectorant
39	Cipro	ciprofloxacin	Quinolone antibiotic	Bacterial infection
40	Claritin	loratadine	H_1 antagonist	Allergies
41	Cleocin	clindamycin	Lincosamide antibiotic	Bacterial infection
42	ClinPro	sodium fluoride	Supplement	Cavity prevention
43	Clobex	clobetasol propionate	Corticosteroid	Dermatoses
44	Cogentin	benztropine mesylate	Anti-Parkinson	Parkinson's disease
45	Combivent	albuterol/ipratropium	Anticholinergic/beta-2 agonist	Asthma
46	Concerta	methylphenidate	Central nervous system stimulant	ADHD
47	Coreg	carvedilol	Beta-blocker	Hypertension
48	Cortef	hydrocortisone	Corticosteroid	Inflammatory disorders
49	Coumadin	warfarin	Vitamin K antagonist	Anticoagulation
50	Cozaar	losartan potassium	ARB	Hypertension
51	Crestor	rosuvastatin calcium	HMG-CoA reductase inhibitor	Hyperlipidemia
52	Cymbalta	duloxetine	SNRI	Depression
53	Deltasone	prednisone	Corticosteroid	Inflammation
54	Depakote ER	divalproex sodium	Neurologic	Bipolar disorder, migraine headache, seizure disorder
55	Desyrel	trazodone hydrochloride	Serotonin reuptake inhibitor	Insomnia, depression
56	Diflucan	fluconazole	Antifungal	Fungal infection
57	Dilantin	phenytoin	Hydantoin	Status epilepticus
58	Diovan	valsartan	ARB	Hypertension
59	Diovan HCT	hydrochlorothiazide/ valsartan	ARB/thiazide combination	Hypertension
60	Ditropan	oxybutynin	Antispasmotic	Overactive bladder
61	Dramamine	meclizine hydrochloride	H_1 antagonist	Motion sickness
62	Effexor	venlafaxine hydrochloride	SNRI	Depression
63	Elavil	amitriptyline	TCA	Depression
64	Esidrix	hydrochlorothiazide	Thiazide diuretic	Hypertension
65	Flexeril	cyclobenzaprine hydrochloride	Muscle relaxant	Skeletal muscle relaxant
66	Flomax	tamsulosin hydrochloride	Alpha-blocker	BPH
67	Flonase	fluticasone	Corticosteroid	Allergic rhinitis

	Brand Name	Generic Name	Drug Classification*	Indication or Use
			Drugs by Brand, Generic, Classification, Indication	
68	Focalin XR	dexmethylphenidate hydrochloride	CNS stimulant	ADHD
69	Folic Acid	folic acid	Vitamin	Dietary supplement
70	Fosamax	alendronate	Bisphosphonate	Osteoporosis
71	Gianvi	drospirenone/ethinyl estradiol	Monophasic oral contraceptive	Oral contraceptive
72	Glucophage	metformin hydrochloride	Biguanide	Type 2 diabetes mellitus
73	Glucotrol	glipizide	Sulfonylurea	Type 2 diabetes mellitus
74	Humalog	insulin lispro	Insulin	Diabetes mellitus
75	Humulin N	insulin NPH	Insulin	Diabetes mellitus
76	Hytrin	terazosin	Alpha-1 blocker	BPH
77	Hyzaar	hydrochlorothiazide/ losartan potassium	ARB/thiazide combination	Hypertension
78	Imdur	isosorbide mononitrate	Vasodilator	Angina
79	Imitrex	sumatriptan	Serotonin 5-HT$_1$ receptor agonist	Migraine headache
80	Inderal	propranolol hydrochloride	Beta-blocker	Hypertension
81	Inderide	hydrochlorothiazide/ propranolol hydrochloride	Beta-blocker/diuretic combination	Hypertension
82	Iron	ferrous sulfate	Supplement	Iron-deficiency anemia
83	Janumet	metformin hydrochloride/ sitagliptin phosphate	Biguanide/DPP-4 inhibitor	Type 2 diabetes mellitus
84	Januvia	sitagliptin phosphate	DPP-4 inhibitor	Type 2 diabetes mellitus
85	Jolessa	ethinyl estradiol/ levonorgestrel	Monophasic oral contraceptive	Oral contraceptive
86	K-Dur, Klor-Con, Klor- Con M, Micro K	potassium chloride	Electrolyte	Potassium supplement
87	Kariva	desogestrel/ethinyl estradiol	Monophasic oral contraceptive	Oral contraceptive
88	Keflex	cephalexin	Cephalosporin antibiotic	Bacterial infection
89	Keppra	levetiracetam	Antiepileptic	Seizure
90	Klonopin	clonazepam	Benzodiazepine	Seizure
91	Lamictal	lamotrigine	Antiepileptic	Bipolar disorder
92	Lanoxin	digoxin	Cardiac glycoside	Arrhythmia, myocardial infarction
93	Lantus	insulin glargine	Insulin	Diabetes mellitus
94	Lasix	furosemide	Loop diuretic	Hypertension
95	Levaquin	levofloxacin	Quinolone antibiotic	Bacterial infection
96	Levemir	insulin detemir	Insulin	Diabetes mellitus
97	Lexapro	escitalopram oxalate	SSRI	Depression
98	Lioresal	baclofen	Muscle relaxant	Spasticity
99	Lipitor	atorvastatin	HMG-CoA reductase inhibitor	Hyperlipidemia
100	Lithobid	lithium	Antimanic	Bipolar disorder
101	Loestrin Fe-24	ethinyl estradiol/ norethindrone, iron	Monophasic oral contraceptive	Oral contraceptive

Continued

		Drugs by Brand, Generic, Classification, Indication		
	Brand Name	Generic Name	Drug Classification*	Indication or Use
102	Lopid	gemfibrozil	Antilipemic agent	Hyperlipidemia
103	Lopressor	metoprolol tartrate	Beta-blocker	Hypertension
104	Loratadine	cetirizine hydrochloride	H₁ antagonist	Allergies
105	Lotensin	benazepril hydrochloride	ACE inhibitor	Hypertension
106	Lotrel	amlodipine besylate/ benazepril hydrochloride	ACE inhibitor/CCB combination	Hypertension
107	Lovaza	omega-3-acid ethyl esters	Esterified fish oils	Hypertriglyceridemia
108	Lyrica	pregabalin	GABA analogue	Neuropathic pain
109	Maxzide or Dyazide	hydrochlorothiazide/ triamterene	Potassium-sparing/thiazide diuretic	Hypertension
110	Medrol	methylprednisolone	Corticosteroid	Inflammation
111	Mevacor	lovastatin	HMG-CoA reductase inhibitor	Hyperlipidemia
112	Micronase or DiaBeta	glyburide	Sulfonylurea	Type 2 diabetes mellitus
113	Mobic	meloxicam	NSAID	Osteoarthritis
114	Motrin†	ibuprofen	NSAID	Inflammation
115	MS Contin	morphine	Opioid analgesic	Analgesic
116	Namenda	memantine hydrochloride	NMDA receptor agonist	Alzheimer's disease
117	Naprosyn	naproxen	NSAID	Inflammation
118	Nasacort AQ	triamcinolone	Corticosteroid	Allergic rhinitis
119	Neurontin	gabapentin	Neurologic	Seizure
120	Nexium†	esomeprazole	PPI	GERD
121	Nitrostat	nitroglycerin	Vasodilator	Angina
122	Norvasc	amlodipine besylate	CCB	Hypertension
123	Novolog	insulin aspart	Insulin	Diabetes mellitus
124	Nyamyc	nystatin	Antifungal	Fungal infection
125	Oraped	prednisolone	Corticosteroid	Inflammatory disorders
126	Ortho-Tri-Cyclen Lo	ethinyl estradiol/norgestimate	Triphasic oral contraceptive	Oral contraceptive
127	Oxycontin	oxycodone	Opioid	Analgesic
128	Pacerone	amiodarone hydrochloride	Antiarrhythmic	Antiarrhythmic
129	Pamelor	nortriptyline hydrochloride	TCA	Depression
130	Paxil	paroxetine	SSRI	Depression
131	Veetids	penicillin VK	Penicillin antibiotic	Bacterial infection
132	Pepcid†	famotidine	H₂ blocker	GERD
133	Phenergan	promethazine hydrochloride	Antihistamine	Antiemetic
134	Plaquenil	hydroxychloroquine sulfate	Aminoquinoline	Antimalarial
135	Plavix	clopidogrel bisulfate	Antiplatelet	Thrombotic event prevention
136	Pradaxa	dabigatran etexilate mesylate	Anticoagulant; DOAC	Thrombotic event prevention
137	Pravachol	pravastatin	HMG-CoA reductase inhibitor	Hyperlipidemia

	Brand Name	Generic Name	Drug Classification*	Indication or Use
			Drugs by Brand, Generic, Classification, Indication	
138	Premarin	estrogens conjugated	Estrogen	Vasomotor symptoms
139	Prevacid†	lansoprazole	PPI	GERD
140	Prilosec†	omeprazole	PPI	GERD
141	Pristiq	desvenlafaxine	SNRI	Depression
142	ProAir HFA, Proventil HFA, Ventolin HFA	albuterol	Bronchodilator	Asthma
143	Procardia	nifedipine	Dihydropyridine CCB	Hypertension
144	Proscar	finasteride	5 Alpha-reductase inhibitor	BPH
145	Protonix	pantoprazole sodium	PPI	GERD
146	Prozac	fluoxetine hydrochloride	SSRI	Depression
147	Pulmicort Respules	budesonide	Corticosteroid	Asthma
148	Remeron	mirtazapine	Antidepressant	Depression
149	Requip	ropinirole hydrochloride	Dopamine agonist	Parkinson's disease
150	Restoril	temazepam	Benzodiazepine	Insomnia
151	Risperdal	risperidone	Antipsychotic	Schizophrenia
152	Robaxin	methocarbamol	Skeletal muscle relaxant	Spasticity
153	Seroquel	quetiapine fumarate	Antipsychotic	Schizophrenia
154	Singulair	montelukast	Leukotriene receptor antagonist	Asthma
155	Slow Mag	magnesium	Supplement	Magnesium deficiency
156	Soma	carisoprodol	Muscle relaxant	Skeletal muscle relaxant
157	Spiriva Handihaler	tiotropium	Anticholinergic	COPD
158	Stool softener	docusate	Laxative	Constipation
159	Symbicort	budesonide/formoterol	Corticosteroid/ beta-2 agonist	Asthma
160	Synthroid	levothyroxine sodium	Thyroid hormone	Hypothyroidism
161	Tenoretic	atenolol/chlorthalidone	Beta-blocker/thiazide combination	Hypertension
162	Tenormin	atenolol	Beta-blocker	Hypertension
163	Tessalon Perles	benzonatate	Antitussive	Cough
164	Thalitone	chlorthalidone	Thiazide diuretic	Hypertension
165	Topamax	topiramate	Antiepileptic	Seizures
166	Travatan	travoprost	Prostaglandin analogue	Glaucoma
167	Tricor	fenofibrate	Fibrate	Hyperlipidemia
168	Trileptal	oxcarbazepine	Antiepileptic	Partial seizures
169	Tylenol	acetaminophen	Nonopioid analgesic	Analgesic
170	Ultram	tramadol hydrochloride	Opioid	Analgesic
171	Vagifem	estradiol	Estrogen	Vulvovaginal atrophy
172	Valium	diazepam	Benzodiazepine	Anxiety
173	Valtrex	valacyclovir	Antiviral	Viral infection
174	Vasotec	enalapril maleate	ACE inhibitor	Hypertension
175	Vibramycin	doxycycline hyclate	Tetracycline antibiotic	Bacterial infection

Continued

Drugs by Brand, Generic, Classification, Indication

	Brand Name	Generic Name	Drug Classification*	Indication or Use
176	Vicodin	acetaminophen/ hydrocodone bitartrate	Opioid combination	Analgesic
177	Victoza	liraglutide	GLP-1 receptor agonist	Type 2 diabetes mellitus
178	Vistaril	hydroxyzine	H_1 antagonist	Allergies
179	Vitamin B_{12}	cyanocobalamin	Vitamin	Vitamin B_{12} deficiency
180	Vitamin D 50,000†	ergocalciferol	Vitamin	Vitamin D deficiency
181	Vitamin D3	cholecalciferol/alpha- tocopherol	Vitamin	Vitamin D deficiency
182	Voltaren	diclofenac	NSAID	Analgesic
183	Vytorin	ezetimibe/simvastatin	HMG-CoA reductase combination	Hypercholesterolemia
184	Vyvanse	lisdexamfetamine	CNS stimulant	ADHD
185	Wellbutrin XL	bupropion	Antidepressant	Depression
186	Xalatan	latanoprost	Prostaglandin analogue	Glaucoma
187	Xanax	alprazolam	Benzodiazepine	Anxiety
188	Xarelto	rivaroxaban	DOAC	Anticoagulant
189	Xyzal	levocetirizine dihydrochloride	H_1 antagonist	Allergies
190	Zanaflex	tizanidine	Alpha-2 agonist	Muscle relaxant
192	Zestoretic	hydrochlorothiazide/lisinopril	ACE inhibitor/thiazide combination	Hypertension
193	Zestril or Prinivil	lisinopril	ACE inhibitor	Hypertension
194	Zetia	ezetimibe	Cholesterol absorption inhibitor	Hyperlipidemia
195	Zithromax	azithromycin	Macrolide antibiotic	Bacterial infection
196	Zocor	simvastatin	HMG-CoA reductase inhibitor	Hyperlipidemia
197	Zofran	ondansetron	$5-HT_3$ receptor antagonist	Antiemetic
198	Zoloft	sertraline hydrochloride	SSRI	Depression
199	Zovirax	acyclovir	Antiviral	Viral infection
200	Zyloprim	allopurinol	Xanthine oxidase inhibitor	Gout

ACE, Angiotensin-converting enzyme; *ADHD*, attention deficit/hyperactivity disorder; *ARB*, angiotensin II–receptor blocker; *BPH*, benign prostatic hypertrophy; *CCB*, calcium channel blocker; *CNS*, central nervous system; *COPD*, chronic obstructive pulmonary disease; *COX*, cyclooxygenase; *DPP-4*, dipeptidyl peptidase 4; *DOAC*, direct-acting oral anticoagulant; *DVT*, deep vein thrombosis; *GERD*, gastroesophageal reflux disease; *GLP*, glucagon-like peptide; *GU*, genitourinary; *HMG-CoA*, 3-hydroxy-3- methylglutaryl/coenzyme A; *NMDA*, N-methyl-D-aspartate; *NSAID*, nonsteroidal antiinflammatory drug; *PDE-5*, phosphodiesterase type 5; *PPI*, proton pump inhibitor; *SERM*, selective estrogen receptor modulator; *SNRI*, serotonin-norepinephrine reuptake inhibitor; *SSRI*, selective serotonin reuptake inhibitor; *TCA*, tricyclic antidepressant.

*According to Epocrates.
†Prescription.
Modified from Mizner JJ: Mosby's review for the Pharmacy Technician Certification Examination, ed 3, St Louis, 2014, Mosby.
Davis, K., Guerra, A: Mosby's Pharmacy Technician, Principles and Practice, ed 6, Elsevier

Top Herbal Remedies

Common Name	Scientific Name	Common Reported Uses
Aloe vera (leaf)	*Aloe* spp.	Wound and burn healing
Bilberry (berry)	*Vaccinium myrtillus*	Eye and vascular support
Black cohosh (root)	*Cimicifuga racemosa*	Menopause, premenstrual syndrome (PMS)
Cascara sagrada (aged bark)	*Rhamnus purshiana*	Laxative
Cat's claw (root, bark)	*Uncaria tomentosa*	Antiinflammatory, immune system support
Chondroitin	Chondroitin 4- and 6-sulfate	Osteoarthritis
Dong quai (root)	*Angelica sinensis*	Energy (females), menopause, dysmenorrhea, PMS
Echinacea (flower, root)	*Echinacea purpurea, Echinacea angustifolia*	Support of common cold, immunostimulant
Evening primrose (seed oil)	*Oenothera biennis*	PMS, menopause
Feverfew (leaf)	*Tanacetum parthenium*	Antiinflammatory, migraine prevention
Fish oils	Nutraceutical	Lower triglycerides, heart health
Garlic (bulb)	*Allium sativum*	Lower blood pressure, lower cholesterol
Ginger (root)	*Zingiber officinale*	Antiemetic, gastrointestinal distress, dyspepsia
Ginkgo (root)	*Ginkgo biloba*	Support of memory, increased blood flow to brain, prevention of dementia
Ginseng (American)	*Panax quinquefolius*	Increase physical endurance and concentration, lessen fatigue, support energy, stress, immune system
Glucosamine	3-Amino-6-(hydroxymethyl) oxane-2,4,5-triol sulfate or (3R,4R,5S,6R)-3-Amino-6-(hydroxymethyl)oxane-2,4,5- triol hydrochloride	Osteoarthritis
Goldenseal (root)	*Hydrastis canadensis*	Chest congestion
Grape seed (seed, skin)	*Vitis vinifera*	Support circulation
Green tea (leaf)	*Camellia sinensis*	Improve cognitive performance and mental alertness
Kava (root)	*Piper methysticum*	Anxiety, sedation
Melatonin	N-Acetyl-5-methoxytryptamine	Insomnia, jet lag
Milk thistle (seed)	*Silybum marianum*	Antioxidant, liver support
Saw palmetto (berry)	*Serenoa repens*	Diuretic
Siberian ginseng (root)	*Eleutherococcus senticosus*	Athletic performance, stress, immune system builder
St. John's wort (flowering buds)	*Hypericum perforatum*	Depression, anxiety
Valerian (root)	*Valeriana officinalis*	Sedative, muscle spasms, insomnia
Wild yam (tuber)	*Dioscorea villosa*	PMS, infertility

Davis, K., Guerra, A: Mosby's Pharmacy Technician, Principles and Practice, ed 6, Elsevier.

Glossary

Absorption pharmacokinetic process of medications entering the bloodstream, generally associated with the small intestine

Active Metabolite the active form of a drug or compound that has an effect on the receptor

Addiction inability to control their use of a substance

Adenomatous adjectival form of adenoma, a benign tumor

Adipose body tissue used for the storage of fat

Adjunct (medicine) medication that can reduce or prevent certain adverse effects

Affinity attraction between a receptor and drug

Agonist molecule that activates a receptor, stimulating an action; a substance that stimulates a receptor

Alcohol use disorder abuse of alcohol despite the harm the addiction causes

Allergenic causes an allergic reaction

Amide local anesthetics anesthetics with an amide group, often less allergenic

Aminoglycoside traditional Gram-negative antibacterials that inhibit protein synthesis

Anaerobic absence of oxygen

Anaphylaxis an acute allergic reaction to an antigen (e.g., a bee sting)

Angina pectoris literally means "strangling chest"—chest pain often caused by a lack of enough blood to the heart

Antagonist molecule or other substance that blocks a receptor or action

Antibacterials drugs that destroy bacteria or suppress their growth or reproduction

Anticholinergic inhibiting acetylcholine, synonym for antimuscarinic; literally, anti-acetylcholine, a neurotransmitter; use the ABDUCT mnemonic to remember anhidrosis (reduced sweating or absence of perspiration), blurry vision, dry mouth, urinary retention, constipation, and tachycardia as anticholinergic effects

Antidepressants medicines that improve symptoms of mood

Antidiabetics drugs used in diabetes that lower blood glucose levels

Antiemetic a medicine to prevent vomiting

Antifungals drugs that kill or inactivate fungi

Antigen a foreign substance that induces antibodies

Antihistamines drugs that block H1 receptor sites responsible for sneezing and itching

Antimetabolite interferes with metabolic processes

Antimuscarinic a synonym for anticholinergic; the name comes from the muscarine found in a particular mushroom

Antipsychotics medication primarily used to manage psychoses in schizophrenia and bipolar disorder

Antipyretic fever reducer

Antivirals medications that inhibit viruses

Anxiolytic antianxiety agent

Arrhythmia a change from normal cardiac electrical impulses; literally, no cardiac rhythm but often used as a synonym for dysrhythmia, an abnormal rhythm

Artery blood vessel moving away from the heart

Atherosclerosis arterial disease characterized by plaque buildup

Atrial fibrillation an irregular and rapid heart rate that can increase stroke and heart failure risk

Atrioventricular node (AV node) a part of the heart's electrical conduction system, between the atrium and ventricles

Axon slender projection of a nerve cell

Axonal conduction a mechanism of action of local anesthetics, contrast to synaptic transmission

Autoimmune the body attacking itself

Autoimmune disease a condition in which the body attacks itself

Beers Criteria for Potentially Inappropriate Medication Use in Older Adults is a series of tables reviewed by the American Geriatrics Society for medication safety in the elderly population

Behind-the-counter drugs that have limitations on their use (e.g., pseudoephedrine), thus, are not on open, accessible shelves in commercial pharmacies

Benign prostatic hyperplasia (BPH) a prostate growth that squeezes the urethra, inhibiting urine flow

Benzodiazepines used for anxiety and sleep disorders

Beta-blocker used to control heart rhythm, treat angina, and reduce high blood pressure

Beta-lactamases bacterial enzymes that inactivate penicillins and cephalosporins by hydrolyzing them

Beta-lactam ring a four-membered ring found in penicillins

Biguanide the drug class of metformin (Glucophage); the antidiabetic class in which metformin (Glucophage) belongs

Bisphosphonates drugs that limit bone density loss in osteoporosis and similar conditions; class of drugs to reduce bone density loss

Bradycardia abnormally slow heart rate, below 60 beats per minute

Bradykinesia slow movement

Brand name trade name of a medication

Bronchioles branches off the larger bronchi that form smaller branches in the lungs

Buccal dosage form that involves the cheek

CAD coronary artery disease

Calcium channel blocker (CCB) can lower blood pressure by allowing blood vessels to vasodilate from calcium blockade

Candidiasis oral or vaginal thrush

Cardiovascular involving heart and blood vessels

Cationic positively charged ion

Cations positively charged ions

CCB calcium channel blocker

CDC Centers for Disease Control and Prevention

Centers for Disease Control and Prevention (CDC) helps investigate, prevent, and control diseases

Central nervous system (CNS) the brain and spinal cord

Cephalosporins broad-spectrum antibiotics resembling penicillin

Chemical name the formal name of a medication describing the molecular structure

Chemokine cytokines that attract white blood cells

Chemoreceptor trigger zone (CTZ) an area of the brain that initiates vomiting

Chronic obstructive pulmonary disease (COPD) a chronic inflammatory lung condition

Clark's rule a formula to estimate the dosage for a child by using the adult dose times the child's weight in pounds over 150

CNS central nervous system

CNS depressant a class of drugs that slows down brain activity

Cognitive behavioral therapy intervention to improve mental health by focusing on those thoughts and behaviors contributing to addiction

Competitive antagonist binds to the same site as an agonist but does not activate it

COPD chronic obstructive pulmonary disease

Coronary artery disease (CAD) narrowing or obstruction of coronary arteries

Cosubstrate second substrate or coenzyme

Creatinine clearance rate amount of creatinine per unit time, a sign of kidney health

Crystalluria crystals found in the urine

CTZ chemoreceptor trigger zone

Cubic centimeter is equal to 1 milliliter

Cytoplasmic membrane cell membrane

Demyelinating causing the loss of myelin (in nerve tissue)

Deprescribing the removal of a medication from a patient's regimen

Detrusor muscle contracts and relaxes to control bladder function

Diabetes mellitus a disease of abnormal carbohydrate metabolism and sustained elevated glucose

Dihydrofolate reductase inhibitor (DHFR inhibitor) molecule that inhibits the function of dihydrofolate reductase, sulfamethoxazole, and trimethoprim

Dimensional analysis method unit-factor method or factor-label method using conversion factors to change from one unit to another

Distal convoluted tubule a part of the nephron farther from the proximal convoluted tubule

Distribution pharmacokinetic process of moving a drug through the body, usually the blood

Disulfiram supports chronic alcoholism treatment by inhibiting acetaldehyde dehydrogenase, causing nausea and vomiting

Diuretics medicines that increase the amount of urine, also called water pills

DNA deoxyribonucleic acid

Dopamine a neurotransmitter

Drug Enforcement Administration (DEA) law enforcement agency that combats drug trafficking and distribution, and regulates controlled substances

Drug schedules a drug classification as to its addictive potential

Dysmenorrhea painful menstruation

Dysphonia hoarseness that can come from inhaled corticosteroids (ICS)

Dysrhythmia an abnormal cardiac rhythm

Emesis vomiting

Empiric therapy therapy based on experience, a clinical educated guess

Enantiomers mirror-image pairs of molecules

Endogenous internal cause or origin

Enteral medications passing through the intestine

Enteric-coated an acid-resistant coating to prevent dissolution in the stomach

Ergosterol a compound in fungi, target of antifungal drugs

Ester local anesthetics anesthetics with an ester group, often more allergenic

Estrogen the primary female hormone

Euphoria a feeling of intense excitement

Exacerbate increasing a problem's severity

Excretion removal of a drug from the body, often via the kidneys

Extrapyramidal side effects (EPSE) movement disorders often related to antipsychotic medications

Extrapyramidal symptoms (EPS) drug-induced movement disorders that include acute and tardive symptoms

Familial adenomatous polyposis a hereditary condition that includes polyps that line the intestinal mucosa (particularly the colon)

Fat-soluble dissolves in fat

FDA U.S. Food and Drug Administration

Fibrates (fibric acid derivatives) drug class that lowers blood triglyceride levels

First-pass effect also referred to as first-pass metabolism; drug metabolism and reduction of concentration before it reaches the systemic circulation

Fluoroquinolones antibiotic class that includes ciprofloxacin and levofloxacin

Food and Drug Administration (FDA) responsible for drug approvals in the United States

Formula method desired over have method; allows for conversion of factors if the ordered dose, amount on hand, and quantity of medicine are known

Full agonist molecule that causes a maximal response

Fungicidal a chemical that destroys fungus

Fungistatic inhibiting fungal growth

GABA Gamma-aminobutyric acid

Gamma-aminobutyric acid (GABA) inhibitory neurotransmitter

Gastrostomy a surgically made opening into the stomach from the abdominal wall for food

General anesthetic a medication that will render the patient unconscious

Generic name nonproprietary single name for a medication

GFR glomerular filtration rate

Glomerular filtration rate (GFR) estimate of blood flow through the glomeruli, a part of the nephron

Glomerulus network of capillaries in the nephron

Glucocorticoids a type of steroid with anti-inflammatory action

Glycopeptides vancomycin class

Gram (g) 1/1000 of a kilogram

Health Insurance Portability and Accountability Act of 1996 (HIPAA) federal law that governs how patient information is shared in the United States

Hematologic adjectival form of hematology, the study of blood

Hemodynamic regarding the blood circulation

Hemodynamics dynamics of blood flow

Hemolytic anemia anemia due to the abnormal breakdown of red blood cells

Heparin a fast-acting blood thinner

Herd immunity immunity of a larger number of people because most are vaccinated or due to prior Illness

HIPAA Health Insurance Portability and Accountability Act of 1996

Histamine-2 antagonists drugs that block stomach acid production

Homeostasis stable condition

Hormones signaling molecules produced by glands

Hydrolyzing breaking down a compound with water

Hyperplasia organ or tissue enlargement

Hypertension high blood pressure

Hypoglossal under the tongue, synonym of sublingual

Hypomagnesemia a deficiency of magnesium in the blood

Idiopathic unknown origin of a symptom

Immunomodulators substances that affect the immune system

Inhaled corticosteroids (ICS) also known as inhaled steroids or (asthma) controller medicines

Insomnia sleeplessness

Integrase strand transfer inhibitors blocks integrase, a viral enzyme of human immunodeficiency virus

Interstate commerce buying, selling, or moving products, services, or money across two or more states

Irreversible antagonist a drug that stays with the receptor indefinitely

Islets of Langerhans the pancreatic islets that contain hormone-producing cells

Kernicterus bilirubin-induced brain dysfunction

Kilogram (kg) base unit of mass in the metric system

Kinesiology the study of body movements

Lactic acidosis buildup of lactate in the body, a form of metabolic acidosis

Lethal dose a dose that causes death

Leukotrienes chemical cell messengers (released by mast cells) involved in the asthmatic response process

Lincosamides antibiotics that inhibit bacterial protein synthesis

Liphophilicity literally means "lipid loving"

Liter (L) one kilogram of water in standard conditions; base unit of liquid volume in the metric system

Loading dose a larger initial medication dose

Local anesthetic medication that will numb a specific area

Local effect the therapeutic or toxic effect limits itself to a single site

Loop of Henle located in part of the nephron connecting the proximal and distal convoluted tubules, named after the German anatomist Friedrich Gustav Jakob Henle

Macrolides antibiotics containing a lactone ring (e.g., erythromycin)

Maintenance dose the dose required to keep the therapeutic level of a medication

Mast cells cells responsible for releasing histamine and other substances during inflammatory and allergic reactions

Mechanism of action (MOA) how a drug produces its pharmacological effect; how a drug works biochemically to create a therapeutic effect; biochemical interaction through which a drug produces its effect; how therapeutic agents act (e.g., blocking receptors, stimulating hormones)

Metabolite substance formed in, or necessary for, metabolism

Metabolism the chemical processes that change drug products in the body; the breakdown or change of a medication, usually through the liver

Microgram (mcg or μg) 1/1000 of a milligram

Milligram (mg) 1/1000 of a gram

Milliliter (mL) 1/1000 of a liter

Mnemonic a memory device

Monoclonal forming a clone that is derived asexually from a single individual or cell

Muscarinic a synonym for cholinergic or activating acetylcholine

Mycobacteria common cause of tuberculosis and leprosy

Mycolic acids causative agent of tuberculosis

Myocardial cardiac muscle

Myocardial infarction a heart attack

Naloxone opioid antagonist that can reverse overdose

Narrow therapeutic index small gap between the safe and dangerous dose of a drug

Nasogastric reaching the stomach via the nose

Nasopharyngitis upper respiratory inflammation of the nose and pharynx

Necrosis cell death

Neonate a baby less than 4 weeks old

Nephrons functional units of the kidney

Neuraminidase inhibitors antiviral drug class

Neurons basic units of the nervous system

Neuropharmacology study of how drugs work in the nervous system

Neurotransmitter a chemical agent that stimulates neighboring neurons

Nicotine replacement therapy (NRT) the use of small doses of nicotine to ease the transition to abstinence

Nociceptor a sensory receptor for pain

Noncompetitive antagonist binds to what we call an allosteric or nonagonist site to prevent receptor activation

Noncompliance failure to take a medication on time or correctly

NPH insulin neutral protamine Hagedorn (Humulin N, Novolin N), an intermediate-acting insulin

NRT nicotine replacement therapy

Nucleic acid DNA or RNA

Nucleotide building blocks of DNA and RNA

OBRA 90 Omnibus Budget Reconciliation Act, a pioneering law that required pharmacists to counsel patients and review for medication interactions

Obligate organism that can survive only under certain conditions

Obligate anaerobes cannot survive in normal atmospheric oxygen concentrations

Opioid analgesics narcotic analgesics, strong pain relievers

Osmotic diuretics act on the early part of the nephron

Osteoblasts a cell responsible for bone formation, deposition, and mineralization of the collagen matrix of bone

Osteoclasts cells that break down bone, responsible for bone reabsorption

Otic relating to the ear

Otitis media an inflammation of the middle ear usually secondary to infection

Over-the-counter drugs that do not require a prescription

Oxazolidones class of antibacterial antibiotics

PABA para-aminobenzoic acid

Parenteral administered other than the mouth and alimentary canal

Patent drug drug advertised to cure illnesses often without speaking to its actual effectiveness

Pathophysiologic physiology of abnormal states

Pathophysiology the physiology of disease in living organisms; physiologic processes associated with disease; the physiologic processes of disease; the study of physiologic processes with disease and/or injury

PCT proximal convoluted tubule

Pediatrics a patient group between 4 weeks of age and adolescence

Peripheral nervous system (PNS) nerves and ganglia outside the brain and spinal cord

Phagocyte cell within the immune system that consumes or ingests other cells

Pharmacodynamics the study of drug actions

Pharmacokinetics the pharmacology branch concerning drug movement through the body

Pharmacology the study of drugs and their actions

Pharyngitis sore throat

PHI Protected Health Information

Phocomelia the absence of full limbs in a child

Phosphodiesterase-5 inhibitor (PDE-5) drug class often used for erectile dysfunction

Placebo harmless pill or procedure prescribed for psychological benefit and used as control in clinical trials

PNS peripheral nervous system

Polyp abnormal noncancerous growth that protrudes from a mucus membrane

Polypharmacy the use of many medications and/or many pharmacies

Polyposis multiple noncancerous (benign) growths

PPI Proton pump inhibitor

Prescription drugs (Rx) require a prescription for use

Progestin a hormone that maintains pregnancy and prevents further ovulation

Proportion an equation stating that two fractions across from each other are equivalent

Prostaglandins any of a group of compounds with varying hormone-like effects

Protease inhibitor drug that inactivates the protease enzyme

Protected Health Information (PHI) the data that is covered under HIPAA

Proton pump inhibitor (PPI) reduces stomach acid production by blocking H+/K+ ATPase

Proximal convoluted tubule (PCT) tubular structure in the nephron closer to the glomerulus than the distal convoluted tubule

Psychotherapeutic treatment of mental disorder psychologically rather than with medicines

QT interval an electrocardiographic measurement—the time from the Q wave to T wave; prolongation is dangerous

RAAS renin-angiotensin-aldosterone system

Rare disease a disease that affects less than 200,000 people for orphan drug production purposes

Rate of diffusion how quickly molecules move into a space, affected by ionization

Ratio comparison expressed as a fraction

Receptor a protein or drug that relays a message; a structure that binds to a specific substance; chemical signal acceptor that responds to specific cells, neurotransmitters, hormones, etc.

Receptor antagonist chemical that blocks the action at receptors, sometimes called a blocker

Refractory a case in which the gated channel is inactivated

Renin-angiotensin-aldosterone system (RAAS) involved in regulating blood pressure and renal blood flow

Reuptake the reabsorption of a neurotransmitter

Reverse transcriptase an enzyme encoded from retroviruses

Reversible antagonist a drug that can move away and act at a later time

Reye syndrome a disorder that can come about by giving children aspirin or aspirin-like products

Rhinitis inflammation of the nose

Ribonucleic acid (RNA) a nucleic acid

RNA Ribonucleic acid

Salicylism condition resulting from excess salicylates (aspirin) that manifests as ringing in the ears, nausea, and vomiting

Schizophrenia a mental condition of delusions, hallucinations, and/or disorganized speech

Senna a type of stimulant laxative

Serotonergic stimulated by serotonin

Serotonin a neurotransmitter important in antidepressants and antinausea medications

Sinoatrial node (SA node) specialized heart muscle fibers that initiate the heartbeat

Somnolence drowsiness

Stepwise gradual, distinct stages, but not continual

Steroids Drugs often used to reduce inflammation

Stevens-Johnson syndrome serious disorder of the skin and mucous membranes

Subarachnoid space space between the arachnoid mater and pia mater in the central nervous system

Sublingual applied under the tongue

Sulfamethoxazole antibiotic for bacterial infections such as urinary tract infections, bronchitis, and prostatitis

Sulfanilamide the first sulfa drug

Sulfonamides also called sulfa drugs

Sulfonylureas antidiabetic medicines that stimulate insulin release from the pancreatic beta cells

Superficial mycoses fungal infections in the outermost layers of the skin and hair

Sympathomimetic producing physiologic effects characteristic of the sympathetic nervous system

Synapse a gap between nerve cells

Synaptic transmission communicating with other neurons at a synapse

Systemic effect an effect that affects the body as a whole; the therapeutic or toxic effect does not limit to a single site

Systemic mycoses fungal infections affecting internal organs

Tetracyclines four-ring antibiotics

The Harriet Lane Handbook a trusted resource for treating pediatric diseases

Therapeutic healing of disease

Therapeutic index difference between where a drug will help the patient (therapeutic effect) or hurt the patient (toxic effect)

TNF tumor necrosis factor

Tobacco use disorder inability to stop smoking despite health or social problems

Toxic dose a dose that causes adverse effects

Transcriptase an enzyme that catalyzes RNA from DNA

Tumor necrosis factor (TNF) a promoter of the inflammatory process

Varicella zoster viruses herpesviruses that cause chickenpox (varicella) and shingles (herpes zoster)

Vasoconstrictor a substance, such as epinephrine, that contracts blood vessels

Viscosity how thick or sticky a substance is

Water soluble dissolves in water

Weight-based dosing determining the proper dosage by using a child's weight

Wide therapeutic index larger gap between a safe and dangerous dose

Young's rule a formula that uses the age of a child to determine the dose multiplying the adult dose times the age over the age plus 12 [Age/(Age + 12)] × Recommended Adult Dose = Pediatric Dose]

Index

A

Abatacept (Orencia), 60
Absorption, 1b, 13–14
 changes, 14, 14f
 pharmacokinetic changes and aging, 145
 site of action, 13–14, 14f
 small intestine, 14
 stomach, 14
Acetaminophen (tylenol), 56, 56f, 56b, 99
Acetaminophen/diphenhydramine (Tylenol PM), 99
Acetylcholinesterase inhibitor, 112
Acetyl, drug names, 3
Acetylsalicylic acid (ASA), 6
Active secretion, 116
Acute otitis media, 143–144
Acyclovir (Zovirax), 90–91
Addiction, 157
Adjuncts, anesthesia, 155–156
Administration types, drugs, 28–30, 29f
Adrenaline, 122
Adverse drug reactions, 7, 8f
Affinity, 8–9, 8f
Agonists, 9, 10b
 full, 9, 10f
 partial, 9, 10f
Albuterol (ProAir HFA), 72–73
Alcohol, drug names, 3
Alcoholics Anonymous (AA), 157
Alcohol use disorder, 157, 157b
 prevalence, 157
 treatments, 157
 withdrawal symptoms, 157
Alendronate (Fosamax), 60–61
Alfuzosin (Uroxatral), 139
Allergic rhinitis, 40
Allergy, 40
Allopurinol (Zyloprim), 62
Alpha-blockers, 121–123, 122f, 122t, 123b
Alpha-1 blockers, 139, 140f
5-Alpha reductase inhibitors, 139, 140f
Alprazolam (Xanax), 104
Alzheimer disease, 111–112, 112f

Amide, drug names, 3
Amide local anesthetics, 150
 vs. esters, 150, 153f
Amikacin (Amikin), 83
Amine, drug names, 3
Aminoglycosides, 83–84
Amitriptyline (Elavil), 102
Amlodipine (Norvasc), 121
Amoxicillin (Amoxil), 78, 78f
Amoxicillin/clavulanate (Augmentin), 78
Amphotericin B (Fungizone), 86
Amphotericin B lipid complex (Abelcet), 87
Anabolism, 13
Analgesics
 and first-generation antihistamine, 99
 non-opioid, 54t
 NSAID
  aspirin, 53–55, 55b
  first-generation nonaspirin, 55
  second-generation nonaspirin, 55–56, 56f
 opioid, 56–58, 56f
Anaphylaxis, 74–75
AndroGel, 135
Anesthetics, local, 97–98
Angel dust, 159
Angina pectoris, 126–127, 127b
Angiotensin-converting enzyme inhibitors (ACEIs), 41, 119, 120f
Angiotensin II receptor blockers (ARBs), 41, 119–120, 120f
Antacids, 44–45
Antagonists, 9–10, 10f, 10b
 competitive, 10, 10f
 irreversible, 10
 noncompetitive, 10
 reversible, 10
Antianxiety medicine, 155
Antiarrhythmics, 155
Antibiotics affecting cell walls, 78–81
 cephalosporins, 79–80, 79f
 glycopeptides, 80–81, 80f
 penicillins, 78–79
Anticholinergic agents, 73–74, 112–113, 155

Page numbers followed by *b* indicates boxes, *f* indicates figures and *t* indicates tables.

plain